Communication Skills for Dental Health Care Providers

D1478185

Communication Skills for Dental Health Care Providers

Lance Brendan Young, PhD, MBA
Assistant Professor
Department of Communication
Western Illinois University-Quad Cities
Moline, Illinois

Cynthia Rozek O'Toole, MS, RDH
Assistant Clinical Professor
Department of Preventive and Community Dentistry
The University of Iowa College of Dentistry
Iowa City, Iowa

Bianca Wolf, PhD, MPH
Associate Professor
Department of Communication Studies
University of Puget Sound
Tacoma, Washington

Quintessence Publishing Co, Inc

Chicago, Berlin, Tokyo, London, Paris, Milan, Barcelona, Istanbul,
Moscow, New Delhi, Prague, São Paulo, Seoul, and Warsaw

Library of Congress Cataloging-in-Publication Data

Young, Lance Brendan, author.
  Communication skills for dental health care providers / Lance Brendan
Young, Cynthia O'Toole, and Bianca Wolf.
      p. ; cm.
  Includes bibliographical references and index.
  ISBN 978-0-86715-690-4 (softcover)
  I. O'Toole, Cynthia, author. II. Wolf, Bianca, author. III. Title.
  [DNLM: 1. Communication. 2. Dentist-Patient Relations. 3. Attitude
of Health Personnel. 4. Clinical Competence. 5. Cultural Competency.
WU 61]
  RK28.3
  617.6001'4--dc23
                                    2015018425

© 2015 Quintessence Publishing Co, Inc

Quintessence Publishing Co, Inc
4350 Chandler Drive
Hanover Park, IL 60133
www.quintpub.com

5 4 3 2 1

Editor: Leah Huffman
Design: Ted Pereda
Production: Angelina Sanchez

Printed in the USA

Contents

Preface

Over the past 10 years, the three authors of this book have taught patient-provider communication skills to the dental students at the University of Iowa College of Dentistry. In addition to our academic training, each of us has different real-world experience, ranging from clinical dentistry (O'Toole) to health insurance (Wolf) to business marketing (Young). We therefore recognize the value of basing practical decisions on sound research. Recent years have seen tremendous growth in research on communication between dental professionals and their patients. Individually and collectively, however, we have been frustrated by the lack of a single resource presenting the most reliable and recent evidence to suggest how dental providers should interact with their patients.

In developing and refining our curricula at the university, we located four books published within the previous 30 years that address communication in the dental setting.[1-4] Although each text has its strengths, they all lack recent, evidence-based findings to support the communication practices they recommend. The communication patterns and expectations of patients have changed over time, so research conducted in the 1970s and 1980s may be less reliable than research conducted more recently. Further, demographic changes have resulted in patient diversity unknown to previous generations of oral health professionals. Diversity challenges current dental providers to develop flexible communication skills; scripted communication will not work.

The lack of a dental communication textbook left us scouring research journals for information we believed our students should know before they began practicing on patients. Having received positive feedback on the curricula we developed, we wrote this manual so that other dental professionals may benefit from our work.

Because we exclusively teach future dentists, our focus in writing has been patient-dentist communication. We can think of few instances, however, in which the evidence-based communication skills described in this book do not also apply to dental auxiliaries, including dental hygienists, dental therapists, and dental assistants. We are familiar with one text addressing communication for dental auxiliaries,[3] but it was published 30 years ago and is long out of print. Until another such book is published, we feel comfortable recommending our manual for dental auxiliaries who want to improve their skills in communicating with patients. Throughout this manual, we typically refer to dental or oral health providers and professionals, implying every member of the dental team but particularly the dentist.

The dental students we teach have completed an undergraduate degree, so most of them have taken at least one course in communication studies. Similarly, dental auxiliaries may have taken a communication course during or after high school. Therefore, this manual is written for readers with a basic understanding of communication theory and skills. We assume, for instance, that a reader advised to "make eye contact" does not need to be told how many seconds of eye contact are appropriate. We encourage readers who need more basic instruction in culturally appropriate communication to take an introductory course in communication.

Research into dental provider–patient communication is growing rapidly, yet it still lags behind research into physician-patient communication. The two contexts share many similarities, yet we are aware that they are not identical. In seeking research to support the skills we advocate for dental professionals, we attempted to locate recent articles using dentists or dental hygienists as participants. When such research has not been conducted, we relied on communication research using other medical professionals (eg, physicians or nurses). All such research is cited. In areas where research has not been conducted or is inconclusive, recommendations are based on clinical experience, observation, and feedback from dentists, professors, and students. Such recommendations are experience based and have no citation.

All three authors have completed extensive coursework in public health and highly value the behavioral change theories in which so much patient-provider communication research is grounded. We have introduced our students to the more popular theoretical models (eg, the transtheoretical model, the health belief model, and the parallel processing model). Results were mixed. Although students appreciate that these models provide a valid conceptual framework for encouraging patients toward healthy dental behaviors, they prefer that limited class time be devoted to specific recommendations for interacting with patients.

Given the considerable demands on the time of the dental students and professionals to whom this book is targeted, we have opted to write it as a practical manual instead of a comprehensive textbook. We therefore focus on specific communication skills and strategies rather than on the theory underlying them. The research cited throughout the book includes material that will appeal to those interested in exploring theories on health behavior.

Research suggests that much patient-provider communication training is not grounded in evidence.[5] We wrote this book as a practical manual introducing dental students and professionals to evidence-based suggestions for effective patient communication. Readers vary in their communication skill level, and dental colleges vary in their instructional emphasis, so we have written each chapter to be comprehensible even if the other chapters are not read.

The manual consists of four parts. Part I presents fundamental communication skills for dental professionals. Part II presents those skills as they are applied in specific types of patient interactions. Part III presents chairside strategies to facilitate communication with patients during each stage of a regular appointment. Part IV presents situations that sometimes challenge dental professionals and offers communication strategies for managing such challenges.

This book reviews broad skills and presents specific strategies for optimal patient-provider communication. To enhance comprehension and retention of the material, each chapter includes activities such as exercises, discussion topics, and self-tests. In addition, because patient communication involves professional ethics, common ethical dilemmas are included throughout the text in a feature called "Question of ethics." This feature fosters ethical behavior by enabling readers to consider how to respond to ethical dilemmas before they happen. Finally, checklists are now the state of the art in health care, so in lieu of chapter summaries we have included a checklist near the end of each chapter to provide a quick summary of the recommended communication strategies.[6,7]

References

1. Geboy MJ. Communication and Behavior Management in Dentistry. Philadelphia: Decker, 1984.
2. Jameson C. Great Communication Equals Great Production, ed 2. Tulsa: PennWell, 2002.
3. Wiles CB, Ryan WJ. Communication for Dental Auxiliaries. Reston, VA: Reston, 1982.
4. Chambers DW, Abrams RG. Dental Communication. Sonoma, CA: Ohana Group, 1992.
5. Veldhuijzen W, Ram PM, Van Der Weijden T, Wassink MR, Van Der Vleuten C. Much variety and little evidence: A description of guidelines for doctor-patient communication. Med Educ 2007;41:138–145.
6. Gawande AA. The Checklist Manifesto: How to Get Things Right. New York: Holt, 2009.
7. Weiser TG, Haynes AB, Lashoher A, et al. Perspectives in quality: Designing the WHO Surgical Safety Checklist. Int J Qual Health Care 2010;22:365–370.

About the Authors

Lance Brendan Young, PhD, MBA

Dr Young is an assistant professor at Western Illinois University. He earned a master of business administration from Tulane University and worked in marketing for 14 years before enrolling at the University of Iowa, where he earned his doctorate in communication studies with an emphasis on health communication. He completed a 2-year postdoctoral fellowship with the Veterans Health Administration. He has also been a visiting assistant professor at the University of Iowa College of Dentistry, teaching patient-provider communication to dental students. His research has appeared in the *Archives of Internal Medicine, Culture and Psychology*, the *Journal of Gerontological Nursing*, and the *Journal of Telemedicine and Telecare*.

Cynthia Rozek O'Toole, MS, RDH

Ms O'Toole has worked at the University of Iowa College of Dentistry for 29 years. In addition to her clinical duties, for several years she has taught the communication curriculum to first-, second-, and third-year dental students. She contributed to the development of the communication curriculum for the first- and second-year students and single-handedly redesigned the standardized patient curriculum for the third-year students. She has secured several grants to implement innovative curricular enhancements through technology (eg, videotaping of patient interactions) and through diversity training (eg, Hispanic and deaf/hard-of-hearing patient awareness).

Bianca Wolf, PhD, MPH

Dr Wolf earned a master of arts in communication from Arizona State University and worked in the health insurance field for several years before entering the University of Iowa, where she earned a doctorate in communication studies and a master of public health degree, focusing on community and behavioral health. She taught patient-provider communication at the University of Iowa College of Dentistry. She is currently an associate professor of communication studies at the University of Puget Sound. She has presented her research on patient communication about cancer and other illnesses at regional, national, and international conferences. Her research has also appeared in *Qualitative Health Research*, the *Journal of Social and Personal Relationships*, and the *Journal of Family Communication*.

Part I

Communication Fundamentals

This first section introduces key concepts that are fundamental to effective chairside communication with patients. Individuals who develop communication skills without first understanding communication or their audience may express themselves in a way that sounds insincere or even aggressive. Effective communicators understand how communication functions and can anticipate how it might function with a specific patient in context. This section provides an overview of health communication and its importance to patient-centered care (chapter 1), describes patients' perceptions of dentistry (chapter 2), and discusses cultural influences that shape patients' communication patterns (chapter 3).

Understanding Communication

Why Communication Matters

This initial chapter provides a rationale for studying patient-provider communication. However, this manual is focused on skill acquisition, so we feel it is best to present the rationale as a competence to master instead of simply listing the reasons why you should read our book. The rationale-as-skill concept becomes clearer to us the longer we teach dental students. Let us explain.

When people ask what we do, we reply that we teach patient-provider communication skills to future dentists. Usually, the responses fall into one of two categories. Some people are completely baffled and ask to know what we mean. Others make a lame attempt at humor: "It should be pretty easy to communicate with dental patients because they can't talk back!" We have heard many variations of this theme and try to smile every time.

In truth, the fact that dental patients are often restricted in their verbal expression makes instruction in communication more important, not less so. Communication is far more than rattling off the latest sports scores while manipulating dental instruments in a patient's mouth. The quality of patient-provider communication determines a wide range of outcomes, including satisfaction, treatment adherence, information comprehension and recall, and ultimately oral health.[1] For this reason, we have developed a skill of explaining and illustrating the importance of effective communication with dental patients. Those who work in a dental office—as a dentist, hygienist, assistant, or receptionist—should master this skill so that all of the practice's employees will better understand the value of effective patient communication.

The fundamental communication lesson professionals must learn is that they cannot assume that everyone understands a message in the same way. To apply this lesson to the task at hand, we will explain and explore four key concepts: (1) communication, (2) health communication, (3) patient-provider communication, and (4) patient-provider communication in dentistry. For each concept, we will define the key term and analyze its implications and associated goals.

What Communication Is

Definition of communication

People from varying disciplines have defined **communication** in vastly different ways, from the mechanical definition that relates communication to audiology and broadcast transmission, to the philosophic definition that ties it to ontology and epistemology.[2,3] Between mechanics and philosophy is a social science discipline, which acknowledges both the concrete realities of message transmission and the varied ways humans interpret the meaning of messages. A good working definition has been provided by Stoner et al[4]: "Communication can be defined as the process by which people share ideas, experiences, knowledge and feelings through the transmission of symbolic messages." Four aspects of this definition are particularly important for dental professionals to keep in mind: (1) communication is a process, (2) communication is multifunctional, (3) communication is multichanneled, and (4) communication is not always intentional.

Communication is a process

Often, communication is understood as individual expression. However, when people view communication as a singular act of self-expression, they risk treating other individuals as mere witnesses or audience members, rather than people with whom they are building a relationship. The working definition on page 4 clarifies that communication **occurs only when two or more people are mutually involved in a process of sharing**. Dental professionals must remember that **effective communicators cannot rely on a script** to build relationships.

Communication is multifunctional

The messages shared when providers and patients communicate perform many functions, often simultaneously[5] (Table 1-1). Because communication is a process, achieving those functions depends on both the way a message is sent and the way it is received. Dental professionals must remain aware of their communication goals and listen to patients for indications that the goals are being achieved.

Table 1-1 Functions of communication

Function	Example
Psychologic	Establishing your professional role in patient introductions
Social	Cultivating patient trust through conversation
Informational	Explaining to patients the condition of their oral health
Influential	Urging patients to stop smoking

Communication is multichanneled

Too often, people think that *communication* is synonymous with *speech*, but messages are transmitted through multiple channels, both verbal (speech and writing) and nonverbal (appearance, gesture, and facial expression, among others). Those channels usually operate simultaneously. Dental professionals must remember that some channels are better suited to certain messages than others and that messages sent through one channel should not contradict messages sent through another.

Communication is not always intentional

Another misconception is that communication is restricted to messages we intend to send. While it is true that intentional communication is valuable, any behavior can transmit a message, regardless of intent. Even complete passivity—the refusal to act—communicates, leading some to argue that humans cannot help but communicate. Further, the definition suggested by Stoner et al[4] acknowledges that we communicate with others through symbols (such as words or gestures), and symbolic messages are effective only insofar as they hold similar meaning for both sender and receiver. This is perhaps the hardest lesson: Dental professionals are constantly communicating, and they have limited control over how messages are received. However, the chance that patients will receive the intended message can be improved if dentists enhance their skills of expression and patient monitoring.

Health Communication

Definition of health communication

The study of communication contains numerous subfields. Some of those subfields are differentiated based on message context or subject matter, such as family communication and environmental communication. **Health communication** is a subfield that has expanded tremendously in recent decades, as researchers and clinicians observed its impact on patient health. Definitions of *health communication* vary widely.[6] The Centers for Disease Control and Prevention provides a useful definition: "Health communication is the crafting and delivery of messages and strategies, based on consumer research, to promote the health of individuals and communities."[7]

Health communication can be further divided based on the number of people involved in the communication: mass communication, organizational communication, small group communication, and interpersonal communication. In this manual, we will address interpersonal communication in the patient-provider dyad (or pair).

Activity 1-1

Alone or with your peers, draft a list of qualities possessed by a competent and effective dental professional. Then, briefly survey several people who are not dental professionals and ask them what qualities they value in a dentist or dental auxiliary. Note where the two lists overlap or diverge. Pay particular attention to those qualities indicating clinical competence and those indicating communication competence.

Healthy People 2020

Healthy People is a government-sponsored initiative that uses scientific research to identify national health needs, establish benchmarks and 10-year goals, and monitor progress toward those goals.[8] Healthy People 2020 has identified numerous measurable goals in 42 topic areas. The topic area of "health communication and health information technology" includes 13 goals (Box 1-1).

Box 1-1	Health communication and health information technology goals of Healthy People 2020*

- Improve the health literacy of the population.
- Increase the proportion of persons who report that their health care providers have satisfactory communication skills.
- Increase the proportion of persons who report that their health care providers always involved them in decisions about their health care as much as they wanted.
- Increase the proportion of patients whose doctor recommends personalized health information resources to help them manage their health.
- Increase the proportion of persons who use electronic personal health management tools.
- Increase individuals' access to the Internet.
- Increase the proportion of adults who report having friends or family members whom they talk with about their health.
- Increase the proportion of quality health-related websites.
- Increase the proportion of online health information seekers who report easily accessing health information.
- Increase the proportion of medical practices that use electronic health records.
- Increase the proportion of meaningful users of health information technology.
- Increase the proportion of crisis and emergency risk messages intended to protect the public's health that demonstrate the use of best practices.
- Increase social marketing in health promotion and disease prevention.

*Reprinted from the US Department of Health and Human Services.[8]

Patient-Provider Communication

Definition of patient-provider communication

Health communication contains numerous domains, including public health campaigns, social influences on health, and communication between medical professionals. The domain of **patient-provider communication** is communication between two people assuming the roles of patient and health care provider. Typically, it involves the face-to-face exchange of medical information. Recently, however, advances in communication technology have challenged providers to develop communication skills outside of the office through media such as email, text messages, and instant messages. As cultural emphasis shifts away from formality and privacy, providers must determine appropriate boundaries between professional and personal communication while adhering to the requirements of the federal Health Insurance Portability and Accountability Act of 1996 (HIPAA).[9]

Activity 1-2

Communication requires the participation of at least two people. Discuss with your peers whether patients have an obligation to participate in provider encounters by disclosing information and asking questions. What level of patient participation is helpful? What level of participation becomes burdensome? Do providers differ in their preferences for patient participation in health care?

The patient-centered health care delivery model has focused on the importance of patient-provider communication.[10,11] Often promoted as evidence-based medicine, the traditional model is "diseased-centered" care, emphasizing diagnosis, symptoms, and treatment, rather than the patient.[12,13] Three characteristics distinguish patient-centered care from disease-centered care.[14] First, in addition to biologic influences, patient-centered care acknowledges psychologic and social influences on health.[15] Second, patient-centered care entails decision-making that involves both the patient and the provider.[16,17] Third, patient-centered care encourages an ongoing relationship between the patient and the provider.[18,19]

Patients with a regular care provider rate provider relationships more positively than do those without consistent sources of care.[20] An ongoing relationship between a provider and a patient is associated with multiple advantages for the patient, including enhanced satisfaction, treatment plan adherence, and trust.[19,21] In turn, the health care provider benefits from long-term patient relationships because accurate diagnosis and treatment are easier to accomplish when a patient's history and behavioral habits are well known. Further, loyal patients enhance a practice's financial stability.

Question of ethics: Patient-centered health care acknowledges the patient's right to determine treatment, but the treatment plan selected by the patient may not be the plan endorsed by an evidence-based health care approach. When such a conflict arises, what options are available to the health care provider? How does the provider proceed ethically?

American Dental Association guidelines

Patient-centered care and evidence-based care increasingly overlap in formal research studies of patient-provider communication. Innovative research designs—measuring interaction and its impact on patient health—have given rise to a large and growing evidence base of effective ways of engaging patients. Consequently, interest in this subfield is likely to increase.[22] The communication style practiced by a health care provider is now recognized to have a significant influence on patients' health outcomes. Therefore, simply assuming a lackluster "bedside (or chairside) manner" is no longer acceptable.

In 2009, the American Dental Association's Council on Ethics, Bylaws and Judicial Affairs drafted the Dental Patient Rights and Responsibilities to guide dentist-patient relationships. The statement lists 9 patient responsibilities and 13 patient rights. The statement highlights the centrality of communication to the relationship between patients and dental professionals. Of the nine patient responsibilities, the first four address communication directly: providing accurate information, providing feedback, participating in decisions, and asking about treatment options. The list of patient rights includes even more communication-related elements, indicating the high expectations for a variety of communication skills among dental professionals (Box 1-2).[23]

Box 1-2	American Dental Association Statement of Dental Patient Rights*

1. You have a right to choose your own dentist and schedule an appointment in a timely manner.
2. You have a right to know the education and training of your dentist and the dental care team.
3. You have a right to arrange to see the dentist every time you receive dental treatment, subject to any state law exceptions.
4. You have a right to adequate time to ask questions and receive answers regarding your dental condition and treatment plan for your care.
5. You have a right to know what the dental team feels is the optimal treatment plan as well as a right to ask for alternative treatment options.
6. You have a right to an explanation of the purpose, probable (short- and long-term) results, alternatives, and risks involved before consenting to a proposed treatment plan.
7. You have a right to be informed of continuing health care needs.
8. You have a right to know in advance the expected cost of treatment.
9. You have a right to accept, defer, or decline any part of your treatment recommendations.
10. You have a right to reasonable arrangements for dental care and emergency treatment.
11. You have a right to receive considerate, respectful, and confidential treatment by your dentist and dental team.
12. You have a right to expect the dental team members to use appropriate infection and sterilization controls.
13. You have a right to inquire about the availability of processes to mediate disputes about your treatment.

*Adapted from the Council on Ethics, Bylaws and Judicial Affairs, American Dental Association.[23]

Patient-Provider Communication in Dentistry

Similarities to other medical contexts

Patient-provider communication in dentistry shares many similarities with patient-provider communication in other medical contexts. For instance, the primary relationship is between the dental or medical professional and the patient, although secondary relationships are sustained with others such as auxiliaries on the team, specialists, patient caregivers, and significant others. Also, the primary communication environment is the dental operatory or physician's office, although advances in communication technology are expanding the options of both time and place at which providers can communicate with patients. Finally, the primary goal of the communication is the health of the patient.

In addition to the three similarities noted above, it is worth considering the ways in which disclosure in both dentistry and other medical contexts differs from typical dyadic (two-person) communication within social relationships. All medical professionals must become accustomed to three particular characteristics that are quite different from usual interpersonal communication. First, patient-provider communication is characterized by asymmetric disclosure. In social interactions, communicators expect to contribute equally to the conversation, but in medical encounters, patients disclose more than the provider. Second, high-level disclosure characterizes these interactions.[24,25] Doctors should be prepared for patients to reveal information to their doctors that their closest friends may not know. Third, rapid disclosure is a feature of patient-provider communication. Within minutes of meeting a provider, patients may quickly report details on their health and habits.

 Question of ethics: Research indicates that provider communication influences patient satisfaction. Is it ethical for a provider to communicate poorly with challenging patients, patients with financial problems, or patients with difficult personalities in the hopes they will find another provider?

Differences from other medical contexts

Patient-provider communication in dentistry does differ from communication in other medical contexts in four important ways. First, patient encounters with dental professionals are more physically intrusive than typical medical encounters. The accepted normal amount of personal space for Americans and Europeans is about 20 inches.[26] During a routine examination, a physician may invade that space for a brief time, but a dental professional usually stands very close to—and above—a reclining patient for a substantial length of time. Second, dental examinations are routinely more invasive than most physical examinations. Physicians and medical specialists typically explore body cavities briefly, but dental professionals spend much of the appointment examining, cleaning, or repairing features of the oral cavity. Third, patients are more aggressive during dental visits than in other medical encounters in which their bodies are examined and manipulated. Inevitably, dental visits require patient activity (holding the mouth open, swishing water, spitting, etc). Often this activity can make patients feel uncomfortable and ultimately more difficult to manage. Finally, dental visits hold more potential for pain than other medical encounters. Dental professionals focus on the head and mouth, two of the most vulnerable and sensitive parts of the body. As a result, even a simple dental examination can cause pain in a way physical examinations rarely do. Taken together, these distinguishing features may explain why 1 in 10 people suffers from dental anxiety.[27]

Criteria for training in communication skills

In 2008, the American Dental Education Association issued revised competencies for the new general dentist.[28] These 39 competencies fall into 6 domains: *(1)* critical thinking, *(2)* professionalism, *(3)* communication and interpersonal skills, *(4)* health promotion, *(5)* practice management and informatics, and *(6)* patient care. Fifteen of those competencies relate—either directly or indirectly—to communication with patients (Box 1-3). Training in communication skills is now required in all US colleges of dentistry. The Commission on Dental Accreditation[29] now includes two behavioral science standards entailing patient communication training:

- **2-15** Graduates must be competent in the application of the fundamental principles of behavioral sciences as they pertain to patient-centered approaches for promoting, improving, and maintaining oral health.
- **2-16** Graduates must be competent in managing a diverse patient population and have the interpersonal and communications skills to function successfully in a multicultural work environment.

Benefits and Challenges of Enhanced Communication Skills

Value of communication skills

In dentistry, how important are interpersonal skills relative to clinical skills? Given the tremendous amount of work and resources dental professionals commit to their clinical training and the significant time and skill required at a dental practice, does proficiency in patient communication justify the extra effort required to learn and implement those skills? Patients indicate that it does. Perhaps surprisingly, practicing dentists agree. A 1998 study determined that dentists rated interpersonal skills, stress tolerance, and administrative skills as the most important determinants of professional success.[30] Moreover, although dental professionals might believe patients evaluate them solely on their clinical skills, patients tend to assume professionals are clinically competent and therefore base their evaluations on communication skills.[31,32]

Measurable benefits of effective communication

Effective patient-provider communication supports patient-centered health care and is associated with specific, measurable benefits. Patient-provider communication is associated with **greater patient satisfaction with care**,[33–35] **greater patient adherence to treatment plans**,[34,36,37] and **fewer medical errors and mistakes**.[38,39] Skilled communication may even be associated with **fewer malpractice claims**.[40–44] Ultimately, effective patient-provider communication leads to **better health outcomes for the patient**.[45–47] Skilled communication yields a complementary benefit for the provider: Along with monetary reward and respect, positive patient relationships are a primary contributor to dentists' job satisfaction.[48,49]

| Box 1-3 | Communication-related competencies for the new general dentist* |

1. Critical thinking
　　1.3 Evaluate and integrate best research outcomes with clinical expertise and patient values for evidence-based practice.

2. Professionalism
　　2.1 Apply ethical and legal standards in the provision of dental care.

3. Communication and interpersonal skills
　　3.1 Apply appropriate interpersonal and communication skills.
　　3.2 Apply psychosocial and behavioral principles in patient-centered health care.
　　3.3 Communicate effectively with individuals from diverse populations.

4. Health promotion
　　4.1 Provide prevention, intervention, and educational strategies.
　　4.2 Participate with dental team members and other health care professionals in the management of and health promotion for all patients.
　　4.3 Recognize and appreciate the need to contribute to the improvement of oral health beyond those served in traditional practice settings.

5. Practice management and informatics
　　5.3 Apply principles of risk management, including informed consent and appropriate record keeping in patient care.
　　5.6 Comply with local, state, and federal regulations including OSHA and HIPAA.

6. Patient care
　　6.3 Obtain and interpret patient/medical data, including a thorough intraoral/extraoral examination, and use these findings to accurately assess and manage all patients.
　　6.6 Formulate a comprehensive diagnosis, treatment, and/or referral plan for the management of patients.
　　6.8 Prevent, diagnose, and manage pain and anxiety in the dental patient.
　　6.18 Recognize and manage patient abuse and/or neglect.
　　6.19 Recognize and manage substance abuse.

*Adapted from the American Dental Education Association[28] with permission.

Measure your social style using the instrument below,* scoring each item from 1 ("poor") to 5 ("very good"). Sum your score on the subscales and the total instrument, and then compare your scores with your peers. Do your personal scores reflect the strengths and weaknesses you perceive in your communication skills? Take the test again after you have completed your communication training and note any changes.

Initiating relationships
1. How good are you at asking someone new to do things together, like go to a ball game or a movie?
2. How good are you at going out of your way to start up new relationships?
3. How good are you at carrying on conversations with new people whom you would like to know better?
4. How good are you at introducing yourself to people for the first time?
5. How good are you at calling new people on the phone to set up a time to get together to do things?
6. How good are you at going places where there are unfamiliar people in order to get to know new people?
7. How good are you at making good first impressions when getting to know new people?

Providing emotional support
8. How good are you at making someone feel better when he or she is unhappy or sad?
9. How good are you at making others feel like their problems are understood?
10. How good are you at helping people work through their thoughts and feelings about important decisions?
11. How good are you at helping people handle pressure or upsetting events?
12. How good are you at showing that you really care when someone talks about problems?
13. How good are you at helping others understand their problems better?
14. How good are you at giving suggestions and advice in ways that are received well by others?

Asserting influence
15. How good are you at getting people to go along with what you want?
16. How good are you at taking charge?
17. How good are you at sticking up for yourself?
18. How good are you at getting someone to agree with your point of view?
19. How good are you at deciding what should be done?
20. How good are you at voicing your desires and opinions?
21. How good are you at getting your way with others?

*Adapted from Buhrmester et al[50] with permission.

Barriers to the use of evidence-based communication strategies

The many benefits of enhancing provider communication skills and using those skills when interacting with patients have already been discussed. In addition, a European study indicated that 87% of dentists and 84% of patients support the integration of communication study into dentistry coursework.[47] Yet a recent nationwide survey by the American Dental Association Survey Center found that dentists in private practice routinely engage in only 3.1 of the 7 basic communication techniques, a rate the authors of the study described as "low."[51]

 Question of ethics: Patient-provider communication can determine the level of a patient's access to care. Should providers therefore strive to communicate the exact same information to every patient in the same way? Is it ethical for providers to tailor their message and its delivery to the needs of each patient? Who determines what those needs are?

Given the benefits of effective patient-provider communication and that communication training is now required in US colleges of dentistry, why would dental professionals exclude proven strategies for providing patient-centered care? Three reasons come to mind. First, training in communication skills generally involves a commitment of time and money. A 2007 study found that a single training session did not significantly improve the interpersonal skills of dental students and that a comprehensive communication curriculum was necessary to attain greater gains.[52] Although training is included in colleges of dentistry, we have observed great variation in presentation, the amount of resources and time, and faculty attention devoted to teaching of communication skills.

Second, the practice of adapting communication style to each patient's personality and needs requires a higher level of attention and effort than simply using the same approach with everyone. Patients with challenging clinical, behavioral, or personal characteristics can be particularly frustrating.[53,54] Research documents a decline in emotional empathy over the course of training in dental school, suggesting that the decline is associated with greater exposure to patients.[55,56] This negative association between patient exposure and empathy may carry into the practice. Similarly, "emotional labor" has been identified as a primary occupational stressor for dental hygienists.[57]

Third, providers may perceive that the application of effective communication skills in every encounter takes too much time and interferes with scheduling.

Chapter Checklist ✓

Why communication matters
❏ Understand that communication determines satisfaction, treatment adherence, information comprehension and recall, and oral health.
❏ Realize that providers cannot assume that everyone understands a message in the same way.

What communication is
❏ Understand that communication is the process by which people share ideas, experiences, knowledge, and feelings through the transmission of symbolic messages.
❏ Process: Understand that communication occurs only when two or more people are mutually involved in a process of sharing.
❏ Process: Acknowledge that effective communicators cannot rely on a script to build relationships.
❏ Multifunctional: Remain aware of your communication goals.
❏ Multifunctional: Listen to patients for indications that you are achieving your goals.
❏ Multichannel: Remember that some channels are better suited to certain messages than others.
❏ Multichannel: Remember that messages sent through one channel should not contradict messages sent through another.
❏ Intention: Realize that you are almost always communicating.
❏ Intention: Realize that you have limited control over how messages are received.

Health communication
❏ Understand that health communication is the crafting and delivery of messages and strategies, based on consumer research, to promote the health of individuals and communities.

Patient-provider communication
❏ Understand that patient-provider communication is communication between two people assuming the roles of patient and health care provider.
❏ Understand that patient-centered care acknowledges psychologic and social influences on health.
❏ Understand that patient-centered care entails decision-making that involves both the patient and the provider.
❏ Understand that patient-centered care encourages an ongoing relationship between the patient and the provider.
❏ Understand the 13 patient rights outlined by the American Dental Association.

Patient-provider communication in dentistry
❏ Understand that the primary relationship is between the dental professional and the patient.
❏ Understand that the primary communication environment is the dental operatory.
❏ Understand that the primary goal of the communication is the health of the patient.
❏ Understand that patient-provider communication is characterized by asymmetric, high-level, and rapid disclosure.
❏ Understand that patient-provider communication in a dental context differs from other medical contexts because it is more intrusive and invasive and because patients are more aggressive and more vulnerable to pain.

Benefits and challenges of enhanced communication skills

❑ Benefits: Understand that communication is associated with greater patient and provider satisfaction and treatment adherence, fewer errors and malpractice claims, and better health outcomes.

❑ Challenges: Understand that development and implementation of communication skills demands time, money, attention, and effort, and tailoring messages may interfere with scheduling.

For More Information

Patient-provider communication
- http://www.health.gov/communication/
- http://www.patientprovidercommunication.org/
- http://www.chcf.org/~/media/MEDIA%20LIBRARY%20Files/PDF/P/PDF%20PatientProviderCommunicationTools.pdf
- http://healthcarecomm.org/

Healthy People 2020
- https://www.healthypeople.gov/2020/topics-objectives/topic/health-communication-and-health-information-technology
- https://www.healthypeople.gov/2020/topics-objectives/topic/oral-health

American Dental Education Association competencies
- http://www.adea.org/about_adea/governance/Pages/Competencies-for-the-New-General-Dentist.aspx
- http://www.adea.org/about_adea/governance/Documents/ADEA-Competencies-for-Entry-into-Alied-Dental-Professions.pdf

Commission on Dental Accreditation standards
- http://www.ada.org/en/coda/current-accreditation-standards

Health communication associations
- http://www.aachonline.org/
- http://www.hesca.org/

References

1. Ong LM, de Haes JC, Hoos AM, Lammes FB. Doctor-patient communication: A review of the literature. Soc Sci Med 1995;40:903–918.
2. Dance FEX, Larson CE. The Functions of Human Communication: A Theoretical Approach. New York: Holt, Rinehart & Winston, 1976.
3. Miller K. Communication Theories: Perspective, Processes, and Contexts, ed 2. Boston: McGraw Hill, 2002.
4. Stoner JAF, Freeman RE, Gilbert DR. Management, ed 6. Englewood Cliffs, NJ: Prentice-Hall, 1995.
5. Gamble TK, Gamble MW. Contacts: Interpersonal Communication in Theory, Practice, and Context. Boston: Houghton Mifflin, 2004.
6. Parrott R. Emphasizing "communication" in health communication. J Commun 2004;54:751–787.
7. Roper WL. Health communication takes on new dimensions at CDC. Public Health Rep 1993;108:179–183.
8. Objectives. Health Communication and Health Information Technology. US Department of Health and Human Services. Office of Disease Prevention and Health Promotion. Healthy People 2020. Washington, DC. http://www.healthypeople.gov/2020/topics-objectives/topic/health-communication-and-health-information-technology/objectives. Accessed 6 January 2015.
9. Health Insurance Portability and Accountability Act of 1996, Pub L No 104-191, 110 Stat 1936 (1996). http://www.gpo.gov/fdsys/pkg/PLAW-104publ191/html/PLAW-104publ191.htm. Accessed 12 January 2015.
10. Ponte PR, Conlin G, Conway JB, et al. Making patient-centered care come alive: Achieving full integration of the patient's perspective. J Nurs Adm 2003;33:82–90.
11. Balint E. The possibilities of patient-centered medicine. J R Coll Gen Pract 1969;17(82):269–276.
12. Iqbal A, Glenny AM. General dental practitioners' knowledge of and attitudes towards evidence based practice. Br Dent J 2002;193:587–591.
13. Bensing J. Bridging the gap: The separate worlds of evidence-based medicine and patient-centered medicine. Patient Educ Couns 2000;39:17–25.
14. Golin CE, Thorpe C, DiMatteo MR. Accessing the patient's world: Patient-physician communication about psychosocial issues. In: Earp JE, French E, Gilkey M (eds). Patient Advocacy for Health Care Quality: Strategies for Achieving Patient-Centered Care. Burlington, MA: Jones & Bartlett Learning, 2007:185–213.
15. Mead N, Bower P. Patient-centredness: A conceptual framework and review of the empirical literature. Soc Sci Med 2000;51:1087–1110.
16. Chewning B, Bylund CL, Shah B, Arora NK, Gueguen JA, Makoul G. Patient preferences for shared decisions: A systematic review. Patient Educ Couns 2012;86:9–18.
17. Keirns CC, Goold SD. Patient-centered care and preference-sensitive decision making. JAMA 2009;302:1805–1806.
18. Yedidia MJ. Transforming doctor-patient relationships to promote patient-centered care: Lessons from palliative care. J Pain Symptom Manage 2007;33:40–57.
19. Fuertes JN, Mislowack A, Bennett J, et al. The physician-patient working alliance. Patient Educ Couns 2007;66:29–36.
20. DeVoe JE, Wallace LS, Fryer GE Jr. Measuring patients' perceptions of communication with healthcare providers: Do differences in demographic and socioeconomic characteristics matter? Health Expect 2009;12:70–80.
21. Thom DH, Hall MA, Pawlson LG. Measuring patients' trust in physicians when assessing quality of care. Health Aff (Millwood) 2004;23:124–132.
22. Makoul G. The interplay between education and research about patient-provider communication. Patient Educ Couns 2003;50:79–84.
23. Council on Ethics, Bylaws and Judicial Affairs, American Dental Association. Dental Patient Rights and Responsibilities Statement. 2009. http://www.ada.org/~/media/ADA/About%20the%20ADA/Files/statements_ethics_patient_rights.pdf. Accessed 4 March 2015.

24. Hall MA, Dugan E, Zheng B, Mishra AK. Trust in physicians and medical institutions: What is it, can it be measured, and does it matter? Milbank Q 2001;79:613–639.

25. Veatch RM. The Patient-Physician Relation: The Patient as Partner, Part 2. Bloomington, IN: Indiana University, 1991.

26. Ting-Toomey S, Chung LC. Understanding Intercultural Communication. Los Angeles: Roxbury, 2005.

27. Doerr PA, Lang WP, Nyquist LV, Ronis DL. Factors associated with dental anxiety. J Am Dent Assoc 1998;129:1111–1119.

28. American Dental Education Association. Competencies for the New General Dentist. Washington, DC: American Dental Education Association, 2008.

29. Commission on Dental Accreditation. Accreditation Standards for Dental Education Programs. Chicago: American Dental Association, 2010.

30. Kulich KR, Rydén O, Bengtsson H. A descriptive study of how dentists view their profession and the doctor-patient relationship. Acta Odontol Scand 1998;56:206–209.

31. Logan HL. The patient and the shifting health-care paradigm. J Am Coll Dent 1997;64:16–18.

32. Mazzei A, Russo V, Crescentini A. Patient satisfaction and communication as competitive levers in dentistry. TQM Journal 2009;21:365–381.

33. Wanzer MB, Booth-Butterfield M, Gruber K. Perceptions of health care providers' communication: Relationships between patient-centered communication and satisfaction. Health Commun 2004;16:363–384.

34. Beach MC, Sugarman J, Johnson RL, Arbelaez JJ, Duggan PS, Cooper LA. Do patients treated with dignity report higher satisfaction, adherence, and receipt of preventive care? Ann Fam Med 2005;3:331–338.

35. Williams S, Weinman J, Dale J. Doctor-patient communication and patient satisfaction: A review. Fam Pract 1998;15:480–492.

36. DiMatteo MR. Enhancing patient adherence to medical recommendations. JAMA 1994;271:79, 83.

37. Stewart MA. Effective physician-patient communication and health outcomes: A review. CMA J 1995;152:1423–1433.

38. Woolf SH, Kuzel AJ, Dovey SM, Phillips RL Jr. A string of mistakes: The importance of cascade analysis in describing, counting, and preventing medical errors. Ann Fam Med 2004;2:317–326.

39. Bartlett G, Blais R, Tamblyn R, Clermont RJ, MacGibbon B. Impact of patient communication problems on the risk of preventable adverse events in acute care settings. CMA J 2008;178:1555–1562.

40. Kraman SS, Hamm G. Risk management: Extreme honesty may be the best policy. Ann Intern Med 1999;131:963–967.

41. Schwartz B. Errors in dentistry: A call for apology. J Am Coll Dent 2005;72(2):26–32.

42. Gallagher TH, Waterman AD, Ebers AG, Fraser VJ, Levinson W. Patients' and physicians' attitudes regarding the disclosure of medical errors. JAMA 2003;289:1001–1007.

43. Duclos CW, Eichler M, Taylor L, et al. Patient perspectives of patient-provider communication after adverse events. Int J Qual Health Care 2005;17:479–486.

44. Lester GW, Smith SG. Listening and talking to patients. A remedy for malpractice suits? West J Med 1993;158:268–272.

45. Street RL Jr, Makoul G, Arora NK, Epstein RM. How does communication heal? Pathways linking clinician-patient communication to health outcomes. Patient Educ Couns 2009;74:295–301.

46. Stewart M, Brown JB, Donner A, et al. The impact of patient-centered care on outcomes. J Fam Pract 2000;49:796–804.

47. Woelber JP, Deimling D, Langenbach D, Ratka-Krüger P. The importance of teaching communication in dental education. A survey amongst dentists, students and patients. Eur J Dent Educ 2011;16:e200–e204.

48. Logan HL, Muller PJ, Berst MR, Yeaney DW. Contributors to dentists' job satisfaction and quality of life. J Am Coll Dent 1997;64(4):39–43.

49. Shugars DA, DiMatteo MR, Hays RD, Cretin S, Johnson JD. Professional satisfaction among California general dentists. J Dent Educ 1990;54:661–669.

50. Buhrmester D, Furman W, Wittenberg MT, Reis HT. Five domains of interpersonal competence in peer relationships. J Pers Soc Psychol 1988;55:991–1008.
51. Rozier RG, Horowitz AM, Podschun G. Dentist-patient communication techniques used in the United States. J Am Dent Assoc 2011;142:518–530.
52. Cannick GF, Horowitz AM, Garr DR, et al. Use of the OSCE to evaluate brief communication skills training for dental students. J Dent Educ 2007;71:1203–1209.
53. Bodner S. Stress management in the difficult patient encounter. Dent Clin North Am 2008;52:579–603.
54. Groves JE. Taking care of the hateful patient. New Engl J Med 1978;298:883–887.
55. Sherman JJ, Cramer A. Measurement of changes in empathy during dental school. J Dent Educ 2005;69:338–345.
56. Yarascavitch C, Regehr G, Hodges B, Haas DA. Changes in dental student empathy during training. J Dent Educ 2009;73:509–517.
57. Sanders MJ, Turcotte CM. Occupational stress in dental hygienists. Work 2010;35:455–465.

Preparing for Patient Communication

Why Preparation Matters

Five decades of research on source credibility indicates that the way a message is received, interpreted, and recalled is influenced by variables in five domains: source, message, channel, receiver, and destination.[1,2] The source's task of crafting a message, selecting a channel, addressing a receiver, and accounting for features of the destination are complicated by the fact that the source of messages is simultaneously a receiver of messages. Although many communication guides focus on individual expression, the challenge for dental professionals is to craft appropriate messages at the same time as they are receiving messages from the patient.

Effective message transmission depends on the source's ability and willingness to understand the perspective of the receiver. Before patients ever meet a dental professional face to face, they have formed expectations based on the role of the health care provider and the context of the dental office or practice. Those expectations guide patients' communication behavior, so an understanding of common perceptions, expectations, and responses can help dental professionals to prepare messages tailored to achieve treatment goals. This book devotes three chapters explicitly to the skills involved in understanding patients. This chapter provides guidance on anticipating the common perceptions and expectations of dental patients. Chapter 3 provides guidance on the perceptions and expectations of patients from various cultural groups. Chapter 4 advises clinicians about how to listen to and monitor patients while they are in the dental chair.

Stereotypes of Dentists

A **stereotype**, according to Davis and Palladino,[3] is "a set of socially shared beliefs that we hold about members of a particular group." Because stereotypes offer a shortcut for defining ourselves while evaluating others, they can be useful for reducing the stress of cognitive processing.[4,5] Although stereotypes are useful and often accurate, several characteristics of such categorization can lead to inaccurate assumptions. As generalizations, stereotypes describe an average or norm and work less well when applied to a specific individual within the stereotyped category. Further, stereotypes are culture specific, so stereotypes in one culture may not apply in another. Finally, stereotypes develop over time but often become outdated when they do not evolve to reflect changes in the stereotyped group.

Stereotypes are pervasive and often operate outside awareness.[6] In the United States, stereotypical characteristics of dentists tend to be negative rather than positive. Thibodeau and Mentasti[7] reviewed a century of portrayals of dentists in film and concluded that "Dentists often still are portrayed in the movies in a comedic role or as incompetent, sadistic, immoral, disturbed or corrupt." They noted that previously underrepresented groups (eg, women and racial minorities) are now cast in the role of dentist, but the negative stereotypes attaching to the role persist. Film portrayals reflect, reinforce, and shape attitudes of the audience, so in the absence of empirical research on popular stereotypes of dentists, popular films serve as useful indicators of the characteristics attributed to dentists (Box 2-1).

Six stereotypes hold particular relevance for patient-provider communication: *(1)* Dentists are rejected physicians; *(2)* dentists are sadistic; *(3)* dentists are greedy; *(4)* dentists are lecherous; *(5)* dentists are attractive; *(6)* dentists are trustworthy.

Box 2-1	Films featuring dentists

- *Laughing Gas* (1914)
- *Greed* (1924)
- *The Dentist* (1932)
- *The Strawberry Blonde* (1941)
- *The Little Shop of Horrors* (1960)
- *Rudolph the Red-Nosed Reindeer* (1964)
- *Marathon Man* (1976)
- *10* (1979)
- *The In-Laws* (1979)
- *Little Shop of Horrors* (1986)
- *Eversmile, New Jersey* (1989)
- *The Dentist* (1996)
- *Schizopolis* (1997)
- *The Secret Lives of Dentists* (2002)
- *Snow Dogs* (2002)
- *Finding Nemo* (2003)
- *Good Luck Chuck* (2007)
- *Wild Hogs* (2007)
- *Ghost Town* (2008)
- *The Spirit* (2008)
- *The Hangover* (2009)
- *Horrible Bosses* (2011)

Dentists are rejected physicians

One persistent stereotype is that dentists go into dentistry because they were unable to enter and complete medical school. Dental students indicate that they sometimes must defend the decision to pursue dentistry to people who ask why they did not instead go to medical school. Medical students do not generally report explaining why they did not pursue dentistry. The stereotype of dentists as rejected physicians likely derives from the cultural elevation of physicians in the United States and a poor understanding of the education and training required of dentists.[8] Other medical professionals (eg, pharmacists, physician assistants, and nurses) likewise are sometimes perceived as rejected physicians. This hierarchy of prestige may also persist in the research community.[9] A running joke in *The Hangover* involves the dentist's claim that he is a doctor. A physician in the film provides the typical response: "You said that several times last night, but really you're just a dentist."

When communicating with patients, dentists should remain aware that many patients do not understand the relationship between oral health and systemic health, much less where dentists and other dental professionals fit in the confusing constellation of health care delivery. Without sounding defensive or patronizing, dental professionals should make it a priority to educate patients about the significance of oral health and the role of the dentist as a doctor specializing in oral health. Through such education, patients may take more seriously both their oral health and the dentist who advises them. Dentists can further reinforce their medical qualifications in the minds of patients by consulting with patients' primary care physician and other health care providers whenever possible.

Dentists are sadistic

Pain is a motivator for a dental visit, and dental treatments are historically associated with pain.[10] Olav[11] found that 20% to 30% of adults rated their previous visit to the dentist as "moderately painful" (or worse) and 60% reported at least one "very painful" experience. Pain and the associated anxiety are sometimes unavoidable, but in the popular imagination, some dentists inflict pain intentionally, and some even enjoy doing so. This stereotype is so pervasive that audiences quickly perceived why dentists were selected to employ "enhanced interrogation" techniques in *Marathon Man* and *The Spirit. Little Shop of Horrors* dropped all pretense of pain as a means to an end: The patient's torture was its own reward for that dentist.

Dental professionals should remain aware of these stereotypes, acknowledge a patient's pain, and provide accurate information about the "discomfort" a procedure will entail. Patients expect some pain and are generally willing to endure it, but they react negatively when a dentist disregards it. Clinicians should avoid laughing and appearing unconcerned when examining patients in pain or performing procedures that are causing pain. Providers who arrange a system for patients to signal when pain becomes unbearable, and then stop the procedure promptly, are unlikely to be perceived as sadistic.

Dentists are greedy

A third persistent stereotype is that dentists are motivated primarily by money. Several factors contribute to this stereotype. First, 38.2% of the US population has no dental insurance, and patients may be more aware of charges because they are more likely to pay out of pocket.[12] Second, patients often may not perceive the multiple costs involved in running a dental practice, such as training, continuing education, overhead, and insurance.[13] When patients mistakenly believe that they are paying only for appointment time, they may believe they are paying too much. Third, evidence suggests that dentists may be reluctant to serve lower-income patients, fostering the stereotype that dentists are interested mainly in collectable fees from financially secure patients.[14,15]

A testament to the endurance of the stereotype of the greedy dentist is a 1924 Erich von Stroheim film in which the main character becomes a dentist and steals his friend's girlfriend for her lottery winnings. The title? *Greed*. In communicating with patients, today's dentists must be sensitive to perceptions of greed and excessive wealth. When building rapport with patients, providers should avoid discussions of their expensive cars, upscale neighborhood, exotic trips, or private schools.

In addition, when presenting treatment plans, today's dentists must be truthful regarding the necessity and cost of services.[16] Patient-centered care allows patients to collaborate with providers in determining services and treatment, so providers should listen to patients' concerns about costs when reviewing treatment options.[17] It is unethical to pressure patients to accept an expensive treatment and then pass them off to a billing clerk to arrange payment. Even with good clinical results, patients who feel pressured to undergo an expensive treatment may thereafter suspect a dentist's motives.

Persuasion, not pressure, is simultaneously more ethical and more satisfactory for the patient. Whenever possible, patients should be provided a choice of treatments at different price points. Dental professionals can (and should) offer an opinion on the best option, given the patient's concerns (eg, cost, appearance, and durability). The patient ultimately makes the choice, however, and given that the patient will live with the results, that choice should be respected. Information on communicating treatment options is presented in chapter 9.

Dentists are lecherous

A fourth negative stereotype is that dentists are prone to take sexual advantage of patients, including sexual harassment, abuse, and assault. One possible explanation for this stereotype is the publicity surrounding high-profile cases of dentists engaging in sexual misconduct with patients.[18-20] Another explanation is the potential for misinterpretation of intrusive nonverbal behaviors (eg, proximity and touch) required in dentistry[21] (see chapter 1). A third explanation is the potential for sexual hallucinations in patients emerging from anesthesia.[22,23] Whatever the reason for the stereotype, it appears to endure, as it was a plot point in the 2011 film *Horrible Bosses*. Curiously, in that movie the sexually predatory dentist was a woman, although female dentists are rarely accused of sexual misconduct.

Dental professionals can reduce the potential for misperceptions of sexual aggressiveness by following a few communication strategies. First, social touch should be restricted to the hands and arms, and professional touch should be confined to the oral cavity as much as possible. Second, if the operatory has a door, it should be closed for privacy during the health history interview but otherwise left ajar. Third, during examinations or procedures, another professional should be in the operatory—either a dental hygienist or a dental assistant. If the patient would like a relative or friend in the operatory, and if that request can be reasonably accommodated, the request should be honored. Finally, providers should announce what they are doing and why, guiding interpretation so that the patient will be less likely to attribute proximity and touch to lecherous motives.

 Question of ethics: Communication researchers have documented that flirting often is not an invitation to sexual coupling but can instead serve other functions and provide benefits such as tension reduction and relationship building. Is it ethical to flirt with patients? Does your answer change if the patient is receptive to flirting behavior? Does your answer change if the patient initiates flirting behavior?

Dentists are attractive

A couple of positive stereotypes of dentists go far toward counteracting the negative impression of dentists as sadistic, greedy, lecherous, physician wannabes. One positive stereotype is that dentists are physically attractive. One reason for this stereotype is that—other physical characteristics notwithstanding—dentists tend to have good teeth, and good teeth are an indicator of attractiveness, particularly when evaluated by the opposite sex.[24,25] Further, physical attractiveness exhibits a halo effect in which attractive people are also assumed to be more competent.[26] Another reason is that dentists work on patient's mouths, and it has been noted that "the oral cavity has an erogenous potential."[27] Yet another reason is that arousal of fear and anxiety responses can be misinterpreted by individuals as sexual attraction.[28,29] Films often reinforce the attractiveness stereotype by casting attractive actors in the dentist role in films such as *Snow Dogs* and *Eversmile, New Jersey*.

Dentists can, and should, benefit from the attractiveness stereotype but also must be careful to maintain professional boundaries. Dentists' teeth and breath advertise the quality of their work, so they should be in excellent condition. Dental professionals should encourage mutual trust and liking in the patient relationship but must also sensitize themselves to indicators of danger. Dangerous dentist behaviors include consistently treating patients of one sex differently than patients of the other sex or treating one patient much differently than other patients. Dangerous patient behaviors include inappropriate verbal disclosures, questions, touching, and gift giving.

Mutual attractions sometimes do lead to relationships, but dating patients can lead to multiple practical and ethical problems, particularly if the relationship ends.[30,31] Providers who find themselves interested in a patient should refer the patient to a colleague before pursuing a romance.

Dentists are trustworthy

Seemingly incompatible with the negative stereotypes discussed is a positive stereotype that may compensate for all the negative associations: People trust dentists. In Gallup polls on the ethics and honesty of various professions, dentists consistently place in the top 10.[32] In the 2009 poll, 57% of respondents rated the honesty and ethical standards of dentists "high" or "very high."[33] This rating placed dentists sixth, behind nurses (83%), pharmacists (66%), physicians (65%), police officers (63%), and engineers (62%). The ranking is high but below the 62% rating achieved in 2006 and continues a declining trend.[34] Christensen[35] attributed that trend to several factors, relating primarily to dentists' focus on financial concerns to the neglect of patients' needs.

Even so, trust remains high, probably for the same reasons that so many of the most trusted professions are in the medical field. Patients seeking medical care are physically vulnerable, often weak and uncomfortable, and frequently do not fully understand the details of their diagnosis and treatment. As a result, they can appreciate that medical professionals hold a great deal of power to heal or harm. When professionals avoid harming patients or taking advantage of their vulnerability, they are rewarded with trust. The dentists in *Wild Hogs* and *Eversmile, New Jersey* are portraits of honesty and trustworthiness.

The primary communication strategy for fostering trust is to avoid any verbal or nonverbal messages that would undermine the honesty and fairness patients generally ascribe to the profession. Our culture typically promotes an idealistic portrait of dentistry to young children to facilitate visits and encourage lifelong dental care. Therefore, dentists are assumed to have positive qualities until personal experience indicates otherwise. The negative stereotypes are perhaps given more credibility only after a dentist causes pain (sadistic), overcharges (greedy), or makes an inappropriate comment (lecherous). Avoiding those messages is the best way to cultivate trust. The second best way is to apologize for such messages, whether they were intentional or misconstrued by the patient.

Activity 2-1

Consider portrayals of dentists in popular culture—film, television, and books. Do you think these portrayals are more likely to reflect popular attitudes about dentists or shape those attitudes? Discuss with your peers or instructors the influences on your decision to enter dentistry. Were you influenced primarily by personal experiences and relationships or by popular portrayals? Which experiences or portrayals?

Preappointment Perceptual Influences

In addition to stereotypes reinforced by the mass media, other types of influence shape patient perceptions of dentistry and dental professionals. By developing an awareness of these influences and understanding how they might affect the patient-provider relationship, providers can prepare themselves to correct misperceptions and reinforce positive perceptions. We will consider three influences on patient perceptions: (1) advertising and promotions, (2) word of mouth, and (3) websites and social media.

Advertising and promotions

Until the 1970s, advertising by dentists and other professionals was restricted or prohibited by professional organizations. After the US Supreme Court prohibited such restrictions, dentists began employing increasingly sophisticated advertising and marketing techniques to attract patients, and the distinction between a patient and a customer blurred. Such commercialization has remained controversial and prompted ongoing arguments about the ethics of marketing medical care.[36,37] Most dentists—particularly the older ones—initially opposed dental services advertising, but their views have moderated in the intervening years.[38,39] Consumers are generally more accepting of advertising than dentists are and value the information advertising provides, although patients also believe selection of a dentist should not be based on advertising.[38,40]

Advertising dental practices will continue via traditional media: television, radio, print, billboards, and direct mail. Because these are mass media, they potentially influence everyone. Whether or not a dentist chooses to advertise, patients will be exposed to the advertising of others. Only 9.2% of dentists advertise on television, but 46.7% of consumers report exposure to these advertisements.[38] Only 3.1% of dentists use billboards, but 31.7% of consumers report seeing billboard advertisements for dentists.

The public's exposure to mass media messages (including advertising) likely contributes to the high degree of agreement regarding standards of dental attractiveness.[41] Dental advertising also likely shapes patient expectations about the appointment experience and the possible results.[42,43] For instance, "pain-free dentistry" is a catchphrase often used to attract patients. Dental techniques can be less painful than they once were, and advances in pain management have further reduced the pain most procedures entail. Yet, contrary to the premise of pain-free dentistry, the potential for discomfort and pain remains. To correct misperceptions about pain-free dentistry, providers must be prepared to engage patients in an honest discussion of the pain involved and their pain threshold.

> **Q** **Question of ethics:** List three arguments for the right of dental practices to advertise and three arguments against. Do you feel dentists should have any restrictions on their advertising? If so, what are the limits?

Dental professionals must also be prepared to respond when patients show up for appointments with photographs ripped from magazines and before-and-after dental product advertisements showing "perfect" smiles. First, providers should discuss with the patient whether the outcome portrayed is achievable, given the condition of the patient's mouth and teeth. Second, providers should discuss whether the outcome is desirable. Patients may not understand the disadvantages of some procedures (eg, the installation of tooth jewelry or "grills" or unnaturally white teeth), and the dentist should be careful to explain the drawbacks without insulting the patient's knowledge or taste. Third, if the outcome is both achievable and desirable, providers should explain whether they are willing to do the procedure and, if so, the commitment of money, discomfort, and time the procedure requires.

In addition to advertising, dentists sometimes resort to marketing promotions to draw clients, and these strategies can distort a patient's perceptions of the cost of dental care. Garretson and Clow[44] found that coupons for dental care did increase the intention to purchase but at the expense of negative impacts on perceived quality and risk. Raghubir and Corfman[45] found that negative associations are more likely in service industries (such as dentistry) in which price promotions are traditionally uncommon. Whether those negative effects extend beyond the dental practice offering the discount or free trial is unknown.

What is known is that price promotions often list rates for specific procedures (eg, "$495 porcelain crown"), and these rates likely influence what patients expect to pay their own dentist. Therefore, dentists should remain aware of current local pricing levels for standard procedures. They should also be prepared to account for discrepancies between the lower rates advertised by other dentists and their own rates. Clinicians should explain to patients if procedures or materials differ or if a higher price includes more service.

Word of mouth

A 2009 study identified the implicit communication deriving from successful dental treatment as the key communication factor determining patient satisfaction.[46] The secondary factors, however, were the dentist-provider relationship and referrals by previous patients. Word-of-mouth referrals by patients are the most cost-effective form of marketing a dental practice.[47] A 2008 survey asked about the influences on respondents' selection of an orthodontist.[48] Fifty percent noted recommendations by family and friends, and 57% noted professional referrals. Very few respondents were influenced by Yellow Pages advertising (4%) or websites (1%). Dentists believe lay referral is the major source of new patients.[49]

Word of mouth can also negatively influence a practice. Reichheld[50] suggested that several positive comments would be necessary to overcome a single negative evaluation a patient disclosed. Other researchers, however, dispute this claim, although they acknowledge that negative word of mouth can drive away potential patients.[51,52]

Question of ethics: Assume the role of a patient instead of a health care provider. Is it ethical for patients to tell family and friends of negative experiences with a health care provider? Is it ethical to post such experiences on the Internet?

Dental professionals have limited control over what is said to whom after patients leave the office. Yet the reputation of a practice is largely built—or destroyed—by social network communication, which is now magnified by the availability of digital communication and social media. Dental professionals should realize that new patients may already have formed a strong opinion of them before ever sitting in the chair.

Developing an awareness of your reputation is essential to strengthening it or defending it. Satisfied patients can be explicitly encouraged to refer friends and family members to the practice. All patients should be encouraged to express any dissatisfaction to their dentist first, to offer an opportunity to fix problems. If they make a good-faith effort to address patient dissatisfaction and a patient continues to complain to others about service, providers have few options beyond referring the patient to a colleague. Such providers might console themselves with the assumption that the friends and family of the former patient are accustomed to hearing his or her complaints and therefore discount the evaluation.

Websites and social media

As an influence on patient perceptions, digital communication bridges mass media advertising and word of mouth. It also remains a frontier. A 2007 study found that 71.5% of dentists market their practice using a website, but only 11.7% of consumers reported viewing their dentist's website.[38] These numbers may increase, however, as more practices make use of Internet portals to schedule appointments, document a patient's health history, and provide information and follow-up for procedures.

Practices increasingly use the Internet for promotional purposes. For instance, dental practices have begun offering discounts through Internet sites such as Groupon and LivingSocial. Some professional organizations suggest that these promotions should be prohibited because they represent compensation for referral.[53] The Internet will continue to raise provocative issues that the entire dental profession must confront.

Even those practitioners who do not have a website or market themselves via the Internet must contend with two particular influences. First, patients now have access to an enormous amount of information on dental health and the latest developments in dental care. The Internet has simultaneously expanded access to information and democratized information flow, allowing anyone to attract an audience. A second important development is the rise of social media such as Facebook and Twitter, which permit real-time interaction with enormous networks. As a result of these two influences, before they arrive for an appointment, patients may have formed strong beliefs and attitudes regarding dental health (eg, mercury in restorations), dental procedures (eg, tooth whitening), and even specific dentists.

Not all of these beliefs may be accurate, nor may all the attitudes be justified. Dental professionals, however, have an obligation to listen to patients and validate their concerns. Dentists should always begin by praising the initiative patients have shown in researching or investigating an issue. When patients are misinformed, providers should use patients' misperceptions as an opportunity to educate them. Clinicians should encourage patients to pursue their interest in dental care but suggest some specific, credible resources—perhaps their own practice's website or the American Dental Association's excellent site, which includes an enormous amount of information in its Public Programs section (http://www.ada.org/en/public-programs).

Social media may be a source for information and misinformation, but it serves an additional function in allowing patients to disseminate opinions about their recent procedure or provider encounter. An increasing number of patients are taking to the Internet to air complaints against medical professionals.[54] However, unlike nonmedical service providers, medical professionals are typically prohibited by federal law (Health Insurance Portability and Accountability Act of 1996[55]) from disclosing patient information, thus preventing response to a patient's complaint in an online forum. Dentists should periodically conduct an Internet search of their name to ensure that no such complaints are floating around. If such complaints are found, the complaining patient can be contacted directly to arrange a resolution involving the removal of the online complaint. In some cases, legal action may be necessary.

Dental Anxiety

Odontophobia, **dental phobia**, **dental fear**, and **dental anxiety** are defined differently by various researchers. We refer to both **dental fear** and **dental anxiety** to describe the negative reactions of some patients toward dental treatment. Those reactions may be cognitive and emotional or they may be behavioral, but every dentist will encounter patients who are dentally anxious; interacting with such patients usually induces stress in the dentist.[56]

Poor anxiety management may lead patients to change dentists.[49] As with patient-provider communication in general, no single approach works best in every circumstance, so concurrent treatment of dental anxiety must be tailored to the patient.[57,58] To accomplish this, providers should understand what causes dental anxiety and what types of treatment are effective.

Causes of dental anxiety

An extensive research literature has developed around the causes and treatment of dental anxiety. Older patients and women are more likely to exhibit dental anxiety, which is often a consequence of a negative experience.[59] A 1996 study found more than three-quarters of the population reports direct negative dental experiences: painful (71%), frightening (23%), or embarrassing (9%).[60] Further, the relationship between dental anxiety and such experiences is strong. Patients can also develop dental anxiety vicariously through the experience of others—anxious parents or friends who had a painful procedure.[61] A more recent study by Armfield[62] found that previous negative dental experiences are weaker predictors of anxiety than are perceptions of uncontrollability, unpredictability, dangerousness, and disgustingness.

Regardless of cause, anxiety can have clinical consequences. For instance, anxious patients are significantly more likely to have caries lesions and to be edentulous.[63,64] Dental anxiety is also related to reductions in oral health–related quality of life.[65]

Diagnosis of dental anxiety

Although validated instruments have been developed to diagnose dental anxiety and dental fear, they are inconvenient in a clinical setting.[66–69] Recently, Jaakkola et al[70] developed a one-question screening tool that can be used chairside and has shown promise in determining the level of a patient's fear (Table 2-1). If a screening instrument is used, we advise against revealing a diagnosis of "anxious" or "fearful," which could label the patient with a condition that may be situational or temporary.

Of course, the provider can always simply ask, perhaps during the health history interview, whether the patient has delayed or canceled previous appointments or is worried about the present appointment.[71] The goal is to identify specific fears so they can be addressed.

Table 2-1 The Short Dental Fear Question and clinical classification*

Question: The last time you visited your dentist, how did it go?	Classification of fear
1. I was totally relaxed during the treatment.	Relaxed
2. I was nervous, but the treatment was carried out successfully.	Slightly frightened
3. I was nervous; the treatment could only just be carried out.	Moderately frightened
4. I was so frightened and nervous that...	
a. Treatment was difficult.	Severely frightened
b. The treatment didn't succeed.	Severely frightened
c. I totally missed my appointment.	Severely frightened

*Reprinted from Jaakkola et al[70] with permission.

The four anxiety classifications identified in the study by Jaakkola et al[70] are similar to the four types of anxious patient described in a study by De Jongh et al[72]:

1. Patients with mild anxiety
2. Patients fearful of specific dental procedures or situations
3. Patients with psychiatric symptoms
4. Patients with a high treatment need

Communication strategies with anxious patients

The De Jongh et al[72] study identified three chairside approaches effective in reducing anxiety. First, the progress of the appointment should be highly predictable for the patient. At the beginning, providers should preview the agenda by describing the goals of the appointment and the procedures required to meet those goals. Predictability can be enhanced by previewing and narrating the procedures as they occur.

Second, the teaching of coping skills to anxious patients reduces their anxiety. Such skills can include thought-stopping, deep breathing, meditating on positive affirmations, imagery, and holding a comforting object.[73] Milgrom and Weinstein[61] indicated that the acquisition of coping skills can enhance trust and feelings of control. A meta-analysis of behavioral interventions to reduce dental fear indicated a medium to large effect, and the results seem to be long-lasting.[74]

Third, desensitization to stimuli is an effective way to reduce anxiety. A European study ranked 67 stimuli by the degree of patient anxiety that they evoked.[75] Stimuli that scored higher included seeing the needle and other dental instruments, hearing the handpiece, and several sensations—the needle, the handpiece, and cold air on a tooth. Anxious patients who are prepared for these stimuli through a show-and-tell approach may become desensitized to the objects and experiences that they associate with anxiety.

In their review of psychologic (nonpharmaceutical) techniques for treating dental anxiety, Jerjes et al[76] included the suggestions made by De Jongh et al[72] and added a few more. A few of the communication strategies warrant emphasis. Ultimately, the dentist should aim to create a positive dental experience to counteract anxiety that has resulted from previous painful and negative dental experiences. To this end, a dental professional should never ignore dental anxiety, treat it as irrational, or try to argue a patient out of anxiety.

One easy strategy is to distract the anxious patient during a procedure by talking, playing music, or allowing the patient to listen to an MP3 player (such as an iPod or smartphone) on low volume.[73,77] The provider can allow the patient to select the type of music he or she wishes to hear during the appointment. To accomplish this, the provider can keep a variety of compact discs on hand, sort music by genre on an MP3 player, or select a type of streaming music from an online service such as Pandora.

Another easy strategy to alleviate anxiety is to allow the patient to pause the procedure by signaling when a break is needed. This approach enhances an anxious patient's perceived sense of control.

Patient Preferences

A growing body of research documents patient preferences and patient perceptions of the ideal dentist. Despite broad agreement across various demographic categories, however, patients often differ from one another in their preferences for many attributes and behaviors.[78] Furthermore, patients often differ from their provider in their expectations. Zimmerman[79] found a strong positive relationship between patient satisfaction and patient-provider agreement on expectations for interaction during an appointment.[80] Thus, providers should remain aware of the trends in patient preferences but should always clarify with specific patients their expectations for the consultation.[80]

The following sections discuss communication-relevant preferences that have emerged in the literature, supplemented by anecdotal and observational reports that have emerged in our discussions with students and patients.

Communicative and honest

A research team led by Lahti[81,82] reported strong preferences among Finnish patients for communicative and informative dentists. Behaviors associated with this attribute include telling patients why procedures are being done, asking if patients have specific concerns, encouraging patient questions, and telling what procedures are included in the treatment. A follow-up study indicated that patients prefer that dentists give accurate information regarding pain.[83]

A survey by Rankin and Harris[78] likewise found that patients want accurate information regarding pain and discomfort. Those patients also preferred full explanations of treatment, equipment, and behavioral expectations of the patient.

A study of patient loyalty found that patients indicate that the primary reason they remain with a dental practice is the honesty of their dentist.[84] In that study, quality of work and knowledge of dentistry were noted but were secondary to honesty, suggesting the importance of trust. A 1994 study found that 61% of patients indicated that explanations of procedures are very important, but only 39% of dentists agreed.[85]

Patients also tell us that they prefer being informed about the wait time for appointments and about the progress of the consultation. Regarding language use, they report a preference for explanations in lay terminology that they can understand rather than medical or dental jargon. Patients dislike the tendency of providers to leave the operatory without any explanation or estimated time they will be gone.

Activity 2-2

This chapter references film portrayals of dentists, but several television shows have also featured dentists prominently: *Friends*, *The Bob Newhart Show*, *The Carol Burnett Show*, *Seinfeld*, *Beverly Hills 90210*, *M*A*S*H*, *The Swan*, *Extreme Makeover*, and *John and Kate Plus 8*. Can you think of others? How do TV dentists compare to movie dentists? Discuss with your peers whether any of these portrayals reinforce the negative and positive stereotypes mentioned in this chapter.

Sensitive

A 1993 study found that sensitivity is considered by patients as the most important attribute when selecting a dental practice.[86] Specifically, patients prefer providers who are responsive to their pain and willing to discuss and overcome their fears. A survey of dentists indicates that they believe patients most frequently leave a practice due to external circumstances (such as relocation), but they also noted that patient turnover increases when patients are dissatisfied with the way they are treated and with quality of care.[49] Patients do not like being blamed by their dentist, criticized for the condition of their teeth, or scolded for poor oral hygiene.[78,82,83] In addition, 53% of patients say it is very important that providers not rush through an appointment, but only 32% of dentists agreed.[85]

Our own research confirms these findings and indicates that patients dislike negativity in general and alarming comments in particular. We have also been told repeatedly that patients dislike being neglected or ignored, as when members of the dental team converse as if the patient were not there. Perhaps because it interferes with their ability to perceive the progress of the appointment, patients also dislike reclining so far that their feet are above their head.

Collaborative

A study of decision-making preferences found that most patients prefer collaboration between provider and patient, although patients perceive that they play a passive role.[87] A minority of patients preferred a more passive role, citing their lack of knowledge, trust in their provider, and time constraints as reasons to place decisions in the provider's hands. A recent systematic review of decision-making in physician-patient relationships found that 50% of studies completed before 2000 reported a preference for shared decision-making compared with 71% after 2000, suggesting a generational shift toward collaboration.[88] When asked what dentist behaviors they dislike, patients in Rankin and Harris's survey[78] said that they did not like dentists who began treatment without a full explanation.

Our research indicates that patients prefer to have treatment options presented to them but also like knowing which option the dentist advocates. They report a strong dislike for feeling pressured to make a treatment decision.

Supportive

One study found that, in addition to professional skill, patients believe that the ideal dentist should be friendly and able to put patients at ease.[89] However, there are limits to supportive behaviors. Patients prefer that providers refrain from excessive touch, especially patting or caressing.[83] Patients dislike the failure of providers to comment on patient cooperation.[78]

Our research reveals a patient preference for compliments and positive reinforcement. They also like to be greeted by name, and they like it when the provider recalls personal details about them. Patients report a strong preference for eye contact. Patients dislike a lack of tact—as when providers take a condescending tone or curtly command, "Open!" Although patients like providers to be friendly and supportive, more than a few have reported that they dislike flirting.

Professional in appearance

Patients also report preferences regarding their provider's appearance. Actually, the strongest appearance-related preferences relate to smell rather than looks or dress. Patients prefer that their providers not smell of smoke or perfume.[83] They also prefer that their dentist not have bad breath.[90]

Our research confirms these preferences, and our patients also report liking their providers to have a nice appearance and clean clothes. A few reported disliking beards, but our dental students indicate that most patients likely have no beard preference, and in some cultures beards might actually be preferred.

Chapter Checklist ✔

Addressing stereotypes
- ❏ Failed-doctor stereotype: Prioritize education of the patient.
- ❏ Failed-doctor stereotype: Emphasize the role of dentist as a doctor specializing in oral health.
- ❏ Failed-doctor stereotype: Coordinate care with the patient's other health care providers.
- ❏ Sadistic stereotype: Remain aware of the stereotype.
- ❏ Sadistic stereotype: Acknowledge a patient's pain.
- ❏ Sadistic stereotype: Provide accurate information about the nature of discomfort a procedure will entail.
- ❏ Sadistic stereotype: Avoid laughing or appearing unconcerned when a patient is in pain.
- ❏ Sadistic stereotype: Arrange a signaling system for a patient in pain.
- ❏ Sadistic stereotype: Stop when a patient requests a break.
- ❏ Greedy stereotype: Remain sensitive to perceptions of greed and excessive wealth.
- ❏ Greedy stereotype: Avoid discussions of expensive cars, homes, etc.
- ❏ Greedy stereotype: Be truthful regarding the necessity and cost of services.
- ❏ Greedy stereotype: Listen to the patient's concerns about costs.
- ❏ Greedy stereotype: Do not pressure the patient to accept expensive treatments.
- ❏ Greedy stereotype: Provide a range of treatments at different price points.
- ❏ Greedy stereotype: Offer an expert opinion, but respect the patient's choice.
- ❏ Lecherous stereotype: Restrict social touch to the patient's hands and arms.
- ❏ Lecherous stereotype: Restrict professional touch to the oral cavity.
- ❏ Lecherous stereotype: Leave the operatory door ajar after the health history interview and update.
- ❏ Lecherous stereotype: Announce what is happening and why, to prevent misinterpretation.
- ❏ Attractive stereotype: Maintain professional boundaries with the patient.
- ❏ Attractive stereotype: Maintain your teeth and breath in excellent condition.
- ❏ Attractive stereotype: Encourage mutual trust and liking, but be sensitive to indicators of danger, such as treating one sex or one patient differently than others.
- ❏ Attractive stereotype: Refer patients to a colleague before pursuing a romance.
- ❏ Trustworthy stereotype: Avoid messages that would undermine perceptions of honesty.
- ❏ Trustworthy stereotype: Apologize for intentional or unintentional messages that undermine patient trust.

Addressing preappointment influences
- ❏ Pain: Prepare to discuss pain and the patient's pain threshold.
- ❏ Patient requests: Discuss whether the outcome is achievable and desirable.
- ❏ Patient requests: Explain commitments of money, discomfort, and time required to achieve results.
- ❏ Local promotions: Remain aware of local pricing levels for standard procedures.
- ❏ Local promotions: Address pricing discrepancies, noting differences in procedures, materials, and included services.
- ❏ Word of mouth: Realize that the patient may have well-formed opinions before a face-to-face meeting.
- ❏ Word of mouth: Encourage the patient to express any dissatisfaction to you first.
- ❏ Websites and social media: Listen to the patient and validate his or her concerns.
- ❏ Websites and social media: Praise the patient's initiative in researching oral health.

❑ Websites and social media: Use misinformation as an opportunity for education, referring the patient to credible sources of online information.
❑ Websites and social media: Periodically conduct an Internet search to identify online complaints against your practice.
❑ Websites and social media: Contact any complaining patient directly to resolve the source of dissatisfaction.

Addressing dental anxiety
❑ Understand the causes of dental anxiety: negative experiences; vicarious experiences; and perceptions of uncontrollability, unpredictability, dangerousness, and disgustingness.
❑ Diagnose dental anxiety through a validated instrument or by asking about dental fear during the health history interview.
❑ Make the appointment predictable by previewing and narrating procedures.
❑ Teach coping skills, such as thought-stopping, deep breathing, meditating on positive affirmations, imagery, and holding a comforting object.
❑ Desensitize the patient to stimuli through a show-and-tell approach.
❑ Create a positive dental experience to counteract negative past experiences.
❑ Never ignore anxiety, treat it as irrational, or argue over the rationality of anxiety.
❑ Use distractions such as talking and playing music.
❑ Allow the patient to pause procedures by signaling.

Accommodating patient preferences
❑ Communicative and honest: Tell the patient why procedures are being done, ask if the patient has specific concerns, encourage questions by the patient, and tell what procedures are included in the treatment.
❑ Communicative and honest: Using lay terms, provide full explanations of treatment, equipment, and behavioral expectations of the patient.
❑ Communicative and honest: Inform the patient of the wait time for appointments and the progress of the consultation.
❑ Communicative and honest: Avoid leaving the operatory without explaining or estimating the length of the absence.
❑ Sensitive: Respond to the patient's pain and show willingness to discuss dental fears.
❑ Sensitive: Avoid negativity; alarming comments; and blaming, criticizing, and scolding the patient.
❑ Sensitive: Avoid rushing through appointments or giving the appearance of rushing.
❑ Sensitive: Avoid neglecting or ignoring the patient.
❑ Sensitive: Avoid over-reclining the patient in the chair.
❑ Collaborative: Exhibit a willingness to collaborate.
❑ Collaborative: Begin treatment with a preview of the appointment.
❑ Collaborative: Provide treatment options and a professional recommendation, but avoid pressure.
❑ Supportive: Put the patient at ease.
❑ Supportive: Refrain from excessive touch.
❑ Supportive: Greet the patient by name, recall personal details, and make eye contact.
❑ Supportive: Compliment the patient and comment on his or her cooperation.
❑ Supportive: Show tact and avoid flirting.
❑ Professional appearance: Maintain a nice appearance with clean clothes.
❑ Professional appearance: Avoid bad smells such as smoke, perfume, and bad breath.

For More Information

Professional codes of ethics
- http://www.ada.org/en/about-the-ada/principles-of-ethics-code-of-professional-conduct/
- http://www.adha.org/bylaws-ethics

Questions patients ask
- http://www.ahrq.gov/questions
- http://www.ihs.gov/healthcommunications/index.cfm?module=dsp_hc_toolkit
- http://www.mouthhealthy.org/en/dental-care-concerns/questions-about-going-to-the-dentist
- http://www.npsf.org/?page=askme3

Dental advertising
- http://www.crookedbrains.net/2009/10/advertising.html
- http://www.healthpromotionsnow.com/browse/Dental-Promotions-and-Practice-Marketing_149/default.aspx

The Joint Commission's Speak Up Program
- http://www.jointcommission.org/speakup.aspx

Dental anxiety
- http://www.sitalchauhan.pwp.blueyonder.co.uk/dentalanxietyassessment/Index.htm
- http://www.dentalfearcentral.org
- http://www.dentalphobia.co.uk
- http://www.hatedentists.com/1112/fear-dentists-dental-anxiety

Lists of films featuring dentists
- http://www.amazon.com/ (search "Dentists in movies")
- http://www.classicfilmguide.com/index2f36.html
- http://www.chiprowe.com/videorev/dentist.html
- http://www.listal.com/list/movie-dentists

References

1. Hovland CI, Weiss W. The influence of source credibility on communication effectiveness. Public Opin Q 1951;15:635–650.
2. Pornpitakpan C. The persuasiveness of source credibility: A critical review of five decades' evidence. J Appl Soc Psychol 2004;34:243–281.
3. Davis SF, Palladino JJ. Psychology, ed 5. Upper Saddle River, NJ: Prentice-Hall, 2007:447.
4. Park B, Judd CM. Rethinking the link between categorization and prejudice within the social cognition perspective. Pers Soc Psychol Rev 2005;9:108–130.

5. Fiske ST, Russell AM. Cognitive processes. In: Dovidio JF, Hewstone M, Glick P, Esses VM (eds). The SAGE Handbook of Prejudice, Stereotyping and Discrimination. Thousand Oaks, CA: Sage, 2010:115–130.
6. Nosek B, Smyth F, Hansen J, et al. Pervasiveness and correlates of implicit attitudes and stereotypes. Eur Rev Soc Psychol 2007;18:36–88.
7. Thibodeau E, Mentasti L. Who stole Nemo? J Am Dent Assoc 2007;138:656–660.
8. Christensen GJ. The diversity of dentistry. J Am Dent Assoc 2000;131:83–85.
9. Aleo JJ. Is scientific judgment by a dentist the ultimate indignity? J Dent Res 1989;68:744.
10. Duncan RP, Gilbert GH, Peek CW, Heft MW. The dynamics of toothache pain and dental services utilization: 24-month incidence. J Public Health Dent 2003;63:227–234.
11. Olav V. Anxiety, pain and discomfort associated with dental treatment. Behav Res Ther 1993;31:659–666.
12. Sanmartin C, Ng E, Blackwell D, Gentleman J, Martinez M, Simile C. Joint Canada/United States Survey of Health, 2002-03. Ottawa, Ontario: Statistics Canada and the Centers for Disease Control and Prevention; 2004.
13. Dharamsi S, Pratt DD, MacEntee MI. How dentists account for social responsibility: Economic imperatives and professional obligations. J Dent Educ 2007;71:1583–1592.
14. Lévesque MC, Dupéré S, Loignon C, et al. Bridging the poverty gap in dental education: How can people living in poverty help us? J Dent Educ 2009;73:1043–1054.
15. Wallace BB, Macentee MI. Access to dental care for low-income adults: Perceptions of affordability, availability and acceptability. J Community Health 2012;37:32–39.
16. American Dental Association. American Dental Association Principles of Ethics and Code of Professional Conduct. Chicago, IL: American Dental Association, 2012. http://www.ada.org/~/media/ADA/About%20the%20ADA/Files/code_of_ethics_2012.ashx. Accessed 26 February 2015.
17. Newsome P, Wolfe IS. Value gaps in dental practice: Understanding how differences in core values can adversely affect the practice. J Am Dent Assoc 2003;134:1500–1504.
18. Day A. Fifteen infamous dentists. Milwaukee: Clarity Digital Group, 2009.
19. Lee HK. Patient-fondling dentist pleads no contest. San Francisco Chronicle, May 5, 2009.
20. Ross B. Dentist found guilty of fondling patients. New York Daily News, October 1, 1997.
21. Baseheart JR. Nonverbal communication in the dentist-patient relationship. J Prosthet Dent 1975;34:4–10.
22. Balasubramaniam B, Park GR. Sexual hallucinations during and after sedation and anaesthesia. Anaesthesia 2003;58:549–553.
23. Strickland RA, Butterworth JFI. Sexual dreaming during anesthesia: Early case histories (1849–1888) of the phenomenon. Anesthesiology 2007;106:1232–1236.
24. Eli L, Bar-Tat Y, Kostovetzki I. At first glance: Social meanings of dental appearance. J Public Health Dent 2001;61:150–154.
25. Giddon DB, Anderson NK. The oral and craniofacial area and interpersonal attraction. In: Mostofsky DI, Forgione AG, Giddon DB (eds). Behavioral Dentistry. Oxford: Blackwell Munksgaard, 2006:3–18.
26. Jackson LA, Hunter JE, Hodge CN. Physical attractiveness and intellectual competence: A meta-analytic review. Soc Psychol Q 1995;58:108–122.
27. Derbyshire JC. Patient motivation in periodontics. J Periodontol 1970;41:630–635.
28. Barlow DH, Sakheim DK, Beck JG. Anxiety increases sexual arousal. J Abnorm Psychol 1983;92:49–54.
29. Dutton DG, Aron AP. Some evidence for heightened sexual attraction under conditions of high anxiety. J Pers Soc Psychol 1974;30:510–517.
30. Chiodo GT, Tolle SW. Sexual boundaries in dental practice. 1. Gen Dent 1999;47:456–459.
31. Sfikas PM, George LA. Licensing boards confront sexual misconduct: Consent may not be a defense. J Am Dent Assoc 2004;135:1326–1329.
32. Hamilton J. Gallup and Harris Poll Trends: Dentistry is a trusted profession. Chicago Dental Society, December 3, 2008. http://www.cds.org/Page2Column.aspx?PageID=34&id=514&terms=Dentistry%20is%20a%20trusted%20profession. Accessed 15 January 2015.

33. Saad L. Honesty and ethics poll finds Congress' image tarnished. Washington, DC: Gallup, December 9, 2009. http://www.gallup.com/poll/124625/Honesty-Ethics-Poll-Finds-Congress-Image-Tarnished.aspx. Accessed 15 January 2015.

34. Saad L. Nurses top list of most honest and ethical professions. Washington, DC: Gallup, December 14, 2006. http://www.gallup.com/poll/25888/nurses-top-list-most-honest-ethical-professions.aspx. Accessed 15 January 2015.

35. Christensen GJ. The credibility of dentists. J Am Dent Assoc 2001;132:1163–1165.

36. Jerrold L, Karkhanehchi H. Advertising, commercialism, and professionalism: A history of the ethics of advertising in dentistry. J Am Coll Dent 2000;67(4):39–44.

37. Nisselson HS. What ethical considerations are involved in offering introductory discounts to attract new patients? J Am Dent Assoc 2008;139:769–771.

38. Clow KE, Stevens RE, McConkey C, Loudon DL. Attitudes of dentists and dental patients toward advertising. Health Mark Q 2007;24(1–2):23–34.

39. Hite RE, Bellizzi JA, Andrus DM. Consumer versus dentist attitudes toward dental services advertising. J Health Care Mark 1988;8(1):30–38.

40. Moser HR. How consumers view dental advertising: An empirical analysis. J Med Market 2008;8:229–240.

41. Dunn WJ, Murchison DF, Broome JC. Esthetics: Patients' perceptions of dental attractiveness. J Prosthodont 1996;5:166–171.

42. Golub-Evans J. Unity and variety: Essential ingredients of a smile design. Curr Opin Cosmet Dent 1994:1–5.

43. Pitigoi-Aron G, Geissberger M. Esthetic case design. In: Geissberger M (ed). Esthetic Dentistry in Clinical Practice. Ames, IA: Blackwell, 2010:55–74.

44. Garretson JA, Clow KE. The influence of coupon face value on service quality expectations, risk perceptions and purchase intentions in the dental industry. J Services Market 1999;13:59–72.

45. Raghubir P, Corfman K. When do price promotions affect pretrial brand evaluations? J Market Res 1999;36:211–222.

46. Mazzei A, Russo V, Crescentini A. Patient satisfaction and communication as competitive levers in dentistry. TQM J 2009;21:365–381.

47. Clarkson E, Bhatia S. Management and marketing for the general practice dental office. Dent Clin North Am 2008;52:495–505.

48. Edwards DT, Shroff B, Lindauer SJ, Fowler CE, Tufekci E. Media advertising effects on consumer perception of orthodontic treatment quality. Angle Orthod 2008;78:771–777.

49. O'Shea R, Corah N, Ayer W. Why patients change dentists: Practitioners' views. J Am Dent Assoc 1986;112:851–854.

50. Reichheld F. The microeconomics of customer relationships. MIT Sloan Manage Rev 2006;47:73–78.

51. East R, Hammond K, Lomax W. Measuring the impact of positive and negative word of mouth on brand purchase probability. Int J Res Mark 2008;25:215–224.

52. Uncles MD, East R, Lomax W. Market share is correlated with word-of-mouth volume. Australas Market J 2010;18:145–150.

53. Kharif O. Oregon dentist board says Groupon-like coupons may break rules. Bloomberg Business Week, September 1, 2011.

54. Shivers R, Shivers L. Nothing to smile about. A cautionary tale for dentists about electronic communication. J Okla Dent Assoc 2005;97(3):22–25.

55. Health Insurance Portability and Accountability Act of 1996, Pub L No. 104-191, 110 Stat 1936 (1996). http://www.gpo.gov/fdsys/pkg/PLAW-104publ191/html/PLAW-104publ191.htm. Accessed 12 January 2015.

56. Hill KB, Hainsworth JM, Burke FJT, Fairbrother KJ. Evaluation of dentists' perceived needs regarding treatment of the anxious patient. Br Dent J 2008;204:E13.

57. Weiner AA (ed). The Fearful Dental Patient: A Guide to Understanding and Managing. Ames, IA: Wiley-Blackwell, 2011.

58. Bray A, Chhun A, Donkersgoed R, Hoover S, Levitan S. An Evidence-Based Report Investigating the Most Effective Method to Reduce Dental Anxiety. Toronto: University of Toronto Faculty of Dentistry, 2009.

59. Hittner JB, Hemmo R. Psychosocial predictors of dental anxiety. J Health Psychol 2009;14:53–59.
60. Locker D, Shapiro D, Liddell A. Negative dental experiences and their relationship to dental anxiety. Community Dent Health 1996;13:86–92.
61. Milgrom P, Weinstein P. Dental fears in general practice: New guidelines for assessment and treatment. Int Dent J 1993;43(3 suppl 1):288–293.
62. Armfield JM. Towards a better understanding of dental anxiety and fear: Cognitions vs. experiences. Eur J Oral Sci 2010;118:259–264.
63. Eitner S, Wichmann M, Paulsen A, Holst S. Dental anxiety: An epidemiological study on its clinical correlation and effects on oral health. J Oral Rehabil 2006;33:588–593.
64. Locker D, Liddell AM. Correlates of dental anxiety among older adults. J Dent Res 1991;70:198–203.
65. Mehrstedt M, John MT, Tönnies S, Micheelis W. Oral health-related quality of life in patients with dental anxiety. Community Dent Oral Epidemiol 2007;35:357–363.
66. Corah NL. Development of a dental anxiety scale. J Dent Res 1969;48:596.
67. Corah NL, Gale EN, Illig SJ. Assessment of a dental anxiety scale. J Am Dent Assoc 1978;97:816–819.
68. Kleinknecht RA, Klepac RK, Alexander LD. Origins and characteristics of fear of dentistry. J Am Dent Assoc 1973;86:842–848.
69. Kleinknecht RA, Thorndike RM, McGlynn FD, Harkavy J. Factor analysis of the Dental Fear Survey with cross-validation. J Am Dent Assoc 1984;108:59–61.
70. Jaakkola S, Rautava P, Alanen P, et al. Dental fear: One single clinical question for measurement. Open Dent J 2009;3:161–166.
71. Heaton LJ, Carlson CR, Smith TA, Baer RA, de Leeuw R. Predicting anxiety during dental treatment using patients' self-reports: Less is more. J Am Dent Assoc 2007;138:188–195.
72. De Jongh A, Adair P, Meijerink-Anderson M. Clinical management of dental anxiety: What works for whom? Int Dent J 2005;55:73–80.
73. Lahmann C, Schoen R, Henningsen P, et al. Brief relaxation versus music distraction in the treatment of dental anxiety: A randomized controlled clinical trial. J Am Dent Assoc 2008;139:317–324.
74. Kvale G, Berggren U, Milgrom P. Dental fear in adults: A meta-analysis of behavioral interventions. Community Dent Oral Epidemiol 2004;32:250–264.
75. Oosterink FMD, De Jongh A, Aartman IHA. What are people afraid of during dental treatment? Anxiety-provoking capacity of 67 stimuli characteristic of the dental setting. Eur J Oral Sci 2008;116:44–51.
76. Jerjes W, Hopper C, Kumar M, et al. Psychological intervention in acute dental pain: Review. Br Dent J 2007;202:337–343.
77. Bare LC, Dundes L. Strategies for combating dental anxiety. J Dent Educ 2004;68:1172–1177.
78. Rankin J, Harris M. Patients' preferences for dentists behaviors. J Am Dent Assoc 1985;110:323–327.
79. Zimmerman RS. The dental appointment and patient behavior: Differences in patient and practitioner preferences, patient satisfaction, and adherence. Med Care 1988;26:403–414.
80. Kay E, Nuttall N. Clinical decision making—An art or a science? 5. Patient preferences and their influence on decision making. Br Dent J 1995;178:229–233.
81. Lahti S, Tuutti H, Hausen H, Kääriäinen R. Dentist and patient opinions about the ideal dentist and patient: Developing a compact questionnaire. Community Dent Oral Epidemiol 1992;20:229–234.
82. Lahti S, Tuutti H, Hausen H, Kääriäinen R. Opinions of different subgroups of dentists and patients about the ideal dentist and the ideal patient. Community Dent Oral Epidemiol 1995;23:89–94.
83. Lahti S, Hausen H, Kääriäinen R. Patients' expectations of an ideal dentist and their views concerning the dentist they visited: Do the views conform to the expectations and what determines how well they conform? Community Dent Oral Epidemiol 1996;24:240–244.
84. Kelly MA, Lange B, Dunning DG, Underhill TE. Reasons patients stay with a dentist. J Dent Pract Adm 1990;7(1):9–15.
85. Gerbert B, Bleecker T, Saub E. Dentists and the patients who love them: Professional and patient views of dentistry. J Am Dent Assoc 1994;125:264–272.

86. Chakraborty G, Gaeth G, Cunningham M. Understanding consumers' preferences for dental service. J Health Care Mark 1993;13(3):48–58.
87. Chapple H, Shah S, Caress AL, Kay EJ. Exploring dental patients' preferred roles in treatment decision-making—A novel approach. Br Dent J 2003;194:321–327.
88. Chewning B, Bylund CL, Shah B, Arora NK, Gueguen JA, Makoul G. Patient preferences for shared decisions: A systematic review. Patient Educ Couns 2012;86:9–18.
89. Van Groenestijn MA, Maas-de Waal CJ, Mileman PA, Swallow JN. The ideal dentist. Soc Sci Med 1980;14A:533–540.
90. Lahti S, Verkasalo M, Hausen H, Tuutti H. Ideal role behaviors seen by dentists and patients themselves and by their role partners: Do they differ? Community Dent Oral Epidemiol 1996;24: 245–248.

3

Developing Cultural Competence

Why Cultural Competence Matters

Chapter 2 explored stereotypes and media influences that shape societal perceptions of dentistry. This chapter takes a different approach, examining how perceptions and preferences are influenced within a society by the cultural background of a patient. The American Dental Education Association's (ADEA's) *Competencies for the New General Dentist* include the ability to "communicate effectively with individuals from diverse populations."[1] The ADEA[2] also requires that new dental hygienists be able to "initiate a collaborative approach with all patients when developing individualized care plans that are specialized, comprehensive, culturally sensitive, and acceptable to all parties involved in care planning." The core competence requirement for dental assistants uses similar wording. The current emphasis on developing communication skills with patients from diverse backgrounds reflects a broader movement in health care toward cultural competence among providers.[3–5] The Commission on Dental Accreditation[6] defines **cultural competence** as follows:

> Having the ability to provide care to patients with diverse backgrounds, values, beliefs and behaviors, including tailoring delivery to meet patients' social, cultural, and linguistic needs. Cultural competence training includes the development of a skill set for more effective provider-patient communication and stresses the importance of providers understanding the relationship between diversity of culture, values, beliefs, behavior and language and the needs of patients.

Cultural competence contributes to a patient-centered approach to health care and therefore seems like a nice way to treat patients, but it is more than that. A growing body of research suggests at least four advantages associated with culturally competent providers. First, the United States is becoming ever more diverse. By 2042, the aggregate ethnic "minority" population will become the majority.[7] This diversity is reflected not only among patients but also among providers, suggesting that patients and providers increasingly will come from different cultural backgrounds.

Second, cultural competence may reduce disparities in health care access. Differential access to oral health care is associated with a range of demographic and cultural variables.[8,9] Yet, even after controlling for income, education, age, and dental insurance, data indicate significant disparities in access that may relate to cultural barriers.[10] Deliberate efforts by dental professionals to overcome those barriers could enhance access to care.[11,12]

Third, by reducing communication barriers, culturally competent providers can provide better care. Most explicitly when accommodating patients' language limitations, culturally competent providers hold an advantage in understanding patients' chief complaint and desired outcome.[13]

Fourth, providers who are culturally competent diversify their patient base and enhance patient satisfaction. Patient satisfaction with dental care varies significantly by patient ethnicity and income.[14,15] Because technical competence does not vary by patient ethnicity and income, it can be assumed that patients from different backgrounds perceive their treatment differently. Development of skills in culturally competent communication is a step toward minimizing these perceived differences.

Culture and Context

Definition of culture

Culture is commonly understood in concrete terms—as the collection of symbols that characterize a given population. In other words, culture comprises a people's customs, dress, music, literature, rituals, and so on. This conceptualization is flawed in at least two ways. First, it portrays culture as rigid and unchanging rather than dynamic and evolving. For this reason, some Americans visit the Netherlands expecting the Dutch to wear wooden shoes. Second, this rigid understanding of culture is likewise very narrow, so it fails to account for the wide variation in behaviors among those sharing a given culture. For this reason, many international visitors expect all Americans to carry handguns. Unfortunately, cultural research and education often reflect this flawed approach to culture. Even formal measures of cultural competence often equate culture with possessed traits (usually race and ethnicity) and assume that health care providers are white and Western.[16]

We prefer Wood's communication-oriented definition,[17] which reflects the dynamism and variability of culture by emphasizing meaning rather than artifacts: **Culture** is "the beliefs, understandings, practices, and ways of interpreting experience that are shared by a group of people." Simply put, culture is the worldview of a group of people, which is expressed in communicative behavior. Dental professionals, however, do not treat groups of people; they treat individual patients. Therefore, professionals must bear in mind two points. First, no given patient perfectly represents the culture of a group to which he or she belongs. We all have individual preferences for enacting or rejecting various aspects of the culture to which we belong.

Activity 3-1

What are the elements that distinguish the culture of dentistry? To help you answer this question, imagine that you are asked to educate members of an isolated tribe about their first visit to a US dental practice. Make a list of 10 things they should know so their appointment will be successful. Consider from their point of view which things will seem the most unexpected.

Second, the culture to which we belong is not a single monoculture but rather the overlap of various co-cultures. Wood's definition[17] relates culture to a group of people, but we all belong to various groups simultaneously: nation, school, workplace, religion, service organization, sports team, and so on. The list of overlapping groups is large, and each has its own culture. Therefore, an individual's cultural background is a mix of cultures reflecting the various groups to which he or she belongs.

Further complicating matters, the expression of culture is shaped by individual preferences and the context in which a person is situated. The dental practice is a specific context that can affect a patient's cultural expression; dental professionals should therefore consider the ways they and their environment might be perceived differently, depending on a patient's cultural background.

Patient-provider context

Culture cannot exist in a vacuum, because a person's ways of interpreting experience—or ways they do not interpret experience—take on meaning only when they are compared to alternatives. As a result, the degree of contrast between two cultures suggests how challenging the communication between members of those cultures will be. For instance, health care in the United States has developed a culture of its own. Those who operate within this culture take for granted assumptions about germ theory, the roles of physicians and nurses, the quality of hospital food, and a host of other characteristics that were internalized long ago. In advanced Western societies, even adults who have never been inside a clinic can quickly figure out how the culture works because they are familiar with other bureaucratic institutions. Adults from cultures that are less bureaucratic or practice other types of healing will struggle to understand the US health care system. If dental professionals aim to deliver patient-centered care, they must be culturally competent enough to determine whose cultural background could make the dental practice seem foreign and how to reconcile one culture to another.

The patient-provider dyad is fundamental to the dental context. From a clinical standpoint, the provider can operate only within narrow parameters supported by evidence-based practice. Patients whose cultural background makes them unfamiliar with clinical procedures involved in examination and treatment should be educated because the procedures themselves cannot be changed significantly. On the other hand, nonclinical interaction often can be modified to accommodate cultural expectations and individual preferences.

First, however, providers must gain a full understanding of their own appearance, behavior, and cultural background so they can better understand how patients perceive them. Communication challenges can result from differences between patient and provider, but such challenges are not inevitable. Rather, the challenges tend to emerge when the provider does not meet the patient's cultural expectations about who should be a provider and how they should behave.

Male and female dentists are remarkably similar in the way they approach and practice their profession.[18–20] Yet, research on gender stereotypes indicates that patients believe female dentists are more likely to ensure that patients are relaxed and to take time to discuss symptoms.[21] Patients believe that male dentists are more likely to expect the patient to endure pain without complaint. When presented with photographs of general dentists, participants in one study[22] indicated that female dentists are more caring than their male counterparts, whereas males are more competent, and the participants would more likely choose a male as their dentist in the absence of other information. On the other hand, a study of British patients found that they prefer female dentists to male dentists.[23] These perception studies were conducted with small, nonrepresentative samples, but for that reason they suggest how a patient's cultural background can shape perceptions of the provider based on characteristics unrelated to clinical skill.

Activity 3-2

Interview a dental professional who does not fit cultural or traditional expectations for the role. For instance, talk to a male dental hygienist or a black female dentist. Ask if patients respond to the provider differently than they do to colleagues who match cultural expectations. What sorts of responses has the provider gotten? How has he or she handled such reactions?

Concordance

Concordance is simply the degree of similarity or agreement between two individuals on a given measure. Because culture is variable and dynamic, validated measures are difficult to construct, so researchers have instead attempted to measure the degree of patient-provider concordance on cultural proxies such as race and sex to identify how concordant dyads may differ from nonconcordant dyads on such outcomes as treatment planning and adherence. Such research is important, given that 76.3% of dentists, 88.9% of hygienists, and 69.2% of dental assistants in the United States are white.[24] In each profession, whites are overrepresented relative to their proportion of the US population. Further, 77.8% of dentists are male, and 99% of dental hygienists are female.[25,26] From a communication perspective, such skewed representation is not a problem if the professionals are comfortable and if patients are satisfied and receiving equal treatment. The evidence, however, suggests room for improvement.[27]

A lack of cultural competence could be responsible for some of the frustrations experienced by providers. Milgrom et al[28] developed a measure for frustrating patient visits. Three of the four factors identified are related to frustrations that could have cultural explanations: unpleasant feelings (eg, "The patient was too controlling."), lack of communication (eg, "The patient and I seemed to come from different worlds."), and compliance (eg, "The patient did not accept responsibility for his or her dental health.").

The cultural explanation is supported by a study by Rouse and Hamilton,[29] who found that dentists evaluate patients on three culturally relevant dimensions: compliance, tractability, and likability. Some evidence suggests that more cooperative patients receive higher-quality restorative treatment.[30] Given that knowledge of cultural groups among dental students is low, the potential for frustration and treatment disparities is high.[31]

One solution is for providers simply to treat patients whom they feel comfortable treating. In 1981, Ayer[32] suggested that the patient-provider relationship reflects a mutual selection process in which individuals of similar backgrounds and values are more satisfied than dissimilar dyads. Presumably, patients and, to a lesser degree, providers continue to be drawn to those with whom they feel comfortable. However, in the three decades since the study by Ayer,[32] demographics and expectations have changed among both patients and providers.

The implications of these changes are not entirely clear. A 2007 study by Bender[33] found that most patients report no preference for a dentist of the same race or sex, but among subgroups some differences emerged. Hispanic females expressed a marked preference for both a race- and sex-concordant dentist. A proportion of black and Hispanic patients may prefer a racially concordant dentist, and a proportion of female patients may prefer a female dentist.

Black and white patients report similar satisfaction with white providers, but black patients give lower ratings for how well the white dentist got to know them.[34] Another study found that black dentists are significantly more likely to treat underserved populations, but the reasons for this are unclear.[35] Bare and Dundes[36] discovered that anxious patients preferred male dentists to female dentists, and this tendency was most pronounced among anxious male patients, 91% of whom preferred a male dentist.

Studies from the broader health care environment offer additional insights. A 2009 review of the literature found that 33% of studies documented positive health outcomes for minorities in race-concordant patient-provider dyads.[37] An additional 37% found mixed results. Another report was more conclusive, linking racial and ethnic concordance with greater patient satisfaction and improved health care processes.[38] The authors of that study explicitly called for efforts to recruit minority providers while improving the cultural competence of current providers. A study of patient-provider communication found that, in racially concordant consultations, physicians visited longer and patients rated them as more participatory.[39]

Question of ethics: Practicing dentistry requires a degree of intimacy between patient and provider. Appointments involve questions about health history and personal habits, followed by a physically intrusive examination. Given the sensitivity of these procedures, patients from conservative cultural backgrounds may prefer providers of the same sex. Should you accommodate these cultural preferences? What if the request is for a provider of the same religion or ethnicity? What are your limits for accommodating cultural differences?

Cultural Influences

Because culture is dynamic and variable, instructions on communicating with individuals from specific cultures are prone to error and quickly become outdated. Because such guidelines assume that everyone affiliated with a given culture is identical, they are also offensive. Consider your reaction to instructions on "How to talk to girls" or "How to marry a millionaire." Furthermore, individuals belong to multiple social groups and therefore hold overlapping cultural identities. Some of these identities may be more salient to dental care (eg, Somalian or mixed martial artist) and others less so (eg, Apple user or geocacher). In short, no one can provide worthwhile instruction on how to communicate effectively with people from every culture on earth. Even if such a resource existed, providers could ignore most of it, because the cultural diversity they will encounter in their practice is likely to be limited to the number of cultural groups that populate the community they serve.

What is possible, and far more useful, is sensitizing dental care providers to the ways culture can influence oral health care so they can quickly identify and accommodate challenges and opportunities when they arise. Training for a career in dentistry helps students develop cultural sensitivity in that dental colleges and training institutions often attract a diversity of patients and typically require service learning outreach to underserved populations.[40,41] As noted, however, cultural barriers persist in dental care. For a more comprehensive understanding of health care issues related to diversity, we recommend that providers review some of the excellent books on intercultural communication in health care.[42–46] We also recommend that providers research the cultural beliefs and practices of cultural groups within their practice area. Some resources are listed at the end of this chapter. The final section of this book also includes chapters on intercultural communication with patients likely to visit any practice (eg, the deaf and hard of hearing, those with limited English language skills, and young and old patients).

In addition, there are components of culture that dental providers can notice easily to determine whether a patient's culture might influence care (Box 3-1). Providers should be careful not to stereotype, however, because physical characteristics do not always signify that the patient is a member of a particular culture. For instance, patients with Latino features might claim American heritage stretching back centuries. Patients with Asian features might have been adopted into a non-Asian family and have very little cultural knowledge of Asia, despite the irritating assumptions of others.

In addition, providers should remain aware that many multicultural patients are adept at **code switching**, meaning they are proficient at communicating fluently in at least two different cultures. Refugee and immigrant children, for instance, often behave and speak the "old country way" at home and the "American way" at school or work. Given these cautions, the following discussion will consider the cultural implications of a patient's language, nationality, and ethnicity.

Box 3-1	Ways to determine the cultural background of patients

- **Observe the patient's dress:** A patient who is visiting from another country or a recent immigrant is less likely to buy and wear Americanized clothing.
- **Read the patient's forms:** Lack of response, awkward phrasing, and incorrect spelling can suggest that the patient is not familiar with English.
- **Review the patient's information:** The information the patient provides could yield clues to his or her cultural background.
- **Listen to the patient's language:** If the patient speaks another language with family or friends in the waiting room, he or she may have limited English skills.
- **Listen to the patient's vocabulary:** If the patient uses strange English phrasing or addresses people more formally than native-born Americans usually do, he or she may speak English as a second language or come from a former British colony.
- **Observe the patient's interaction:** If the patient appears uncertain how to respond to the receptionist, he or she may not understand English or appointment procedures.
- **Observe the patient's behavior:** If standard appointment procedures seem foreign to the patient, he or she may not have visited a Western dentist (or any dentist).
- **Consider the community:** Determine whether the community includes social or religious gathering places for people of different cultures.
- **Ask the patient:** The question, "Are you foreign?" is both intrusive and offensive. However, you can often elicit cultural information through polite rapport: "Have you always lived in Springfield?" If communication is not going well, you can ask the patient for help: "I am worried I am not doing what you wanted. Can you tell me what your previous dental visits were like?"

Language

Language and culture are inseparable because language reflects culture, shapes culture, and determines which individuals can verbally interact with a social group. Regarding language, dental professionals have three primary concerns. First, the patient must be able to provide an accurate health history. Second, the patient must be able to understand diagnoses and treatment options. Third, the patient must be able to understand and grant informed consent.

These are ethical concerns, but they are also legal concerns. Title VI of the Civil Rights Act of 1964[47] requires health care providers who accept federal financial assistance such as Medicaid and the State Children's Health Insurance Program to provide and pay for "meaningful access" for patients with limited English proficiency. For deaf patients, the Americans with Disabilities Act[48] requires providers to ensure communication equivalent to that with a hearing patient, regardless of federal financial assistance.

Language barriers are associated with cultural barriers but can present a separate set of challenges. The challenges of delivering care to deaf patients and patients with limited English proficiency (LEP) are complex enough to merit a separate chapter in the final section of this book (see chapter 11). LEP is associated with poorer oral health and fewer preventive dental visits.[49–51] Further, health literacy is a problem for English speakers as well as patients with LEP, and it is addressed in the chapter on verbal skills (see chapter 11).

Nearly every provider can expect to treat patients with LEP. Unfortunately, such treatment can take longer, and some providers alter their treatment recommendations and treatment provided to these patients.[52] Providers perceive that patients with LEP are more difficult to treat, so providers must be on guard to provide adequate care to such patients.[53]

Nationality

Culture is not defined by national boundaries, but prior to the widespread availability of telecommunication technology, culture was necessarily localized and spread by interpersonal contact. Furthermore, nationality frequently is an important component of a group's cultural identity, even when the groups relocate. Consider Americans of Irish or Italian heritage who identify with Ireland and Italy for generations after an ancestor emigrated.

Geert Hofstede[54] is a Dutch social psychologist who developed a theory of cultural dimensions to provide a framework for analyzing cultures across modern nations. Hofstede's analyses are used extensively as resources by international businesses seeking research on cultural preferences of a given nation's population. A consulting website based on his work offers cultural analyses of more than 50 nations: http://geert-hofstede.com/countries.html.

Briefly, the cultural dimensions Hofstede[54] isolates are power distance, individualism, masculinity, uncertainty avoidance, and long-term orientation. These dimensions are presented here as cultural influences for the dental provider to consider when treating someone from a different country. **Power distance** is the degree to which members of a culture accept imbalances of power and authority. Patients from countries where power distance is high might expect those in authority (eg, the dentist or the head of the family) to make treatment decisions for them. **Individualism** is the degree to which members of a culture accept independent (versus collective) action. Patients from less individualistic cultures may wish to confer with family members before making treatment decisions. **Masculinity** is the rigidity or fluidity of gender roles in a society, with implications for the value placed on traditionally masculine traits such as aggression and competitiveness. Patients from less masculine cultures might embrace the relational aspects of patient-provider interaction more than patients from more masculine cultures. **Uncertainty avoidance** is a culture's tolerance for ambiguity. Patients from cultures high in uncertainty avoidance may request more specific information regarding diagnosis, treatment outcomes, and cost. Finally, **long-term orientation** refers to a culture's time horizon. Patients from cultures with a long-term orientation might be more accepting of treatments that require multiple visits and more gradual results.

> **Question of ethics:** The health care culture in the United States places the highest value on curing and symptom relief. Other cultures, however, are more accepting of chronic health problems and pain. If one of your patients refuses a simple restorative treatment, should you feel obligated to find out why? If the reasons are cultural or religious, is it ethical to attempt to persuade the patient to change his or her mind?

Ethnicity

A 2006 review of the research on health care barriers related to ethnicity identified potential barriers at the patient, provider, and system levels.[55] Potential patient-level barriers included health beliefs and attitudes, perceptions of illness, health practices, and social variables and resources. Potential provider-level barriers included provider skills and attitudes. System-level variables related primarily to organization. The multiple variables determining access to and quality of care led the authors to conclude what we previously asserted[55]: "The barriers are all tied to the particular situation of the individual patient and subject to constant adjustment. In other words, generalizations should not be made."

Although providers should tailor communication to individual patients, they should also remain aware of health disparities between ethnic groups and consider the possible cultural reasons for those disparities. Books and online resources provide information on myriad ethnic groups and their health practices. The following is an example of the type of research that is conducted and how it can be applied. Black and Hispanic Americans tend to have poorer oral health than white Americans.[56] Manski and Magder[10] found significant and large differences between dental care utilization between whites and their black and Hispanic counterparts. Those differences in oral health and dental care utilization persisted even after the data were controlled for income and dental insurance, suggesting the influence of other variables.

One cultural explanation is that patient ethnicity seems related to attitudes toward prevention. Whites are more likely to believe in the benefits of preventive dental practices (perhaps as a result of greater access to preventive dental care), and some ethnic groups perceive dental visits in terms of problem solving rather than prevention.[57,58] Other possible explanations for differences include diet and acculturation, although the impact of these cultural factors on oral health has not been adequately studied.[59–61] Detailed information on ethnic disparities in oral health is presented in the 2009 National Healthcare Disparities Report.[24] Research on the oral health beliefs of four ethnic minorities in the United States was discussed in a 2008 review by Butani et al.[62]

Culture is context based. The way a group of people view the world attains meaning only if it can be described as different from another way of viewing the world. Often, minority groups are perceived in cultural terms because their worldview and behaviors are different from those of the majority, whose worldview and behaviors are considered "normal" and therefore not seen in cultural terms. The blog http://stuffwhitepeoplelike.com/full-list-of-stuff-white-people-like/ explores this idea by making the majority culture seem different and worthy of comment. Read some of these entries and discuss with your colleagues whether the observations are accurate and what they say about cultures in our society.

Providers can and should inform themselves about these and other cultural influences on oral health, including education, socioeconomic status, sexual orientation, and even age and sex. In applying such knowledge, however, caution should be emphasized. In a multicultural society, a patient's cultural background can be impossible to determine based on appearances. Even when a provider has accurate information regarding a patient's ethnicity, the patient's health-related values, beliefs, attitudes, and practices may differ markedly from those that are generally associated with his or her cultural heritage.

Furthermore, cultural imperialism can lead Western health care providers to believe in the superiority of evidence-based practice over faith healing, folk remedies, prayer, and refusal of treatment. As members of a distinct health care culture, providers are often perceived as detached and condescending, particularly to patients who do not share their native language, nationality, or ethnicity. To provide patient-centered care, dental professionals must determine a patient's values and goals for care and sensitively collaborate with the patient to deliver the best evidence-based care acceptable to the patient. Developing and sustaining empathy with patients, despite their differences, are crucial aspects of this process.[63,64]

The questions below are adapted from The Jefferson Scale of Physician Empathy.* Respond to each statement with a number from 1 ("strongly disagree") to 7 ("strongly agree") and total your points. Compare your score with those of your peers. Discuss those items that seem to generate the most variability in scores.

1. Dental professionals should try to imagine themselves in their patients' shoes when providing care to them.
2. Dental professionals' understanding of their patients' feelings gives the patients a sense of validation that is therapeutic in its own right.
3. An important component of the patient relationship is the dental professional's understanding of the emotional status of patients and their families.
4. Dental professionals should try to understand what is going on in their patients' minds by paying attention to their nonverbal cues and body language.
5. Dental professionals should try to think like their patients in order to render better care.
6. I believe that empathy is an important therapeutic factor in dental treatment.
7. Empathy is a therapeutic skill without which success as a dental professional would be limited.
8. Patients' problems can be cured by medical treatment, but emotional ties to patients cannot have a significant place in this endeavor.
9. Dental professionals should allow themselves to be touched by intense emotional relationships between patients and their family members.
10. I believe that emotion has no place in the treatment of dental problems.
11. Because people are different, it is almost impossible for dental professionals to see things from their patients' perspectives.
12. Attentiveness to patients' personal experiences is irrelevant to treatment effectiveness.
13. Patients feel better when the dental professional understands their feelings.
14. Dental professionals should have a good sense of humor because I think it contributes to a better clinical outcome.
15. I consider understanding patients' body language as important as verbal communication in patient-provider relationships.
16. Dental professionals should try to pay attention to patients' emotions in interviewing and history taking.

Activity 3-4 (cont)

17. I consider asking patients about what is happening in their lives as an important factor in understanding their physical complaints.
18. It is easy for me to view things from patients' perspectives.
19. I enjoy reading nondental literature and the arts.
20. A dental professional's understanding of how patients and their families feel is a relevant factor in dental treatment.

*Adapted from Hojat et al[63] with permission.

Culturally Competent Communication Strategies

Even without training, health care providers with a natural inclination toward empathy can instinctually understand patients and often know the best way to respond. Balancing empathy with the clinical detachment necessary for effective care, however, can be challenging, particularly when the patient is from a different culture. Box 3-2 lists several adjustments to your standard communication style that may be appropriate when interacting with patients from diverse cultures. These suggestions integrate our own experience with the work of Teal and Street.[65] In addition to these adjustments, this section will present a brief overview of language use, the LEARN model,[66] and the Kleinman questions.[67]

| Box 3-2 | Communication adjustments for patients from diverse cultures* |

- **Greeting:** Always smile and say hello while looking at the patient. A smile is a universal expression of good will.
- **Address:** Always call the patient by his or her title (Mr, Ms, Dr, etc) until granted permission to call the patient something else. Many cultures retain a formality the US culture is rapidly shedding.
- **Patient chaperones:** Patients from some cultures are more likely to bring someone with them to a dental appointment. If this happens, greet the chaperone. If the chaperone wants to observe, attempt to accommodate him or her in the operatory if it will not interfere with procedures.
- **Nonclinical touch:** A handshake is generally appropriate, but in some cultures male-female touching is disapproved, so note the patient's reaction when you extend your hand. Refrain from other nonclinical touch (on arms or the back) until you are certain it will not offend.
- **Rapport:** In some cultures, medical professionals are expected to act authoritarian and detached. If the patient seems unresponsive to friendly rapport building, do not persist in attempting to draw out personal information.
- **Speech:** Speak slowly, facing the patient, to enhance understanding if the patient's first language is not English.
- **Patient response time:** Allow extra time for the patient to respond so he or she can interpret or process what you have asked and formulate a reply.
- **Patient responses:** As you present information and listen to replies, look for signs of incomprehension, such as blank eyes, furrowed brow, shifting gaze, and silence. If the patient appears not to understand, repeat the information with simpler wording, use presentation aids, or enlist the help of the chaperone.
- **Treatment decisions:** In some cultures, decisions regarding treatment are made by someone other than the patient (eg, the health care provider or the head of the family). If the patient seems unwilling to make a treatment decision, clarify which treatment you recommend and ask whether the patient would like to discuss treatment options with someone at home. Send the patient home with written information outlining the treatment options.

*Adapted from Teal and Street[65] with permission.

Vocabulary

Culture is a primary means of identifying and distinguishing social groups. It has therefore been misused for millennia as a way for members of one social group to insult, provoke, and minimize the worth and accomplishments of other social groups. A healthier expression of this human tendency is observable in modern school and sports team rivalries. More malignant expressions remain observable in some of the language that is used to reference social and cultural groups.

Although progress has been made on this front in recent years, changes in language use and preferences stated by social and cultural groups can leave some adults using an outdated or offensive term. Table 3-1 presents several such terms, along with more acceptable alternatives. This information is presented with two cautions. First, providers who commonly refer to a patient's social group may be in danger of placing too much emphasis on affiliation and not enough on the patient's individuality. There are few occasions when dental care providers would be called on to refer to a patient's sexuality or ethnicity, for example. Second, patients should always have the last word in how others refer to them. If a patient corrects the provider, the provider should thank the patient and make a note of this preference in the patient's file.

Table 3-1 Culturally sensitive vocabulary

Insensitive term	More sensitive term	Most sensitive term
Oriental	Asian	Japanese, Korean, etc
American Indian	Native American	Cherokee, Navaho, etc
Chicano	Latino or Hispanic	Mexican, Puerto Rican, Colombian, etc
Colored	Black	African American
Hybrid or mulatto	Mixed race	Multiracial
Hearing impaired	Hard of hearing	Deaf or person with hearing loss
Queer	Homosexual	Gay or lesbian
Midget		Dwarf or little person
Retarded	Developmentally disabled	Person with an intellectual disability
Crippled or handicapped	Disabled	Person with a physical disability
Old	Elderly	Senior
Junkie or drunk	Addict or alcoholic	Substance-dependent person
Crazy		Person with a mental illness
Senile		Person with Alzheimer disease or dementia

The LEARN model

A 1983 report by Berlin and Fowkes[66] presented a framework for cross-cultural communication in family practice. That framework is the **LEARN model**, referring to the actions a provider should take when interacting with a patient from a different culture: **listen**, **explain**, **acknowledge**, **recommend**, and **negotiate**. That model applies equally to the dental setting.

Listening seems an obvious and intuitive activity, but clinical tasks can be distracting, and the routine of interviewing can deceive a provider into thinking he or she is listening when that is not the case, even with a concordant patient. A culturally or linguistically different patient can be even more challenging to listen to, as he or she may be reticent or difficult to understand. Active and reflective listening are crucial.

Explaining the diagnosis and treatment is perhaps even more important with a patient from a different culture. Providers can assume that a patient familiar with Western medicine comprehends examination procedures, typical diagnoses, and standard treatments. A patient from another culture may not understand the words or the concepts that underlie these procedures, so gauging the patient's comprehension level and addressing the patient at that level is very important, particularly with preventive care. If the patient does not understand why the provider wants something done, the patient is unlikely to do it.

Acknowledging when a patient has a different conception of illness and health is as important as explaining the Western model of medicine. The Kleinman questions,[67] discussed in the next section, suggest ways to elicit the patient's model.

Recommending the most appropriate treatment follows learning how a patient perceives health problems and solutions. By integrating the patient's model with the medical model, the provider can address unhealthy practices and encourage appropriate treatment.

Negotiating the final treatment is important, because the provider must not impose a treatment if a patient is unwilling or unable to carry out any part of it. The provider should remain aware that some cultures value harmony and authority, so patience and persistence may be required to elicit a patient's concerns. When such concerns are articulated, the provider should avoid refuting or discrediting them, a sure way to shut down dialogue. The provider should be willing to negotiate the treatment recommendations.

Kleinman questions

A 1978 study by Kleinman et al[67] used anthropologic methods to explore how diverse cultures understand clinical experiences. One outcome was a series of questions providers can ask in order to understand the patient's cultural framework for health and illness. The Kleinman questions (Box 3-3) are therefore a way to address the acknowledging step in the LEARN model. The authors emphasize, however, that question wording should vary based on patient and problem characteristics. They also urge patience and persistence, as patients from other cultures may be hesitant to disclose their cultural frameworks for illness.

| Box 3-3 | The Kleinman questions for eliciting patient illness frameworks* |

Questions related to diagnosis
1. What do you think has caused your problem?
2. Why do you think it started when it did?
3. What do you think your sickness does to you?
4. How severe is your sickness? Will it have a short or long course?

Questions related to treatment and therapeutic goals
5. What kind of treatment do you think you should receive?
6. What are the most important results you hope to receive from this treatment?
7. What are the chief problems your sickness has caused for you?
8. What do you fear most about your sickness?

*Adapted from Kleinman et al.[67]

Stigma

Although **stigma** originally referred to body modifications intended to signify something bad or wrong about the bearer, stigma is now better understood in relational terms as a failure to meet normative social expectations.[68] Because those expectations are social, they are profoundly cultural and therefore variable over time and across cultures. For instance, in the United States, crooked, broken, and rotted teeth are increasingly marks of stigma that alter perceptions about the person the teeth belong to—or do not belong to, in the case of missing teeth. In earlier times and in other cultures, lack of preventive dental care and fluoridated water resulted in a higher prevalence of poor oral health, and less stigma was attached to the appearance of teeth.

What is true of teeth is true of other individual characteristics: The patient, the provider, or both may perceive a given characteristic as stigmatized. Such situations call for cultural competence on the part of the provider to reduce the stigmatized patient's shame, defensiveness, or unwillingness to disclose medically relevant information. Too often, dental professionals report unwillingness or discomfort in addressing patients' stigmatized conditions. Chapter 12 explores stigmatized conditions in more depth, but this section considers two stigmatized conditions that dental professionals may encounter and offers suggestions for dialogue.

Eating disorders

Lifetime prevalence of anorexia nervosa is 0.9% among women and 0.3% among men.[69] Lifetime prevalence of bulimia nervosa is 1.5% among women and 0.5% among men. Symptoms of an eating disorder may appear as erosion of a patient's hard or soft tissue. Groups at elevated risk for these two eating disorders are females, whites, and perhaps Hispanics as they are acculturated.[70] Eating disorders are often accompanied by an inordinate focus on diet and are most prevalent during adolescence and early adulthood. They also tend to occur with comorbid psychiatric disorders.

Burkhart et al[71] researched provider communication with dental patients who have an eating disorder (Box 3-4). As with other forms of stigma, patients may be unwilling to acknowledge a problem. Several organizations, such as the Academy for Eating Disorders and the National Association of Anorexia Nervosa and Associated Disorders, offer information about eating disorders. An online screening program for eating disorders is available through Screening for Mental Health (http://www.mentalhealthscreening.org). These and other online resources, including brochures, are listed at the end of the chapter.

Box 3-4	Communicating with patients with suspected bulimia nervosa*

- **Timing:** Planning the discussion early or late in the day may allow adequate time to explore concerns.
- **Location:** Choose a location that is comfortable for both patient and provider. Ensure that the location is private enough that the discussion will not be overheard. The dental chair may be appropriate.
- **Nonverbal behavior:** Maintain an adequate distance (2.5 to 3.5 feet) and comfortable eye contact. Do not encroach on the patient's personal space or lean so far forward that the patient feels trapped.
- **Slow beginning:** (1) Express concern. (2) Describe changes you have noticed in the patient's mouth and teeth. (3) Ask if the patient knows what might be causing the damage.
- **Possible causes:** If the patient does not volunteer information, suggest various possible causes (eg, gastric reflux, pregnancy, frequent self-induced vomiting, restrictive diets) and ask whether any apply.
- **Food relationship:** Ask whether you can explore the patient's relationship with food. The patient's answer should indicate his or her readiness for change.
- **Body image:** Ask open-ended screening questions such as, "How do you feel about your eating behavior in general?" or "How do you feel about your weight?"
- **Eating behaviors:** State that you will ask some direct questions about eating to determine the cause of the changes you have noticed. For instance, "Do you ever make yourself throw up?" or "Has anyone expressed concern about your eating habits?"
- **Summarize:** Thank the patient, provide literature on eating disorders and local treatment resources, and ask permission to coordinate care with the primary physician.

*Adapted from Burkhart et al[71] with permission.

HIV/AIDS and other sexually transmitted infections

Sexually transmitted infections (STIs) remain highly stigmatized. Estimating the prevalence of STIs is difficult, given that stigma suppresses reporting and that some STIs are curable. In the United States, an estimated 65 million people live with at least one viral STI, most commonly genital herpes.[72,73] Nineteen million new STIs occur annually, and about half of these occur among young people aged 15 to 24.[74]

Perhaps because it is associated with racial and sexual minorities and because it is potentially fatal, HIV is stigmatized more than other STIs. At present, an estimated 1 million people in the United States are living with HIV, and 21% are unaware of their infection.[75] More than 56,000 new infections occur annually. Groups at higher risk for HIV include gay, bisexual, and other men who have sex with men. Although white men who have sex with other men constitute the majority of new infections each year, black Americans represent 46% of those living with HIV and 45% of new infections. Hispanics are also disproportionately infected; the infection rate of Hispanic men is more than double that of white men, and the rate among Hispanic women is more than double that among white women.

In the 1980s and 1990s, a substantial body of research addressed infection control practices and professional attitudes of dental professionals toward patients with HIV and AIDS.[76,77] Fear of infection and differential treatment of infected patients was documented, with some practices refusing altogether to treat patients with HIV/AIDS.[78–80] The past decade has seen a shift in society's attitudes toward those living with HIV/AIDS, as medications have reduced the mortality of HIV. Yet the attitude of dental professionals and HIV/AIDS patients toward each other can reflect the fear and misperceptions cultivated in a previous era.

A 2005 study of hygienists found that 53.9% believed that treating HIV/AIDS patients increased their risk of contracting HIV, and 65.8% would not use an ultrasonic scaler on such patients, indicating differential treatment.[81] More recent studies showed that dentists and hygienists are comfortable treating HIV/AIDS patients and confident in their ability to do so.[41,82] Explicit training in interaction with HIV/AIDS patients is effective.[83] In one study, training-enhanced empathic themes expressed by providers included the importance of maintaining health, reassurance, and hope.[84]

Perhaps as a result of real or perceived stigma from health care professionals, some HIV-positive patients likely remain cautious about seeking care and disclosing their status. A Canadian survey from the mid-1990s found that only 54% of HIV-positive patients always disclosed their status to their dentist, and a significant predictor of disclosure was trust in the dentist's confidentiality.[85] A 2008 UK study indicated that 34.6% of HIV-positive patients who had revealed their status to a dentist believed it negatively influenced the care they received; 6.2% were refused treatment.[86] A study of HIV-positive men documented the communication behaviors of health care professionals that patients perceive as stigmatized (Box 3-5).[87] A participant in this study told of an encounter in which a dental assistant learned the patient had AIDS[87]:

> As I'm sitting there and [the dentist and I were] talking, [the assistant] comes running over. I could tell it was a big emergency. He says, "Wait a minute!" and grabs the manila folder. Because he's writing it so large, I can tell what he's writing across the front of this manila folder on the side that I can't see, and he's writing the word "AIDS!"

Box 3-5	Health care provider behaviors that patients associate with stigma*

- Avoiding eye contact
- Speaking in clipped, flat, or brusque tones
- Standing too far away from the patient
- Expressing irritation or anger
- Displaying nervousness or fear
- Panicking
- Shifting demeanor on learning HIV status
- Taking excessive precautions
- Taking different precautions than usual
- Labeling patient files, rooms, specimens, etc
- Scaring the patient with diagnoses
- Mocking the patient (eg, for sexual practices)
- Blaming the patient (eg, for sexual practices)

*Information compiled and adapted from Rintamaki et al.[87]

Standard infection-control procedures such as labeling biologic specimens and wearing eye protection and masks may be perceived as excessive and stigmatizing by patients with HIV. Providers should therefore good-naturedly explain that these precautions are taken with every patient.

Chapter Checklist

Developing cultural competence
- Examine your own appearance, behavior, and cultural background to understand how the patient may perceive those things.
- Understand how culture can influence oral health care in order to identify and accommodate challenges and opportunities.
- Read books on intercultural communication in health care.
- Research beliefs and practices of cultural groups within the practice's market area.
- Avoid cultural stereotyping based on physical or behavioral characteristics.
- Remain aware that the multicultural patient may be adept at code switching.

Determining cultural background
- Observe the patient's dress, behavior, and interactions.
- Read the patient's forms and review the information they contain.
- Listen to the patient's language and vocabulary.
- Consider which cultural communities are nearby.
- Inquire politely.

Addressing cultural barriers
- Language: Overcome reluctance to treat a patient with limited English proficiency or hearing problems.
- Nationality: When developing intercultural communication strategies, consider power distance, individualism, masculinity, uncertainty avoidance, and long-term orientation of the patient's country of origin.

❑ Ethnicity: Avoid generalizations and tailor communication to the individual patient.
❑ Ethnicity: Remain aware of health disparities and possible reasons for those disparities among people of different cultures, education levels, socioeconomic status, sexual orientations, age, and sex.
❑ Ethnicity: Avoid basing cultural assumptions on appearance alone.
❑ Ethnicity: Acknowledge that health-related values, beliefs, attitudes, and practices may vary widely even among patients who share a common culture.
❑ Ethnicity: Determine a patient's values and goals for care and sensitively collaborate with the patient to deliver the best evidence-based care acceptable to the patient.
❑ Ethnicity: Avoid the detached and condescending behavior often associated with the health care culture.
❑ Ethnicity: Develop and sustain empathy with the patient.
❑ Vocabulary: Use culturally sensitive terminology when referring to a patient's background or characteristics.
❑ Vocabulary: Avoid placing too much emphasis on a patient's background or characteristics.
❑ Vocabulary: Honor the patient's preferences in what he or she is called and how he or she is referred to.

Conversing with patients from other cultures
❑ Greet the patient with a smile, verbal greeting, and eye contact.
❑ Use a title with the patient's name until the patient says otherwise.
❑ Welcome a patient's chaperones.
❑ Minimize nonclinical touch.
❑ If the patient is unresponsive to rapport building, take a more detached approach.
❑ Speak slowly and face the patient.
❑ Allow extra time for responses and monitor the patient for signs of incomprehension.
❑ If the patient seems unwilling to commit to treatment, encourage consultation with the family.

LEARN model
❑ Listen: Employ active and reflexive listening.
❑ Explain: Gauge the patient's comprehension and address the patient at his or her level of comprehension.
❑ Acknowledge: Explore the patient's illness frameworks using the Kleinman questions.
❑ Recommend: Integrate the patient's model with the medical model when suggesting the most appropriate treatment.
❑ Negotiate: Elicit the patient's concerns, address those concerns respectfully, and remain willing to negotiate the treatment recommendation.

Kleinman questions to elicit illness framework
❑ Diagnosis: What do you think has caused your problem?
❑ Diagnosis: Why do you think it started when it did?
❑ Diagnosis: What do you think your sickness does to you?

□ Diagnosis: How severe is your sickness? Will it have a short or long course?
□ Treatment: What kind of treatment do you think you should receive?
□ Treatment: What are the most important results you hope to receive from this treatment?
□ Treatment: What are the chief problems your sickness has caused for you?
□ Treatment: What do you fear most about your sickness?

Addressing the stigma of eating disorders
□ Plan the discussion for early or late in the day.
□ Hold the conversation in a comfortable and private place.
□ Maintain adequate distance and comfortable eye contact.
□ Begin slowly by expressing concern about symptoms and asking the patient if he or she knows what may be causing the problems.
□ Suggest possible causes.
□ Ask about the patient's relationship with food, body image, and eating behaviors.
□ Summarize what was said, thank the patient, provide literature, and ask if you can coordinate care to address the eating disorder.

Addressing the stigma of HIV/AIDS and other STIs
□ Make eye contact.
□ Take normal infection-control precautions and explain that the precautions are routine with all patients.
□ Avoid brusque or clipped speech.
□ Avoid displaying irritation, anger, nervousness, fear, or panic.
□ Avoid changes in demeanor on learning a patient's infection status.
□ Avoid obvious labeling of the patient's files, rooms, specimens, etc.
□ Never scare, mock, or blame the patient.

For More Information

Health and culture
- https://www.thinkculturalhealth.hhs.gov
- http://nccc.georgetown.edu
- http://www.xculture.org
- http://www.diversityrx.org
- http://erc.msh.org/mainpage.cfm?file=1.0.htm&module=provider&language=English
- http://wps.prenhall.com/chet_spector_cultural_7/94/24263/6211431.cw/index.html
- http://www.minorityhealth.hhs.gov/omh/browse.aspx?lvl=1&lvlid=6

Cultural competence assessments
- http://www.aafp.org/fpm/2000/1000/p58.html
- http://nccc.georgetown.edu/resources/assessments.html

Effective and ineffective cultural communication
- http://www.youtube.com/watch?v=pY8QsvAzBcw
- http://www.youtube.com/watch?v=OwmhZNd9uQE&feature=relmfu
- http://www.mdanderson.org/education-and-research/resources-for-profession-als/professional-educational-resources/i-care/ICAREguide_CultComp.pdf

Health care disparities
- http://www.ahrq.gov/research/findings/nhqrdr
- http://www.biomedcentral.com/content/pdf/1472-6831-8-26.pdf

Communicating with specific cultures
- http://depts.washington.edu/pfes/CultureClues.htm
- http://www.mckinley.illinois.edu/multiculturalhealth/index.htm
- http://www.hrsa.gov/culturalcompetence/index.html
- http://www.cvahec.org/resources/cultural-competency
- http://www.deaflinx.com/Services/health.html
- http://www.hispanichealth.org
- http://americanindianhealth.nlm.nih.gov

Sensitive terminology
- http://en.wiktionary.org/wiki/Category:English_politically_correct_terms
- http://www.unh.edu/inclusive/bias-free-language-guide

Screening for eating disorders
- www.mentalhealthscreening.org

Information and brochures on eating disorders
- www.gurze.com
- www.aedweb.org
- www.anad.org

References

1. American Dental Education Association. Competencies for the New General Dentist. Washington, DC: American Dental Education Association, 2008.
2. American Dental Education Association. ADEA competencies for entry into the allied dental professions. J Dent Educ 2010;74:769–775.
3. Betancourt JR, Green AR, Carrillo JE, Park ER. Cultural competence and health care disparities: Key perspectives and trends. Health Aff 2005;24:499–505.
4. Pilcher ES, Charles LT, Lancaster CJ. Development and assessment of a cultural competency curriculum. J Dent Educ 2008;72:1020–1028.
5. American Dental Association. Multicultural Communication in the Dental Office. Chicago: American Dental Association, 2006.
6. Commission on Dental Accreditation. Accreditation Standards for Dental Education Programs. Chicago: American Dental Association, 2010.
7. Vincent GK, Velkoff VA. The Next Four Decades: The Older Population in the United States: 2010 to 2050. Washington, DC: US Census Bureau, 2010.
8. Smedley BD, Stith AY, Nelson AR (eds). Unequal Treatment: Confronting Racial and Ethnic Disparities in Health Care. Washington, DC: National Academies Press, 2002.

9. Agency for Healthcare Research and Quality. 2010 National Healthcare Disparities Report. Rockville, MD: US Department of Health and Human Services, 2011.

10. Manski RJ, Magder LS. Demographic and socioeconomic predictors of dental care utilization. J Am Dent Assoc 1998;129:195–200.

11. Crall JJ. Access to oral health care: Professional and societal considerations. J Dent Educ 2006;70:1133–1138.

12. Formicola A, Stavisky J, Lewy R. Cultural competency: Dentistry and medicine learning from one another. J Dent Educ 2003;67:869–875.

13. Garcia RI, Cadoret CA, Henshaw M. Multicultural issues in oral health. Dent Clin North Am 2008;52:319–332.

14. Reifel NM, Rana H, Marcus M. Consumer satisfaction. Adv Dent Res 1997;11:281–290.

15. Milgrom P, Spiekerman C, Grembowski D. Dissatisfaction with dental care among mothers of Medicaid-enrolled children. Community Dent Oral Epidemiol 2008;36:451–458.

16. Kumas-Tan Z, Beagan B, Loppie C, MacLeod A, Frank B. Measures of cultural competence: Examining hidden assumptions. Acad Med 2007;82:548–557.

17. Wood JT. Communication Mosaics: An Introduction to the Field of Communication, ed 7. Boston: Wadsworth Cengage Learning, 2014:332.

18. Adams TL. Feminization of professions: The case of women in dentistry. Can J Sociol 2005;30: 71–94.

19. del Aguila MA, Leggott PJ, Robertson PB, Porterfield DL, Felber GD. Practice patterns among male and female general dentists in a Washington state population. J Am Dent Assoc 2005;136:790–796.

20. Riley JL, Gordan VV, Rouisse KM, McClelland J, Gilbert GH. Differences in male and female dentists' practice patterns regarding diagnosis and treatment of dental caries. J Am Dent Assoc 2011;142:429–440.

21. Smith MK, Dundes L. The implications of gender stereotypes for the dentist-patient relationship. J Dent Educ 2008;72:562–570.

22. Newton JT, Davenport-Jones L, Idle M, Patel M, Setchell A, Turpin C. Patients' perceptions of general dental practitioners: The influence of ethnicity and sex of dentist. Soc Behav Personal 2001;29:601–606.

23. Swami V, McClelland A, Bedi R, Furnham A. The influence of practitioner nationality, experience, and sex in shaping patient preferences for dentists. Int Dent J 2011;61:193–198.

24. Agency for Healthcare Research and Quality. 2009 National Healthcare Disparities Report. Rockville, MD: US Department of Health and Human Services, 2010.

25. American Dental Association. Distribution of Dentists in the United States by Region and State, 2009. Chicago, IL: American Dental Association, 2011.

26. American Dental Hygienists' Association. Survey of Dental Hygienists in the United States, 2007: Executive Summary. Chicago, IL: American Dental Hygienists' Association, 2009.

27. Mouradian WE, Berg JH, Somerman MJ. Addressing disparities through dental-medical collaborations. 1. The role of cultural competency in health disparities: Training of primary care medical practitioners in children's oral health. J Dent Educ 2003;67:860–868.

28. Milgrom P, Cullen T, Whitney C, Fiset L, Conrad D, Getz T. Frustrating patient visits. J Public Health Dent 1996;56:6–11.

29. Rouse RA, Hamilton MA. Dentists evaluate their patients: An empirical investigation of preferences. J Behav Med 1991;14:637–648.

30. Weinstein P, Milgrom P, Ratener P, Read W, Morrison K. Dentists' perceptions of their patients: Relation to quality of care. J Public Health Dent 1978;38:10–21.

31. Wagner JA, Redford-Badwal D. Dental students' beliefs about culture in patient care: Self-reported knowledge and importance. J Dent Educ 2008;72:571–576.

32. Ayer WA. Dental providers and oral health behavior. J Behav Med 1981;4:273–282.

33. Bender DJ. Patient preference for a racially or gender-concordant student dentist. J Dent Educ 2007;71:726–745.

34. Williams KA, Demko CA, Lalumandier JA, Wotman S. Caring for African-American patients in private practice: Disparities and similarities in dental procedures and communication. J Am Dent Assoc 2008;139:1218–1226.

35. Mofidi M, Konrad TR, Porterfield DS, Niska R, Wells B. Provision of care to the underserved populations by national health service corps alumni dentists. J Public Health Dent 2002;62:102–108.

36. Bare LC, Dundes L. Strategies for combating dental anxiety. J Dent Educ 2004;68:1172–1177.
37. Meghani SH, Brooks JM, Gipson-Jones T, Waite R, Whitfield-Harris L, Deatrick JA. Patient-provider race-concordance: Does it matter in improving minority patients' health outcomes? Ethn Health 2009;14:107–130.
38. Cooper LA, Powe NR. Disparities in Patient Experiences, Health Care Processes, and Outcomes: The Role of Patient-Provider Racial, Ethnic, and Language Concordance. New York: The Commonwealth Fund, 2004.
39. Cooper LA, Roter DL, Johnson RL, Ford DE, Steinwachs DM, Powe NR. Patient-centered communication, ratings of care, and concordance of patient and physician race. Ann Intern Med 2003;139:907–915.
40. Rubin R. Developing cultural competence and social responsibility in preclinical dental students. J Dent Educ 2004;68:460–467.
41. McQuistan MR, Kuthy RA, Heller KE, Qian F, Riniker KJ. Dentists' comfort in treating underserved populations after participating in community-based clinical experiences as a student. J Dent Educ 2008;72:422–430.
42. Rundle A, Carvalho M, Robinson M (eds). Cultural Competence in Health Care: A Practical Guide, ed 2. San Francisco: Wiley, 2002.
43. Srivastava RH (ed). The Healthcare Professional's Guide to Clinical Cultural Competence. Toronto: Elsevier, 2007.
44. Spector RE. Cultural Diversity in Health and Illness, ed 7. Upper Saddle River, NJ: Prentice Hall, 2008.
45. Tseng WS, Streltzer J. Cultural Competence in Health Care: A Guide for Professionals. New York: Springer, 2008.
46. Leavitt R. Cultural Competence: A Lifelong Journey to Cultural Proficiency. Thorofare, NJ: Slack, 2010.
47. Civil Rights Act of 1964, Pub L No. 88-352, 78 Stat 241 (1964).
48. Americans with Disabilities Act of 1990, Pub L No. 101-336, 104 Stat 328 (1990).
49. Wallace S, Gutiérrez V, Castañeda X. Access to preventive services for adults of Mexican origin. J Immigr Minor Health 2008;10:363–371.
50. Flores G, Tomany-Korman SC. The language spoken at home and disparities in medical and dental health, access to care, and use of services in US children. Pediatrics 2008;121:e1703–e1714.
51. Noyce M, Szabo A, Pajewski NM, Jackson S, Bradley TG, Okunseri C. Primary language spoken at home and children's dental service utilization in the United States. J Public Health Dent 2009;69:276–283.
52. Hammersmith KJ, Lee JY. A survey of North Carolina safety-net dental clinics' methods for communicating with patients of limited English proficiency (LEP). J Public Health Dent 2009;69:90–94.
53. Itaya LE, Glassman P, Gregorczyk S, Bailit HL. Dental school patients with limited English proficiency: The California experience. J Dent Educ 2009;73:1055–1064.
54. Hofstede G. Culture's Consequences: Comparing Values, Behaviors, Institutions and Organizations Across Nations, ed 2. Thousand Oaks, CA: Sage, 2001.
55. Scheppers E, van Dongen E, Dekker J, Geertzen J, Dekker J. Potential barriers to the use of health services among ethnic minorities: A review. Fam Pract 2006;23:325–348.
56. Sabbah W, Tsakos G, Sheiham A, Watt RG. The effects of income and education on ethnic differences in oral health: A study in US adults. J Epidemiol Community Health 2009;63:516–520.
57. Nakazono TT, Davidson PL, Andersen RM. Oral health beliefs in diverse populations. Adv Dent Res 1997;11:235–244.
58. Mullen K, Chauhan R, Gardee R, Macpherson LMD. Exploring issues related to attitudes towards dental care among second-generation ethnic groups. Divers Health Social Care 2007;4:91–99.
59. Morales LS, Lara M, Kington RS, Valdez RO, Escarce JJ. Socioeconomic, cultural, and behavioral factors affecting Hispanic health outcomes. J Health Care Poor Underserved 2002;13:477–503.
60. Johnson M. Ethnic Minorities, Health & Communication: A Research Review for the NHS Executive and West Midlands Regional Health Authority. Research Paper in Ethnic Relations. Coventry, England: Centre for Research in Ethnic Relations, University of Warwick, 1996.
61. Mobley C, Marshall TA, Milgrom P, Coldwell SE. The contribution of dietary factors to dental caries and disparities in caries. Acad Pediatr 2009;9:410–414.

62. Butani Y, Weintraub J, Barker J. Oral health-related cultural beliefs for four racial/ethnic groups: Assessment of the literature. BMC Oral Health 2008;8(1):26.
63. Hojat M, Gonnella JS, Nasca TJ, Mangione S, Veloksi JJ, Magee M. The Jefferson Scale of Physician Empathy: Further psychometric data and differences by gender and specialty at item level. Acad Med 2002;77(10 suppl):S58–S60.
64. Hojat M, Mangione S, Nasca TJ, et al. The Jefferson Scale of Physician Empathy: Development and preliminary psychometric data. Educ Psychol Meas 2001;61:349–365.
65. Teal CR, Street RL. Critical elements of culturally competent communication in the medical encounter: A review and model. Soc Sci Med 2009;68:533–543.
66. Berlin EA, Fowkes WC Jr. A teaching framework for cross-cultural health care. Application in family practice. West J Med 1983;139:934–938.
67. Kleinman A, Eisenberg L, Good B. Culture, illness, and care: Clinical lessons from anthropologic and cross-cultural research. Ann Intern Med 1978;88:251–258.
68. Goffman E. Stigma: Notes on the Management of Spoiled Identity. New York: Simon & Schuster, 1963.
69. Hudson JI, Hiripi E, Pope HG Jr, Kessler RC. The prevalence and correlates of eating disorders in the National Comorbidity Survey Replication. Biol Psychiatry 2007;61:348–358 [erratum 2012;72:164].
70. Jacobi C, Hayward C, de Zwaan M, Kraemer HC, Agras WS. Coming to terms with risk factors for eating disorders: Application of risk terminology and suggestions for a general taxonomy. Psychol Bull 2004;130:19–65.
71. Burkhart N, Roberts M, Alexander M, Dodds A. Communicating effectively with patients suspected of having bulimia nervosa. J Am Dent Assoc 2005;136:1130–1137.
72. Cates W Jr. Estimates of the incidence and prevalence of sexually transmitted diseases in the United States. The American Social Health Association Panel. Sex Transm Dis 1999;26(4 suppl):S2–S7.
73. Guttmacher Institute. Facts on Sexually Transmitted Infections in the United States. New York: Guttmacher Institute, 2009.
74. Weinstock H, Berman S, Cates W. Sexually transmitted diseases among American youth: Incidence and prevalence estimates, 2000. Perspect Sex Reprod Health 2004;36:6–10.
75. National Center for HIV/AIDS Hepatitis STD and TB Prevention. HIV in the United States. Atlanta: Centers for Disease Control and Prevention, 2010.
76. Bennett ME, Weyant RJ, Wallisch JM, Green G. Dentists' attitudes toward the treatment of HIV-positive patients. J Am Dent Assoc 1995;126:509–514.
77. Verrusio AC, Neidle EA, Nash KD, Silverman S Jr, Horowitz AM, Wagner KS. The dentist and infectious diseases: A national survey of attitudes and behavior. J Am Dent Assoc 1989;118:553–562.
78. Hastreiter RJ, Roesch MH, Danila RN, Falken MC. Dental health care workers' response to the HIV epidemic. Am J Dent 1992;5:160–166.
79. Rankin KV, Jones DL, Rees TD. Attitudes of dental practitioners and dental students towards AIDS patients and infection control. Am J Dent 1993;6:22–26.
80. Sadowsky D, Kunzel C. Measuring dentists' willingness to treat HIV-positive patients. J Am Dent Assoc 1994;125:705–710.
81. King TB, Muzzin KB. A national survey of dental hygienists' infection control attitudes and practices. J Dent Hyg 2005;79(2):8.
82. Clark-Alexander B. Dental Hygienists' Beliefs, Norms, Attitudes, and Intentions toward Treating HIV/AIDS Patients [thesis]. Tampa: University of South Florida, 2008.
83. Lewis DA, Brain G, Cushing AM, Hall A, Zakrzewska JM. Description and evaluation of an education and communication skills training course in HIV and AIDS for dental consultants. Eur J Dent Educ 2000;4:65–70.
84. Wiltshire AD, Ross MW, Brimlow DL. Empathic communication between dental professionals and persons living with HIV and AIDS. J Dent Educ 2002;66:86–93.
85. Charbonneau A, Maheux B, Beland F. Do people with HIV/AIDS disclose their HIV-positivity to dentists? AIDS Care 1999;11:61–70.
86. Levett T, Slide C, Mallick F, Lau R. Access to dental care for HIV patients: Does it matter and does discrimination exist? Int J STD AIDS 2009;20:782–784.
87. Rintamaki LS, Scott AM, Kosenko KA, Jensen RE. Male patient perceptions of HIV stigma in health care contexts. AIDS Patient Care STDS 2007;21:956–969.

Part II

Interaction Skills

In this section, the components that constitute face-to-face communication are considered separately: listening (chapter 4), verbal communication (chapter 5), and nonverbal communication (chapter 6). Although all three components are necessary for successful patient-centered communication, individuals are often more skilled at one of these than the others. In reading these chapters, providers should consider their own ability to communicate in each of these areas and which skills they can integrate to improve communication with patients.

Enhancing Listening Skills

Why Listening Skills Matter

The previous two chapters built skills in anticipating and responding to patient communication based on media and cultural categories. This chapter narrows the focus, building listening skills in order to understand patients as individuals and to respond to their individual needs. Listening skills are so important that Pikowski[1] stated that "communication with patients is simply listening." This assertion is counterintuitive in a culture that tends to equate communication with expression and increasingly emphasizes verbal expression over both nonverbal expression and listening. Contrast today's reliance on texting, email, instant messaging, MP3 players, and even talk radio with the communication media and patterns of former generations.

We have not abandoned nonverbal and listening as components of communication, but we have developed more ways to express ourselves verbally, with the result that many people now complain they are unable to listen to and absorb so much spoken and written information. We have necessarily developed filters. The risk of filters is that the listener will lose the skill of discerning which information should be ignored or disregarded and which should be acted on. This risk is particularly acute for health care professionals, who are overwhelmed with verbal information.

Healthy People 2020[2] includes the following objective: Increase the proportion of persons who report that their health care provider always listened carefully to them. The baseline of that objective is 59%, the proportion of patients in 2007 who indicated that their health care provider always listened carefully to them. The goal is a 10% increase to 65%. Patient satisfaction with provider communication skills is significantly associated with patient empowerment, and the strongest relationship is found between empowerment and listening.[3] Simply put, patient-centered care is impossible unless a provider possesses adequate listening skills.

Effective listening skills also yield direct benefits to the provider, yielding more comprehensive and accurate information on which to base clinical decisions and indicating what and how to communicate with each patient. In addition, effective listening (including documentation of what the provider heard) is an evidence-based way of reducing the probability of a malpractice claim.[4,5]

The cultivation of listening skills is therefore not simply feel-good advice recommended by researchers, but it is repeatedly given by oral health providers who argue its practical benefits.[6–13] Nevertheless, in patient interactions, dental providers do more than two-thirds of the talking.[14] This chapter considers barriers to listening, describes active listening and various listening strategies, and concludes with a discussion on documentation of what has been heard and observed.

Barriers to Listening

Humans are incapable of listening to everything all the time. People filter incoming messages; the challenge for the dental professional is to determine which messages to listen to actively, which messages to attend to later, and which messages to completely ignore. The first step to developing listening skills is identifying factors that interfere with listening to important messages. Box 4-1 lists 10 barriers to listening faced by dental professionals.[15] This list is not exhaustive, but providers who minimize these 10 barriers will dramatically enhance their listening effectiveness. Several of the barriers deserve additional attention.

Box 4-1	Barriers to effective listening*

- **Time:** Patients vary in the rate they speak and disclose information, and slower patients can frustrate busy dental professionals.
- **Effort:** Listening requires focused attention, which can become tiresome as the workday proceeds.
- **Message overload:** Important information is easily missed within both the operatory and the broader practice because messages are incoming from multiple sources (eg, coworkers, patients, caregivers, and colleagues) and multiple media (eg, face to face, telephone, email, texts, and faxes).
- **Rapid thought:** Providers can process information much more quickly than most patients talk, tempting them to think about other things or anticipate what the patient will say next.
- **Psychologic noise:** Providers cannot completely ignore the intrusion of thoughts unrelated to the current patient, including thoughts about other patients, workplace stressors, and personal concerns.
- **Physical noise:** Dental practices can be loud places, with noise coming from multiple sources, including ringing telephones, handpieces, conversations, and music.
- **Hearing problems:** Dental professionals are as susceptible to hearing loss as others and may be more vulnerable due to prolonged exposure to drills.
- **Faulty assumptions:** New patients can be stereotyped based on behavior or appearance, and long-term patients can be assumed to have the same problems they previously had. Such assumptions interfere with listening.
- **Emphasis on talk:** Western cultures value talking more than listening, perhaps because the talker seems to have more control over the interaction.
- **Cultural differences:** Talking and listening patterns vary by culture, and patients who differ from providers in communication patterns can prove difficult to listen to and understand.

*Information compiled and adapted from Adler et al.[15]

Time

Perhaps the most significant barrier to listening faced by providers is time. A recent observational study of 3,751 patient visits at 120 dental offices found that the average patient contact time for dental hygienist visits is 36.5 minutes.[16] That average includes the 3 to 5 minutes dentists spend with the patient. During dentist visits, patient contact averages a shorter 25.7 minutes.

Field notes from this study indicate the median time dentists and hygienists spend in various interactions. Chatting with patients consumes less than 2.5 minutes for dentists and less than 5.5 minutes for hygienists. The health history interview consumes less than 30 seconds for dentists and less than 1 minute for hygienists. Both dentists and hygienists spend less than 30 seconds on patient questions. The public's growing perception of health care as a profit center may lead them to suspect that dental practices are concerned primarily with patient turnover.[17]

Unsurprisingly, the Healthy People project reported that only 59% of patients believe that health care providers listen carefully and only 49% spend enough time with patients.[18] The figures for dentistry could be worse than those for general health care, because patients are unable to verbalize during a substantial portion of most dental visits. Furthermore, dental practices are busy even on the best days. Schedule changes, late patients, and procedures that take longer than planned increase the time pressure placed on dental professionals. When appointment time is constricted for a given patient, providers often opt to spend the available time on clinical procedures rather than listening to patients.

Yet the argument for investing a little extra time listening parallels the argument providers make advocating preventive care: It can save time and effort in the long run. In the short run, listening for a minute or two to patients during the interview might add only a few minutes to the workday or none at all if those minutes are subtracted from time spent chatting with patients. When listening results in more targeted treatment, appointments may actually be shortened. At the very least, listening for a longer time likely boosts patient satisfaction and referrals.[19]

Q **Question of ethics:** In dental practice, schedules are affected by many events providers have little control over: emergency care, unexpected problems, absent employees, personal crises, late patients, and so on. When schedules are backed up, the provider's commitment to prompt patient service may conflict with the provider's commitment to active listening. When patient appointments are compressed, is it more ethical to allocate the promised time to each patient (pushing back subsequent patient times) or to shorten the time spent with a couple of patients so you can get back on schedule?

Rapid thought

For practitioners, the downside of their ability to think fast is that they think much faster than patients talk. The normal speaking rate is approximately 130 words per minute, but most humans can comprehend speech two to three times that fast.[20–22] One temptation for quick-thinking practitioners is to ponder other issues or problem solve other patient dilemmas while the patient in front of them is attempting to articulate a problem. Another temptation is to assume that they know what a patient will say and therefore not listen to what the patient actually does say. As difficult as it can be, providers should resist both of these temptations and instead focus on listening to what the patient in front of them actually says. This can be difficult with slow-talking or reluctant patients, but it is an element of patient-centered care.

Physical noise

The physical noise present in dental offices is another important barrier to effective listening and may also increase patient anxiety.[23] Some of these sounds are present in any health care setting: conversation in the waiting area, ringing telephones, discussions among colleagues, and noise in hallways. Other sources of noise are specific to dental settings: high-pitched turbines, high-velocity suction, ultrasonic cleaners, laboratory engines, and running water.[24] Noise levels from these sources can vary; laboratory engines are significantly louder than low-speed, angled handpieces.[25] A recent study of pediatric dentistry found that the noise of crying children exceeded the loudness of dental handpieces.[26] Offices and operatories also can vary in their ability to absorb sound. Partitioned operatories with tile floors tend to be much louder than carpeted operatories with permanent walls and doors.

Background music should be carefully considered. It can increase the noise level, but anxious patients find it soothing.[27–30] Technology may provide a compromise. Noise-filtering earplugs have been developed, and patients can now use earbuds or headphones, as long as the sound is low enough for them to hear the clinician.[31] Simply put, if patients or providers exhibit a pattern of inattention, ambient noise is the first listening barrier that should be considered.

Hearing problems

Because listening cannot occur until hearing does, hearing problems can pose a barrier to effective listening. For both providers and patients, the listening barrier of ambient noise is compounded by hearing problems. (The challenge of treating patients with hearing loss is addressed in chapters 10 and 11.)

For decades, practitioners and observers have speculated that exposure to noise from dental tools is a risk factor for hearing loss among dentists. The issue is unsettled.[32] Several well-designed studies have found the prevalence of hearing loss among dentists to be little or no higher than that in a control group.[33–37] Other studies have found significant potential for hearing loss, notably in the ear closest to the handpiece.[38–41] Whether or not exposure to dental tools leads to hearing loss, dental professionals are as susceptible to age-related hearing loss as the general public.[42]

Compromised hearing can lead a provider to absorb an inaccurate or incomplete version of the patient's health history, resulting in compromised examination or treatment. An early sign that listening problems reflect hearing problems is a pattern of asking patients to repeat what they have said or to speak up. Such requests can grow tiresome for the patient. Furthermore, people often make the unfortunate and incorrect association between hearing loss and cognitive deficiency. Thus, hearing loss can quickly affect the reputation of a provider.

Prevention is the best strategy: minimizing noise, wearing earplugs when high-frequency equipment is in use, and seeking regular hearing tests. When hearing loss is significant, hearing aids should be used and adjusted so they facilitate listening in an environment that includes high-frequency equipment.

> **Q** **Question of ethics:** Physical noise and hearing problems can prompt patients to speak louder than they otherwise would. This can become a problem for confidentiality, particularly if operatories are in the open or in cubicles. Is it an ethical problem when others can hear a patient's health history and other disclosures? Is it a legal problem?

Active Listening

Research has long shown that listening is the communication activity engaged in most often by individuals.[43–46] Even the rapid expansion of portable electronic media has not diminished the primacy of listening.[47] Research suggests the following rule for quantifying communication: We listen to a book a day, we speak a book a week, we read a book a month, and we write a book a year.[48] Yet people overestimate their listening comprehension, suggesting that they may not perceive listening as a skill requiring development in the same way that speaking, reading, and writing are skills acquired through instruction, effort, and time.[49] Consideration and minimization of the 10 listening barriers described earlier will establish an environment conducive to listening, but a facilitative environment is not the same as the deliberate effort to develop listening skills. Duck and McMahan[50] describe skills in **active listening** as a four-stage process of receiving, attending, interpreting, and responding (Box 4-2).

Box 4-2	Steps and strategies for active listening*

Step 1: Receiving
- Regularly check your hearing.
- Minimize office noise.

Step 2: Attending
- Minimize multitasking and do not ignore patients.
- Face the patient.
- Make eye contact.

Step 3: Interpreting
- Consider connotative meanings of words.
- Consider relational meanings of communication.
- Consider what the patient is not saying.
- Consider the patient's nonverbal cues.

Step 4: Responding
- Provide backchannel cues.
- Paraphrase to confirm understanding.
- Invite elaboration.

*Information compiled and adapted from Duck and McMahan.[50]

Step 1: Receiving

The first step in active listening is actually passive. The **reception** of auditory stimuli is simply hearing. The previous discussion of listening barriers explicitly addressed the hearing ability of providers and the noise level of the dental office. In general, humans have less control over the reception of auditory stimuli than they do over the stimulation of the other four senses. People can avert their eyes, hold their noses, shut their mouths, and refrain from touching. Avoiding auditory stimuli, however, requires more effort. Earplugs and hands over the ears are not entirely effective, and withdrawing from the source of a sound can involve walking some distance. As a result, the sound environment can undermine the comprehension of even the most skilled listeners.

An extensive review of the research on the effect of irrelevant sounds indicated that noise can have a significant negative impact, particularly on numeric tasks and memory load, including transcription of data.[51] The implications for the dental professional are that noise may be less problematic during clinical procedures (involving manual tasks) than during the health history interview, when the provider is asking about frequencies and dosages and writing or typing the responses.

Step 2: Attending

The reception of auditory stimuli is sufficient in many daily situations that do not demand the effort of active listening. Background music, for instance, is intended to be heard but (by definition) is meant to serve as the background to conversation, which should be the participants' focus. Any music that demands attention, such as heavy metal, Wagner, and gangsta rap, is inappropriate as background music.

Paying attention, or **attending**, to messages requires the listener to identify a sound as more important than other competing sounds and to simultaneously focus on the source of that sound. Individuals seem to vary in their abilities to focus on specific stimuli, as shown by the prevalence of attention deficit disorder, even among adults.[52] However, variations in attending are not entirely explained by characteristics of the listener. Characteristics of the source can also influence attention. Sounds that are repetitive, intense, and contrasting (sirens, for instance) are likely to capture attention.[15] Finally, the relationship between the source and the listener seems to influence attention. For instance, 80% of mothers, but only 45% of fathers, are able to distinguish their baby's cry from the cry of other babies.[53]

Dental professionals have the advantage of clarity in determining when to pay attention: If providers are co-present in an operatory with a patient, they should be attending to the patient. One of the most common complaints of patients, however, is that they are ignored or neglected.[54] In fact, when asked how much various factors influenced their loyalty to a dentist or practice, "care and attention" topped the list, with 90% saying it is very important.[55]

In attending to patients, the provider should resist two temptations: multitasking and ignoring patients. Time constraints make the temptation to multitask particularly appealing: The provider can boost productivity by washing his or her hands, checking email, or reviewing patient records while the patient is describing a complaint. Consider, however, the negative impact on dialogue when one conversational partner is texting or watching television. Regardless of a provider's skill at multitasking, such behaviors signal that the patient's problems are not that important. In response, the patient may grow silent.

During routine procedures, the patient is usually unable to talk but can still see and hear. Both utter silence from the provider and irrelevant conversations with other members of the dental team indicate that the patient is nothing more than a mouth to be fixed. The provider can indicate that he or she is still paying attention to the patient by narrating procedures, periodically addressing the patient directly, and arranging for communication via hand signals.

Activity 4-1

How good are you at multitasking? Write down whether you think you are better or worse than average and then take a multitasking test published by the *New York Times* to compare your skills against the population:

http://www.nytimes.com/interactive/2010/06/07/technology/-20100607-task-switching-demo.html

Then try a different multitasking test and compare your score with those of colleagues:

http://multitaskgames.com

How do your multitasking skills compare with the population, with your colleagues, and with your expectations?

Nonverbal behaviors will be addressed more fully in chapter 6, but two provider behaviors are presented in this discussion because of their relevance to active listening: When listening, the provider should face the patient and make eye contact. These two behaviors are active and require effort. Facing the patient and making eye contact are behaviors that foster attention.

The provider's mind can still wander while thus engaged with a patient. This phenomenon is called **pseudolistening** and has long been familiar to teachers of disengaged students. Yet pseudolistening is less likely while the provider is facing and watching a patient than while the provider attends to other tasks while simultaneously trying to listen. Furthermore, these behaviors place the provider in a position to observe the patient, which is key to interpreting what the patient says.

Step 3: Interpreting

The third step in the active listening process is **interpretation**, or attaching meaning to the messages received and attended to. At a fundamental level, interpreting is simply understanding spoken words. However, because meaning can be more complex and ambiguous, active listening demands a deeper level of interpretation.

When employing active listening, providers should consider two interpretations of the words used (denotation and connotation) and two interpretations of the messages sent (content and relational).[56] **Denotative meaning** is simply the dictionary definition of a word. Patients, however, can have limited dental vocabulary because they are children, have cognitive deficits, are not native speakers of English, have low health literacy, or are simply distracted, perhaps by dental pain. Skilled providers therefore consider the **connotation** of the words a patient uses to interpret what the patient means.

For example, on hearing, "My tooth hurts," an unskilled provider may quickly diagnose the problem and begin treatment. On the other hand, a skilled provider will consider what "hurts" might connote for the specific patient uttering that word. Does it mean a dull ache or a sharp pain? Is it chronic discomfort, or does it occur at certain times? By considering these questions, posing them to patients, and listening to their answers, providers take a step toward understanding patients' complaints and helping patients understand subsequent treatment recommendations.

When interpreting a message, listeners first consider the denotative meaning of the **content** and then perhaps the connotative meaning of the content. Yet messages also have a relational meaning that is too rarely considered but can facilitate interpretation.[57–59] The **relational meaning** of a message considers what the message implies about the relationship between the speaker and the audience.

The patient-provider relationship typically is well understood by adult participants. Children are socialized to communicate with dental professionals in a certain way, so message content is presented in terms more polite and deferential than might be the case in another relationship. A patient may tell her husband, "This tooth is killing me!" To the dentist, she might say, "I'm afraid my tooth may need some attention, doctor." In dentistry, the initial patient-provider relationship is often characterized by formality, fear, or both.

By listening to and observing patients, providers can identify areas of concern. How much pain is the patient suffering? Is the patient anxious or fearful of treatment? Does the patient have specific concerns about esthetics, cost, comfort, or functionality of treatment outcomes? Will the patient accept the provider's treatment recommendation? Asking these questions is recommended when providers suspect specific concerns or barriers, but patients may be unwilling or unable to address them in plain language. Providers skilled in relational message interpretation can gain insight into patient fears and motivations.

In two ways, time is an ally in relational message interpretation. First, as professionals grow more comfortable in their roles as health care providers, they are better able to notice how patients communicate (or not) when certain conditions apply. Second, specific patient-provider relationships tend to grow more trusting and less formal as they evolve. Patients may become more willing to articulate their fears, concerns, and motivations.

Providers should grow more familiar with the communication style of each patient so that variations from a patient's normal communication style can be explored. For instance, mention of "some pain" will be interpreted differently coming from one patient who always complains than from another patient who has rarely complained over several years.

Interpretation of relational messages also can be facilitated by listening to what a patient does not say.[60] A Dutch survey found that dental patients have a strong preference for information yet ask, on average, only 3.8 questions per consultation, and 30.7% ask 0 or 1 question.[61] Several factors can account for patients' reticence to talk, including cultural background, language skills, mood, pain, and fear. Providers who notice a pattern of reticence across patients should request feedback on their communication skills from patients and colleagues.

If a patient avoids discussing a topic or seems reluctant to disclose particular information, the provider should consider a relational explanation and ways to address the reticence. For instance, a male patient may not want to reveal diagnosis and treatment of erectile dysfunction to a female provider. Patients vary dramatically in their notions of privacy and their comfort level with providers of various backgrounds. Providers should not criticize patients for their reticence but instead should explain the reasons specific information is needed and, when possible, offer alternatives to face-to-face disclosure.

In the process of active listening, interpretation goes beyond discovering the meaning of what is said and unsaid to include observation of nonverbal behaviors. Again, interpretation of such behaviors is enhanced when the patient and provider have a longstanding relationship. Furthermore, nonverbal behavior is much more ambiguous than verbal communication, so any conclusions based on nonverbal messages should be considered tentative and perhaps followed up with a question posed to the patient. Even so, the provider who faces the patient and makes eye contact is in an excellent position to interpret relational messages sent through four nonverbal channels: appearance, facial expression, posture and movement, and eye contact.

First, by noticing the general appearance of a patient, the provider can sometimes tell when something is wrong. A patient who appears sleep deprived may be suffering from dental pain that prevents sleep. Facial bruising may indicate oral trauma requiring sensitive questioning to determine whether the source is accidental (eg, a sports injury) or deliberate (eg, intimate partner violence). Second, by noticing facial expressions while a patient is talking, the provider can usually determine whether the patient has an eager or fearful attitude toward the provider. Third, the patient's attitude can also be communicated by posture and movement. A rigid posture or fidgeting may reveal nervousness that the patient does not articulate. Finally, eye behavior can indicate a number of conditions. Wide eyes can indicate fear. Lack of eye contact can indicate nervousness, intimidation, or deception. Dilated eyes can indicate drug use.

Providers should consider all nonverbal cues as invitations to dialogue rather than conclusive evidence of a patient's background or emotional state. A health care provider's job is to notice a patient's physical condition, so patients should generally accept a well-phrased request for more information. An appropriate exchange begins with an observation, followed by an expression of concern: "The way you are gripping the armrests tells me you may be a little nervous. What can I do to put you at ease?"

Step 4: Responding

The steps in active listening increase in activity, from passive hearing to active attending to more active interpreting. The fourth step, **responding**, requires perhaps the most activity and comprises three actions: (1) providing backchannel cues while the patient is speaking and (2) paraphrasing and (3) questioning after the patient has finished speaking. First, as the patient is speaking, the provider should provide **backchannel cues**, which are verbal and nonverbal behaviors that signal attention and encourage the patient to continue talking[62,63] (Box 4-3).

Box 4-3	Backchannel cues

Verbal cues	Nonverbal cues
• "Yeah." • "Uh huh." • "Oh?" • "Oh really?" • "I see." • "Mm hmm." • "You don't say?"	• Eye contact • Smiles • Head nods • Eyebrow raising • Laughter • Facial expressions appropriate to the patient's statement (eg, grimace or eye roll)

Verbal backchannels should not be confused with interruptions. We cannot overemphasize that providers should avoid interruptions. In routine consultations, dentists control the interaction, contributing 71% of the talk compared to 26% contributed by patients.[64] Dental professionals should understand that patients are in a relationship with someone who can cause them pain and they are on that person's home court. Interruptions only reinforce the power imbalance, making the patient less likely to disclose important information.

Providers also should avoid the tendency to overlap, completing the patient's sentences or phrases.[65,66] Although this can be a cooperative form of talk, it can signal impatience to the patient. The provider must create a space and time for the patient to speak freely without being shut down or criticized. This approach does not mandate silence. Instead, while the patient is talking, the provider should limit sounds to brief verbal backchannels that encourage the patient to continue talking. The value of verbal backchannels can easily be understood by considering how long it takes to realize that a mobile telephone connection has been severed.

In addition to verbal backchannels, providers should engage in nonverbal backchannels. If providers are properly paying attention, they should already be making eye contact, perhaps the most important backchannel. Smiling and nodding are similar ways providers signal that they are listening and wish the patient to continue, and both gestures are associated with higher ratings of providers.[67,68] Providers can also encourage the patient with backchannels appropriate to the content of what is being said. Providers should laugh when patients say something funny, grimace a bit when they describe pain, and roll their eyes when patients describe something ridiculous.

One word of caution is in order: Many backchannel cues are culture specific. When providers find that patients are not responding with backchannels that signal interest and approval, the reason may be cultural.

Activity 4-2

To appreciate how important backchannels are to listening, try the following: Ask someone who is not a colleague to give you directions to the library (or bus stop, or stadium, or any place). As they talk, provide no backchannels whatsoever. Indicate no sign of comprehension or incomprehension: no facial expressions, no head nodding, no eye contact. Did the person notice your nonresponsiveness? Did he or she comment or express frustration? Were the directions as accurate and complete as they would have been if you had responded? Was this activity difficult to carry out?

After a patient has finished a statement or completely answered a question, the provider should consider two forms of response. The first is to paraphrase what the patient said, and the second is to follow up with a question. These two are often done together. A **paraphrase** renders what the patient has just said into a summary in the provider's own words.[69–71] A paraphrase should not simply repeat what the patient said but should succinctly rephrase information provided by the patient. It might begin with an introduction such as, "Tell me if I understand you correctly…." Or, "So, in other words…." A paraphrase and question response should include the following elements: *(1)* a brief summary of the factual information; *(2)* an acknowledgement of the patient's attitude, if known; and *(3)* a request for clarification or confirmation. The following is an example:

Patient: I'm always chewing ice, and my wife tells me to stop it, but I think she just says that because the sound irritates her. But anyway, it is just something I've done forever and don't really plan to give up. I guess the only reason I'm mentioning it to you is that lately when I do it I've been feeling some pain back here. *[Patient points to mandible.]*

Provider: So you are saying that you frequently chew ice, have done so for years, and it doesn't bother you except for the recent jaw pain. Is that correct? *[Patient nods.]* Do you also feel pain when you drink something cold?

The paraphrasing and questioning response in active listening has several benefits. This type of response signals to the patient that the provider has been paying attention. It also ensures a level of interpretation, as the provider must consider what is meant as he or she articulates it in different words. Further, the approach enhances accuracy, because patients are invited to correct any misinterpretations. Summarizing what was said also helps the provider commit the patient's background and concerns to memory. Finally, research indicates that paraphrasing enhances the social attractiveness of the listener.[72]

> **Activity 4-3**
>
> Together with one or more colleagues, practice your paraphrasing skills. One colleague mentions the title of a well-known song. Another colleague then paraphrases the factual information of the lyrics and the attitude of the singer and asks for clarification or confirmation. If the song is the theme from the film *Titanic*, for example, the paraphrase might be: "Let me see if I understand. You dream nightly about a loved one who died, and therefore you feel reassured that he remains with you. Is this correct?"

Benefits of active listening

Compared to typical listening behaviors (eg, interrupting patients or listening while multitasking), active listening has the disadvantage of requiring more time, causing providers to relinquish some control over their schedules.[73] Skilled active listeners, however, can minimize the extra time commitment.

This single disadvantage also can be weighed against the multiple benefits resulting from active listening. First, the satisfaction of patients increases when they perceive that their provider is listening.[3,74–77] Satisfied patients ultimately yield a practice management benefit by enhancing the practice's reputation and referring friends and family members. Second, a therapeutic benefit is associated with active listening, particularly for the anxious patient.[78–80] Third, active listening strategies can enhance trust, building what those in the mental health field call a **therapeutic alliance**.[81–84]

Reduced anxiety and enhanced trust can indirectly improve clinical performance, but active listening provides a direct clinical benefit by providing more comprehensive information during the health history interview, including information on patient attitudes.[85,86] Another potential clinical benefit was suggested by a study that found that general medical practitioners who listened more to their patients could reduce their prescription of antibiotics without decreasing patient satisfaction.[87] Finally, because active listening employs standard behaviors, information gathering may be more uniform, minimizing disparities that otherwise result because providers interact differently with patients from diverse backgrounds.[88]

Activity 4-4

Use the Active Listening Observation Scale (Global) to evaluate a provider during a patient consultation. Observe a dentist or dental hygienist during a patient consultation or search "dentist visit consultation" on www.youtube.com to locate a consultation video. Rate active listening behaviors on the 14 criteria listed, indicating the frequency with which each behavior is exhibited by the health care provider: never (1), rarely (2), sometimes (3), frequently (4), or always (5). The sum of the scores will range from 7 to 35, with higher scores indicating more active listening. Given the score of the provider you observed, do you think the benefits of active listening are likely to materialize? What single item would you recommend the provider work on?

Active Listening Observation Scale*

1. **Shows not to be distracted during the consultation:** Score higher if the provider is not distracted during the consultation, for example by the telephone (constantly) ringing, an assistant walking into the room, or the provider staring at the computer screen or looking into the patient's file while ignoring the patient.
2. **Is not off-hand or hasty:** Score higher when the provider adequately responds to the patient's questions, does not talk at high speed, and allows silences in the conversation.
3. **Listens attentively:** Score higher when the provider uses (comfortable) silences in the conversation to give the patient a chance to think or to elaborate, encourages the patient to clarify the problem, notices nonverbal signs from the patient that indicate an emotion, or summarizes the content of the conversation.
4. **Gives the patient time and space to present the problem:** Score higher when the provider allows the patient to finish when he or she is talking and spends more than the usual time on the patient if necessary.
5. **Uses exploring questions:** Score higher when the provider uses exploring or open-ended questions that do not invite any particular answer but open up discussion or elicit a wide range of answers.
6. **Is good in leading the conversation:** Score higher when the provider takes the initiative in the conversation (if necessary), sets an agenda in collaboration with the patient, involves the patient, paraphrases, repeats decisions or future appointments, or evaluates the consultation.
7. **Expresses understanding nonverbally:** Score higher when the provider acknowledges the patient's emotions nonverbally by, for example, nodding, smiling, sympathizing eye contact, supportive humming, or a pat on the shoulder.

*Adapted from Fassaert et al[78] with permission.

Application of Listening Strategies

This chapter so far has addressed listening barriers and active listening strategies; the suggestions apply to general listening contexts, such as rapport building, the health history interview, examination and clinical procedures, and treatment presentation. This section offers additional strategies for listening in specific contexts that are less common but for which the provider should be prepared.

Detecting fear

Dental professionals should listen carefully to anxious patients to determine and address their specific fears. Fear is not limited to fear of pain. Additional fears reported in the research literature include the needle, the handpiece, the anesthesia, the risk of infection, and the loss of teeth.[89–93] Multiple fears are common.[94]

Not everyone suffers from dental anxiety, so the subject should not be introduced routinely, lest fear be triggered in nonanxious patients. ("No, I'm not scared, but your question makes me wonder if I should be!") Instead, when listening to new patients who have not verbally expressed dental anxiety, the provider should monitor nonverbal cues for signs of fear (Box 4-4).

Box 4-4	Nonverbal fear and deception cues	
Fear cues		**Deception cues**
• Distancing from source of fear		• Tension
• Trembling		• Higher vocal pitch
• Crying		• Fidgeting
• Rapid blinking		• Rapid blinking
• Wide eyes		• Eye shifts
• Rapid breathing		• Chin raises
• Throat clearing		• More body animation
• Sweaty palms		• Less pleasant facial expression
• Bristling hair		• More disfluencies (uh, ah, etc)
• Dilated pupils		• Dilated pupils
• Dry mouth		

If the provider suspects a fearful attitude, the subject should be addressed verbally. First, to determine what items, procedures, or prospects provoke the fear, the provider should ask, with a smile, what the patient's fear is: "You seem a little anxious to me. Is there something about visiting the dentist that makes you nervous?" If the patient confirms anxiety, the provider should determine the origin of the fear. Is it based on a negative personal experience? Is it based on something the patient heard from a relative or friend, perhaps as a child? Is it based on something the patient witnessed or read about?

After determining the source of the fear, the provider should, as far as truth will allow, distinguish the prospective procedure from the retrospective experience underlying the fear. Possible reasons the prospective procedure will be different include advances in pain management, advances in infection control, and better skills of the provider. The provider should never misrepresent what the patient will experience; doing so will break any relational trust. Instead, the provider can reassure the patient with the following promise: The provider will *(1)* inform the patient when to expect the fear-inducing stimulus; *(2)* attempt to minimize the fear-inducing stimulus; and *(3)* pause when the patient asks or signals for a break.

By enhancing the patient's perceived control, breaks taken at the patient's request can minimize dental anxiety. However, providers should remember that fear is an automatic and emotional response. The presentation of supporting scientific evidence about a particular procedure or experience can reduce anxiety, but patients are never argued out of their fears, however irrational. Ultimately, positive dental experiences are the best remedy for dental anxiety.

Detecting inaccurate information

When actively listening, providers might suspect that some information patients provide is not correct. Some misinformation may be irrelevant to dental care: the model of the patient's first car, for instance, or the year the patient graduated high school. Other misinformation may be highly relevant to dental care, although the patient may not perceive the relevance: the patient's last physician visit, for instance, or the patient's cardiac health. Patients can provide inaccurate information both unintentionally and intentionally, so providers must provide a rationale for accurate information relevant to dental care: "The drugs we might prescribe or use during dental procedures could potentially interact with other drugs you take or even alcohol. So please answer these drug and alcohol questions accurately so we can avoid any problems on that front."

Patients report incorrect information unintentionally for two reasons. First, they may have forgotten information they once knew. Patients in cognitive decline or with cognitive deficits may be particularly susceptible to providing incorrect information, particularly regarding numeric data (eg, dosages) and dates (eg, their last physical examination). Second, they may use an incorrect term. Mistaken medical terminology can hold significant implications. Canker is very different from chancre, and Xanax is very different from Zantac.

The proliferation of drugs with similar names has become a recognized problem, so an online source to easily confused names is provided at the end of this chapter. When a patient mentions a drug on this list, the provider should ask the patient to confirm easily confused drug names: "You are taking 20 mg of Celexa? That is Celexa, right, and not Celebrex?" If a patient is unsure, the provider can ask the patient for a description of the pill, a copy of the prescription, the actual pill bottle, or permission to contact the patient's physician or pharmacist.

Rather than say, "I don't know," the patient may come up with an answer to provider questions as a way of pleasing an authority figure or to avoid embarrassment. When listening, the provider should remain aware of this tendency and be prepared to verify information.

Patients can also provide inaccurate information deliberately, via deception. In a 2004 WebMD survey of nearly 1,500 people, 13% admitted that they lied to their physician and another 32% said that they "stretched the truth."[95] The most frequent lies related to the following: doctors' orders (38%), diet and exercise (32%), smoking (22%), sex (17%), drinking (16%), and recreational drug use (12%). Dental patients also often lie about the frequency of flossing.[96]

Research suggests that people have trouble detecting lies. Laypersons can detect deception only about 54% of the time.[97] For centuries, researchers and poker players have attempted to identify nonverbal cues that signal deception, but these efforts have largely failed to produce the desired results. In fact, a focus on nonverbal cues can lead to an overestimation of deception.[98]

Activity 4-5

Conduct an ad hoc interview of a colleague, asking about oral health practices: frequency of brushing, flossing, and dental checkups; number of restorations; orthodontics, etc. The colleague should answer some questions truthfully and others deceptively. Try to determine which answers are truthful and which are lies. Can you do better than the 54% average of most people?

Several reasons account for the failure to identify lies. First, people tend to expect others to tell the truth and usually are not on the alert for deception. Second, nonverbal deception cues are ambiguous and easily confused, for instance, with fear cues (see Box 4-4). A comprehensive review of research on deception concluded that many behaviors tested show no links or only weak links to deception.[99] Third, even when statistically significant differences emerge in the use of specific cues, those differences are small and difficult to detect in particular instances. Finally, liars are also aware of deception cues and can modify their behavior to appear more like truth tellers.

Health care providers may be no better than laypersons in detecting lies. In a review of the research on standardized (lying) patients seeking opioids, physicians correctly identified the liars only 10% of the time.[100] The best advice from those in law enforcement and deception research suggests that listeners should deemphasize nonverbal behaviors and instead focus on the information.[99,101]

Information that seems internally inconsistent or inconsistent with the patient's history should be addressed by the provider. Challenges and accusations should be avoided, as the patient retains the right to represent—or misrepresent—personal health information. The provider should, however, provide a rationale for the question and offer a face-saving way for the patient to correct misinformation: "The tartar and calculus buildup I am seeing should not be there if you are brushing and flossing regularly. We may need to do something more drastic if brushing and flossing aren't working. Are you sure you are doing those things at least two times every day?"

> **Q Question of ethics:** Patients sometimes provide inaccurate information. They may do so unintentionally, as when they say they are taking Celexa but are really taking Celebrex. Alternatively, patients may intentionally give false information, as when they insist they do not smoke, despite evidence to the contrary. How should you respond when you believe a patient is providing false information unintentionally? Does your response differ when you believe that the patient is deliberately providing false information?

Detecting incomplete information

In addition to providing inaccurate information, patients may not provide needed information at all. Freeman placed patient needs in three categories: normative, expressed, and felt.[102] Normative needs include treatment needs objectively determined by a clinician. Expressed needs are those articulated by a patient. In an effective and trusting patient-provider relationship, expressed needs will closely track felt needs. However, when the patient has felt needs that he or she does not express, the provider is unable to address the needs, thereby increasing the possibility that the patient will be dissatisfied with care.

Providers who engage in judgment and criticism prompt patients to conceal felt needs: "If you don't stop drinking soda, you are going to lose all your teeth." By scolding patients in this way, providers act like inflexible authority figures, forcing childish responses from patients. Patients either respond petulantly or become reluctant to disclose further information.

By forging ongoing, trusting relationships with patients, the provider can minimize discrepancies between felt and expressed needs. A provider can take three active steps toward enhanced disclosure: *(1)* refraining from criticism; *(2)* emphasizing that the information requested is relevant to dental care; and *(3)* reassuring the patient of confidentiality—"As a health care provider, I am ethically and legally required to hold the information you disclose in confidence." Relationships, however, take time. The reward of close patient relationships will come to providers who are patient.

Determining what patients know and want to know

Effective patient-provider communication should enhance a patient's oral health not only indirectly, through relationship-building approaches (eg, trust and continuity of care), but also directly through dental education. A patient with a greater understanding of oral health can make better decisions regarding preventive and restorative treatment. During examinations and procedures, a dental professional has more opportunity to talk than does the patient, and the provider can use this time to educate the patient on the causes, symptoms, and treatment of dental problems the patient faces or may face. In a sense, the patient is a captive audience, but such information should not be presented as a lecture, which would quickly grow tiresome for an uninterested patient or one who does not understand what is being said.

Before presenting oral health information to the patient, the provider should first listen to what the patient says to determine his or her level of dental knowledge and level of interest in learning more. The vocabulary the patient uses, the restorative procedures he or she has undergone, and the way the patient describes his or her oral health practices should indicate the level of the patient's dental knowledge. The patient's level of enthusiasm and detail when describing home care practices and habits may provide some insights into the patient's level of interest in oral health. A patient who poses more questions is clearly more interested in learning about oral health.

Simply asking a patient if he or she would like to know more about oral health may not be effective, because a patient who is not interested might claim to be, just to be polite to a person wielding a sharp instrument. A more effective way to determine whether a patient would like to learn more about oral health is for the provider to narrate examinations and procedures and present treatment plans with detail and enthusiasm, which can be contagious. Then the provider should notice the patient's reactions. If the patient does not react with obvious interest, the provider should ask if the patient understands what has been said. If the patient indicates that he or she understood the information, then perhaps the patient prefers that the professional handle oral care and make treatment decisions. This is not an optimal situation, and the provider should encourage the patient to take an interest in and responsibility for his or her own oral health. However, the patient cannot be forced to develop an interest in dental care.

Documentation

Because dental professionals often have more than 1,000 patients and may see a dozen of them each day, remembering all the details for each individual is impossible. On average, people immediately forget about half the information they hear.[103] Within 8 hours, only about 35% is retained.[104] Because active listening requires attention, effort, and repetition, the information received from patients is more likely to be remembered than it would be if providers were casually listening or listening while doing something else. Even so, remembering information is often neglected in listening skill acquisition.[105]

Although dental professionals might benefit from instruction in memory enhancement, they already have the advantage of maintaining patient files, which provide a place to document patient information. In addition to recording routine clinical information, providers can enhance their communication with patients by documenting patients' attitudes, preferences and goals, and personal information and by reminding themselves what information to follow up on when patients return.

Attitudes

The provider should remember that patient files will be accessed by others, including the patient, so subjective opinions and unkind evaluations should never be written or typed. Neither should the provider use shorthand others cannot understand. The provider should resist the urge to describe a patient as "difficult" or "uncooperative," even in shorthand. Rather, the main purpose of documenting a patient's attitudes toward dentistry is to identify any patient who has dental anxiety and the degree of that anxiety. Good communication with a willing patient usually leads the patient to reveal his or her anxiety level and specific fear. When fearful attitudes are disclosed, they should be recorded in the patient's file as factual statements: "Pt moderately fears needles." In subsequent appointments, the provider should remain sensitive to the fear but should update the file as the patient's attitudes change. With good care, such attitudes may improve.

Other attitudes worth documenting are any that reflect a positive regard for dentistry: "Pt enthusiastic abt bleaching" or "Pt optimistic abt smoking cessation."

Preferences and goals

Similar to attitudes, patient preferences should be recorded factually and updated as they change. As the relationship builds, a patient may become more comfortable voicing preferences, and the provider should make an effort to remember those preferences: "Pt prefers early morning appts"; "Pt dislikes fruity toothpaste."

Patient preferences sometimes seem idiosyncratic but should be honored if they do not interfere with standard care. In fact, the more idiosyncratic the preference is, the more impressive the provider seems for remembering it. By analogy, waiters who remember where patrons like to sit or what they like to drink typically are perceived as professional and popular.

The provider can also reduce the frustration of patient communication by noting each patient's preferences for personal and educational messages. Some patients like extensive chatting, while others do not. Some patients like learning about prevention and treatment, while others do not. Remembering and honoring preferences fosters patient-centered care, enhances the provider's reputation, and can make the encounter more enjoyable for both the patient and the provider.

A patient's dentistry goals should also be noted. This information is so important to treatment and follow-up that the patient file should include a designated field to record patient goals. A designated field can serve as a reminder to have each patient articulate what is most important, in terms of prevention and procedures. Although there can be additional goals, perhaps the four most common relate to appearance, comfort, functionality, and cost. The patient may not have considered what is most important to him or her, and priorities may change over time, but whenever a patient clarifies main and secondary objectives, the provider should note these priorities, revisiting and discussing them when presenting treatment plans.

Personal information

Providers should also record significant personal information when forgetting such information would prove embarrassing: "Pt married to pt Bob Smith. Children: pt Susan and pt Sam." Patients will vary in their preference for personal conversation, but nobody likes to repeat information they have already disclosed. Patients who have to tell a provider in three consecutive visits that they were born in Lithuania may begin to doubt the cognitive abilities of that provider.

Follow-up reminders

A central aim of effective patient-provider communication is to promote continuity of care. Development of ongoing relationships with patients increases patient satisfaction, fosters trust, reduces patient turnover, and enhances clinical care because the provider can monitor changes in oral health over time. When a provider does not remember a patient from visit to visit, these advantages are compromised.

Listening and documentation are effective means of sustaining continuity of care, but a final strategy worth implementing is always to include a reminder in the patient file to follow up on a specific item. The follow-up reminder for the next appointment can be clinical, such as "Next time: ask abt commitment to flossing 2× daily," or more personal, such as, "Next time: ask abt Bermuda trip." Follow-up reminders spare the provider the frustration of trying to remember what was discussed during the previous appointment and provide an opening topic of discussion when the patient returns.

Chapter Checklist ☑

Barriers to listening
- ❏ Time: Aim to listen to the patient for 1 or 2 minutes during the health history interview.
- ❏ Effort: Focus attention on the patient, particularly as the workday proceeds.
- ❏ Message overload: Learn to filter out competing messages.
- ❏ Rapid thought: Focus thoughts on the patient, resisting temptations to ponder other issues or anticipate what a patient will say.
- ❏ Psychologic noise: Develop methods of avoiding or minimizing distracting thoughts.
- ❏ Physical noise: Minimize ambient noise in the office and operatory.
- ❏ Hearing problems: Minimize noise, wear earplugs, test hearing, and wear hearing aids when necessary.
- ❏ Faulty assumptions: Avoid stereotyping and labeling the patient based on past complaints.
- ❏ Emphasis on talk: Develop an appreciation for listening as integral to communication.
- ❏ Cultural differences: Take the perspective of the patient from a different cultural background.

Active listening
☐ Receiving: Regularly check hearing.
☐ Receiving: Minimize office noise.
☐ Attending: Minimize multitasking and focus on the patient.
☐ Attending: Face the patient.
☐ Attending: Make eye contact.
☐ Attending: During procedures, indicate attention by narrating procedures, addressing the patient directly, and arranging for communication via hand signals.
☐ Interpreting: Consider both connotative and denotative meanings of words.
☐ Interpreting: Consider both relational and content meanings of words.
☐ Interpreting: Consider what the patient is not saying.
☐ Interpreting: Interpret nonverbal cues as invitations to dialogue rather than as conclusive evidence of a patient's background or state of mind.
☐ Interpreting: When addressing nonverbal communication verbally, begin with an observation, followed by an expression of concern.
☐ Interpreting: Grow more familiar with the communication style of each patient so that variations from a patient's normal communication style can be explored.
☐ Interpreting: If a patient is reluctant to disclose information, consider relational explanations, avoid criticizing the patient, provide a rationale for the information request, and offer alternatives to face-to-face disclosure.
☐ Responding: Provide verbal and nonverbal backchannel cues.
☐ Responding: Create a space and time for patient communication by avoiding interrupting, overlapping, or criticizing.
☐ Responding: Paraphrase and question to confirm understanding.
☐ Responding: Summarize factual information by paraphrasing, acknowledge the patient's attitude, and request clarification or confirmation.

Active Listening Observation Scale items
☐ Avoid signs of distraction during consultation.
☐ Avoid appearing off-handed or rushed.
☐ Listen attentively.
☐ Allow the patient time and space for disclosure.
☐ Use questions to explore the patient's disclosures.
☐ Deftly lead the conversation.
☐ Use nonverbal backchannels to indicate understanding.

Applying listening strategies
☐ Fear: Listen carefully to identify and address signs of anxiety.
☐ Fear: Monitor nonverbal cues for signs of fear.
☐ Fear: Ask what the patient's fear is and how it originated.
☐ Fear: Explain how the prospective procedure differs from past procedures and might involve less pain.
☐ Fear: Reassure the patient that he or she will be notified prior to an uncomfortable stimulus, attempts will be made to minimize pain, and the procedure will stop whenever the patient signals.
☐ Fear: Avoid arguing about a patient's fear.
☐ Inaccurate information: Provide a rationale for accurate information relevant to dental care.

❑ Inaccurate information: Remain aware of patients' tendency to provide an answer—any answer—to an authority figure.

❑ Inaccurate information: Ask the patient to confirm easily confused drug names.

❑ Inaccurate information: If the patient is uncertain about a prescription, ask for a description of the pill, a copy of the prescription, the bottle, or permission to contact the prescribing physician or pharmacist.

❑ Deception: Focus on information and not on ambiguous nonverbal cues.

❑ Deception: Address inconsistent or unlikely information.

❑ Deception: Avoid challenges and accusations regarding the truthfulness of information.

❑ Deception: Provide a rationale for the requested information and provide a face-saving way to correct misinformation.

❑ Incomplete information: Avoid criticizing the patient.

❑ Incomplete information: Emphasize the relevance of the information.

❑ Incomplete information: Reassure the patient of confidentiality.

❑ Determining what patients (want to) know: Listen to determine the patient's dental knowledge and interest.

❑ Determining what patients (want to) know: Note the patient's enthusiasm and detail when describing past procedures.

❑ Determining what patients (want to) know: Note the patient's reactions to diagnosis and treatment plan options.

❑ Determining what patients (want to) know: Encourage interest in and responsibility for oral health, but refrain from forcing a patient to take an interest.

Documenting

❑ Attitudes: Avoid subjective opinions and indecipherable shorthand, remaining aware that others will access the patient's file.

❑ Attitudes: Use the patient's file to document attitudes indicating anxiety or enthusiasm for dental care.

❑ Attitudes: Record factual statements and observations of attitudes and update the observations periodically.

❑ Preferences and goals: Record, update, and honor the patient's preferences as much as possible.

❑ Preferences and goals: Note the patient's preferences for personal and educational messages.

❑ Preferences and goals: Note the patient's dentistry goals in a designated field, particularly as they relate to appearance, comfort, functionality, and cost.

❑ Preferences and goals: Revisit dentistry goals when planning treatment.

❑ Personal information: Record any personal information that would be embarrassing to forget.

❑ Follow-up: Always note specific clinical and personal items to address at the beginning of the next appointment.

For More Information

Online listening assessments
- http://psychologytoday.tests.psychtests.com/take_test.php?idRegTest=1605
- http://www.wisc-online.com/objects/ViewObject.aspx?ID=SPH1701
- http://www.wittcom.com/listening_quiz.htm
- http://highered.mcgraw-hill.com/sites/0073381225/student_view0/chapter8/self-assessment_8_3.html
- http://kentblumberg.typepad.com/kent_blumberg/files/active_listening_quiz.doc
- http://www.accc.ca/ftp/es-ce/ACTIVELISTENINGSELF.pdf

Easily confused medical and drug terms
- http://www.ismp.org/tools/confuseddrugnames.pdf
- http://www.mt911.com/site/term/sound_alike_medical.asp

Listening skills
- http://www.listen.org
- http://www.aafp.org/fpm/2005/0400/p68.html
- http://www.ted.com/talks/julian_treasure_5_ways_to_listen_better
- http://www.au.af.mil/au/awc/awcgate/va/practice_listening.htm

Backchannel cues
- http://www.cs.utep.edu/nigel/bc
- http://tcbdevito.blogspot.com/2009/01/listening-and-politeness.html
- http://www.pattiwood.net/article.asp?PageID=2323

Paraphrasing
- http://deepblue.lib.umich.edu/bitstream/2027.42/64983/5/134-3-4UnderstandSkills.mov
- http://compellingconversations.com/blog/2014/07/10/paraphrasing-is-an-essential-conversation-skill

Listening assessments
- http://www.theconsumervoice.org/uploads/files/events/Listening-Self-Evaluation.pdf
- http://www.adamsmithstudent.com/sitebuildercontent/sitebuilderfiles/listening_selfassessment.pdf

Nonverbal behavior
- http://center-for-nonverbal-studies.org/6101.html

References

1. Pikowski EF. Communication with patients is simply listening. Dent Econ 1983;73(6):70,75.
2. Objectives. Health Communication and Health Information Technology. US Department of Health and Human Services. Office of Disease Prevention and Health Promotion. Healthy People 2020. http://www.healthypeople.gov/2020/topics-objectives/topic/health-communication-and-health-information technology/objectives. Accessed 6 January 2015.
3. Rohrer JE, Wilshusen L, Adamson SC, Merry S. Patient-centredness, self-rated health, and patient empowerment: Should providers spend more time communicating with their patients? J Eval Clin Pract 2008;14:548–551.
4. Coy K, Stratton R. Avoiding your greatest fear—Malpractice. J Okla Dent Assoc 2002;93(2):18–27.
5. Harry D. Risk management techniques for the general dentist and specialist. Dent Clin North Am 2008;52:563–577.
6. Lapp CL. Motivation—The key factor for greater productiveness: Are you listening? Are you thinking? Are you willing to change? Greater St Louis Dent Soc Bull 1971;42:143–147.
7. Geier JG. Listening: Motivation and the dentist. Minneap Dist Dent J 1968;52:65–66.
8. St Germain HA Jr. Effective listening: An important tool for dentist. J Indiana Dent Assoc 1982;61(5):25–27.
9. Baker EE Jr. Are you listening, doctor? N Y J Dent 1984;54:201–202.
10. Smith DB. Reflective listening as a marketing force. N Z Dent J 1984;80(361):81–83.
11. Jameson C. Listening: Your key to practice success. J Mass Dent Soc 1993;42:126–129.
12. Coy K. Listening your way to case acceptance. J Okla Dent Assoc 2000;90(4):34–38.
13. Pruett H. Listening to patients. J Calif Dent Assoc 2007;35:183–185.
14. Sondell K, Soderfeldt B, Palmqvist S, Adell A. Communication during prosthodontic treatment—Dentist, patient, and dental nurse. Int J Prosthodont 2000;13:506–512.
15. Adler RB, Rodman G, Hutchinson CC. Understanding Human Communication, ed 11. New York: Oxford University Press, 2011.
16. Wotman S, Demko CA, Victoroff K, Sudano JJ, Lalumandier JA. A multimethod investigation including direct observation of 3751 patient visits to 120 dental offices. Clin Cosmet Investig Dent 2010;2:27–39.
17. Logan HL. The patient and the shifting health-care paradigm. J Am Coll Dent 1997;64(1):16–18.
18. National Center for Health Statistics. Healthy People 2010: Final Review. Hyattsville, MD: US Department of Health and Human Services, 2012:11.1–11.14. http://www.cdc.gov/nchs/data/hpdata2010/hp2010_final_review.pdf. Accessed 27 January 2015.
19. Levin RP. The ABCs of increasing referrals. J Am Dent Assoc 2008;139:351–352.
20. Carver RP. Effects of increasing the rate of speech presentation upon comprehension. J Educ Psychol 1973;65:118–126.
21. Carver RP, Johnson RL, Friedman HL. Factor analysis of the ability to comprehend time-compressed speech. J Lit Res 1971;4:40–49.
22. King PE, Behnke RR. The effect of time-compressed speech on comprehensive, interpretive, and short-term listening. Hum Commun Res 1989;15:428–443.
23. Elmehdi HM. Assessing acoustic noise levels in dental clinics and its link to dental anxiety and fear among UAE population. In: Burgess M, Davey J, Don C, McMinn T (eds). Proceedings of the 20th International Conference on Acoustics (ICA 2010), vol 3. Sydney, Australia: Australian Acoustical Society, 2010:2038–2041.
24. Kilpatrick HC. Decibel ratings of dental office sounds. J Prosthet Dent 1981;45:175–178.
25. Bahannan S, El-Hamid AA, Bahnassy A. Noise level of dental handpieces and laboratory engines. J Prosthet Dent 1993;70:356–360.
26. Jadid K, Klein U, Meinke D. Assessment of noise exposures in a pediatric dentistry residency clinic. Pediatr Dent 2011;33:343–348.
27. Lahmann C, Schoen R, Henningsen P, et al. Brief relaxation versus music distraction in the treatment of dental anxiety: A randomized controlled clinical trial. J Am Dent Assoc 2008;139:317–324.
28. Bare LC, Dundes L. Strategies for combating dental anxiety. J Dent Educ 2004;68:1172–1177.

29. Olszewska I, Zarow M. Does music during a dental treatment make a difference? Presented at the 81st General Session of the International Association for Dental Research, Gothenburg, Sweden, June 28, 2003.

30. Harp H, Hook E, Solberg E, Anderson D. A patient's perspective on how hygienists can decrease patient anxiety. J Dent Hyg 2000;74:322.

31. Chang JR, Cheng HK, Lee SY, Bai MR, Lean RI. A novel earplug system for filtering out dental noise. J Mar Sci Technol (Taiwan) 2003;11:179–188.

32. Hyson JM Jr. The air turbine and hearing loss: Are dentists at risk? J Am Dent Assoc 2002;133:1639–1642.

33. Forman-Franco B, Abramson AL, Stein T. High-speed drill noise and hearing: Audiometric survey of 70 dentists. J Am Dent Assoc 1978;97:479–482.

34. Lehto T. Dentists' hearing and exposure to high speed turbine dental drill noise. Proc Finn Dent Soc 1990;86:115–125.

35. Man A, Neuman H, Assif D. Effect of turbine dental drill noise on dentists' hearing. Isr J Med Sci 1982;18:475–477.

36. Wilson CE, Vaidyanathan TK, Cinotti WR, Cohen SM, Wang SJ. Hearing-damage risk and communication interference in dental practice. J Dent Res 1990;69:489–493.

37. Rahko AA, Karma PH, Rahko KT, Kataja MJ. High-frequency hearing of dental personnel. Community Dent Oral Epidemiol 1988;16:268–270.

38. Barek S, Adam O, Motsch JF. Large band spectral analysis and harmful risks of dental turbines. Clin Oral Investig 1999;3:49–54.

39. Bali N, Acharya S, Anup N. An assessment of the effect of sound produced in a dental clinic on the hearing of dentists. Oral Health Prev Dent 2007;5:187–191.

40. Zubick HH, Tolentino AT, Boffa J. Hearing loss and the high speed dental handpiece. Am J Public Health 1980;70:633–635.

41. Altinoz HC, Gokbudak R, Bayraktar A, Belli S. A pilot study of measurement of the frequency of sounds emitted by high-speed dental air turbines. J Oral Sci 2001;43:189–192.

42. Lehto TU, Laurikainen ET, Aitasalo KJ, Pietila TJ, Helenius HY, Johansson R. Hearing of dentists in the long run: A 15-year follow-up study. Community Dent Oral Epidemiol 1989;17:207–211.

43. Weinrauch JD, Swanda JR. Examining the significance of listening: An exploratory study of contemporary management. J Bus Commun 1975;13(1):25–32.

44. Barker L, Gladney K, Edwards R, Holley F, Gaines C. An investigation of proportional time spent in various communication activities by college students. J Appl Commun Res 1980;8:101–109.

45. Rankin PT. The importance of listening ability. English J 1928;17:623–630.

46. Davis D. Two ears and one mouth: Two eyes and one hand. ILA Listening Post 2001;(77):10–13.

47. Janusik LA, Wolvin AD. 24 hours in a day: A listening update to the time studies. Int J Listening 2009;23:104–120.

48. Loban W. The Language of Elementary School Children. Champaign, IL: National Council of Teachers of English, 1963.

49. Ford WSZ, Wolvin AD, Sungeun C. Students' self-perceived listening competencies in the basic speech communication course. Int J Listening 2000;14:1–13.

50. Duck S, McMahan DT. Communication in Everyday Life. Thousand Oaks, CA: Sage, 2010.

51. Beaman CP. Auditory distraction from low-intensity noise: A review of the consequences for learning and workplace environments. Appl Cognitive Psychol 2005;19:1041–1064.

52. Schoechlin C, Engel RR. Neuropsychological performance in adult attention-deficit hyperactivity disorder: Meta-analysis of empirical data. Arch Clin Neuropsychol 2005;20:727–744.

53. Green JA, Gustafson GE. Individual recognition of human infants on the basis of cries alone. Dev Psychobiol 1983;16:485–493.

54. Lahti S, Tuuti H, Hausen H, Kaariainen R. Comparison of ideal and actual behavior of patients and dentists during dental treatment. Community Dent Oral Epidemiol 1995;23:374–378.

55. Holt V, McHugh K. Factors influencing patient loyalty to dentist and dental practice. Br Dent J 1997;183:365–370.

56. Edwards R. Listening and message interpretation. Int J Listening 2011;25:47–65.

57. Frentz TS, Farrell TB. Language-action: A paradigm for communication. Q J Speech 1976;62: 333–349.

58. Watzlawick P, Beavin J, Jackson DD. Pragmatics of Human Communication. New York: Norton, 1967.
59. Bateson G. Information and codification: A philosophical approach. In: Ruesch J, Bateson G (eds). Communication: The Social Matrix of Psychiatry. New York: Norton, 1951:168–211.
60. Freeman R. The psychology of dental patient care: Communicating effectively: Some practical suggestions. Br Dent J 1999;187:240–244.
61. Schouten BC, Hoogstraten J, Eijkman MAJ. Patient participation during dental consultations: The influence of patients' characteristics and dentists' behavior. Community Dent Oral Epidemiol 2003;31:368–377.
62. Xudong D. Listener response. In: D'hondt S, Ostman JO, Versucheren J (eds). The Pragmatics of Interaction. Amsterdam: John Benjamins, 2009:104–124.
63. Tannen D. Language and culture. In: Fasold RW, Connor-Linton J (eds). An Introduction to Language and Linguistics. New York: Cambridge University Press, 2006:343–372.
64. Coleman H, Burton J. Aspects of control in the dentist-patient relationship. Int J Sociol Lang 1985;1985(51):75–104.
65. Lerner GH. Notes on overlap management in conversation: The case of delayed completion. Western J Commun 1989;53:167–177.
66. Lerner GH. On the syntax of sentences-in-progress. Lang Soc 1991;20:441–458.
67. Harrigan JA, Rosenthal R. Physicians' head and body positions as determinants of perceived rapport. J Appl Soc Psychol 1983;13:496–509.
68. Griffith CH, Wilson JF, Langer S, Haist SA. House staff nonverbal communication skills and standardized patient satisfaction. J Gen Intern Med 2003;18:170–174.
69. Kulich KR, Berggren U, Hallberg LRM. Model of the dentist-patient consultation in a clinic specializing in the treatment of dental phobic patients: A qualitative study. Acta Odontol Scand 2000;58:63–71.
70. Newton JT, Brenneman DL. Communication in Dental Settings Scale (CDSS): Preliminary development of a measure to assess communication in dental settings. Br J Health Psychol 1999;4:277–284.
71. Nazir M. Illuminating communication. Vital 2008;5(Summer):35–37.
72. Weger H, Castle GR, Emmett MC. Active listening in peer interviews: The influence of message paraphrasing on perceptions of listening skill. Int J Listening 2010;24:34–49.
73. Meeuwesen L, Schaap C, van der Staak C. Verbal analysis of doctor-patient communication. Soc Sci Med 1991;32:1143–1150.
74. Wanzer MB, Booth-Butterfield M, Gruber K. Perceptions of health care providers' communication: Relationships between patient-centered communication and satisfaction. Health Commun 2004;16:363–384.
75. Al-Mudaf BA, Moussa MA, Al-Terky MA, Al-Dakhil GD, El-Farargy AE, Al-Ouzairi SS. Patient satisfaction with three dental speciality services: A centre-based study. Med Princ Pract 2003;12:39–43.
76. Anderson R. Patient expectations of emergency dental services: A qualitative interview study. Br Dent J 2004;197:331–334.
77. Cohen LA, Bonito AJ, Eicheldinger C, et al. Comparison of patient centeredness of visits to emergency departments, physicians, and dentists for dental problems and injuries. J Am Coll Dent 2010;77(4):49–58.
78. Fassaert T, van Dulmen S, Schellevis F, Bensing J. Active listening in medical consultations: Development of the Active Listening Observation Scale (ALOS-global). Patient Educ Couns 2007;68:258–264.
79. Getka EJ, Glass CR. Behavioral and cognitive-behavioral approaches to the reduction of dental anxiety. Behav Ther 1992;23:433–448.
80. Bernson JM, Hallberg LRM, Elfström ML, Hakeberg M. Making dental care possible—A mutual affair. A grounded theory relating to adult patients with dental fear and regular dental treatment. Eur J Oral Sci 2011;119:373–380.
81. Levin RP. The interpersonal factor. J Am Dent Assoc 2008;139:986–987.
82. Nash DA. Engaging children's cooperation in the dental environment through effective communication. Pediatr Dent 2006;28:455–459.

83. Quill TE, Brody H. Physician recommendations and patient autonomy: Finding a balance between physician power and patient choice. Ann Intern Med 1996;125:763–769.

84. White JG, Kruger C, Snyman WD. Development and implementation of communication skills in dentistry: An example from South Africa. Eur J Dent Educ 2008;12:29–34.

85. Knopp R, Rosenzweig S, Bernstein E, Totten V. Physician-patient communication in the emergency department. 1. Acad Emerg Med 1996;3:1065–1076.

86. Sonis ST (ed). Dental Secrets, ed 2. Philadelphia: Hanley & Belfus, 1999.

87. Lundkvist J, Åkerlind I, Borgquist L, Mölstad S. The more time spent on listening, the less time spent on prescribing antibiotics in general practice. Fam Pract 2002;19:638–640.

88. Willems S, De Maesschalck S, Deveugele M, Derese A, De Maeseneer J. Socio-economic status of the patient and doctor-patient communication: Does it make a difference? Patient Educ Couns 2005;56:139–146.

89. Kleinknecht RA, Klepac RK, Alexander LD. Origins and characteristics of fear of dentistry. J Am Dent Assoc 1973;86:842–848.

90. Oosterink FMD, De Jongh A, Aartman IHA. What are people afraid of during dental treatment? Anxiety-provoking capacity of 67 stimuli characteristic of the dental setting. Eur J Oral Sci 2008;116:44–51.

91. Hakeberg M, Cunha L. Dental anxiety and pain related to dental hygienist treatment. Acta Odontol Scand 2008;66:374–379.

92. Horowitz LG. Risk communication in dental practice: Responding assertively to AIDS, fear and infection control. J Tenn Dent Assoc 1993;73(3):16–18, 65.

93. Smyth JS. Some problems of dental treatment. 1. Patient anxiety: Some correlates and sex differences. Aust Dent J 1993;38:354–359.

94. Ulf B. General and specific fears in referred and self-referred adult patients with extreme dental anxiety. Behav Res Ther 1992;30:395–401.

95. DeNoon D. WebMD survey: The lies we tell our doctors. MedicineNet, September 21, 2004. http://www.medicinenet.com/script/main/art.asp?articlekey=46985. Accessed 29 January 2015.

96. Dworkin-McDaniel N. The lies women tell their doctors. Redbook, September 25, 2008. http://www.redbookmag.com/body/health-fitness/advice/a3965/women-health-lies/. Accessed 29 January 2015.

97. Bond CF Jr, DePaulo BM. Individual differences in judging deception: Accuracy and bias. Psychol Bull 2008;134:477–492.

98. Vrij A. Nonverbal dominance versus verbal accuracy in lie detection. Crim Justice Behav 2008;35:1323–1336.

99. DePaulo BM, Lindsay JJ, Malone BE, Muhlenbruck L, Charlton K, Cooper H. Cues to deception. Psychol Bull 2003;129:74–118.

100. Jung B, Reidenberg MM. Physicians being deceived. Pain Med 2007;8:433–437.

101. Mann S, Vrij A, Bull R. Detecting true lies: Police officers' ability to detect suspects' lies. J Appl Psychol 2004;89:137–149.

102. Freeman R. The psychology of dental patient care: Reflections on professional and lay perspectives of the dentist-patient interaction. Br Dent J 1999;186:546–550.

103. Nicholas RG, Stevens LA. Listening to people. Harvard Bus Rev 1957;35:90–97.

104. Barker LL. Listening Behavior. Englewood Cliffs, NJ: Prentice Hall, 1971.

105. Wintersteen LR. Listening techniques. How to break through patient sound barriers. Dent Teamwork 1994;7(4):19–21.

5

Improving Verbal Skills

Why Verbal Skills Matter

Verbal communication is simply any form of communication relying on words—spoken or written. The presence of words distinguishes verbal and nonverbal communication, but the difference is even more profound. Words are always arbitrary symbols associated with a particular meaning by a particular social group. Verbal communication skill therefore requires learning words, learning their associated meaning, and learning how to put them together in a comprehensible way. By contrast, nonverbal communication also includes biologically based, nonarbitrary signs (such as perspiring with fear), making it more spontaneous than verbal communication.[1] In short, because all verbal communication must be learned, people vary widely in their ability to understand and express verbal messages.[2,3]

The educational requirements for a career in dentistry ensure that providers have high verbal comprehension skills, but they can vary in their ability to express themselves verbally and adjust their verbal expression to match the comprehension level of a given patient.

Research is lacking on any association between oral health and the verbal skills of either patient or provider. Research does, however, indicate significant positive associations between education and oral health and oral health literacy.[4,5] Compared to those with some college education, adults with less than a high school education can face a threefold increase in caries and untreated periodontal disease.[6] Research also documents that health care is less effective when patients and providers do not share the same language.[7] These findings suggest that patients with poorer verbal skills may have less access to dental care and may receive less effective care when they do have access.

By speaking to patients at a level they can comprehend and by providing information that ultimately increases patients' oral health literacy, dental professionals can enhance patient care and minimize the patient and provider frustrations that arise from limited mutual understanding. This chapter first presents the goals of verbal communication, then discusses the significance of oral health literacy, and concludes with a variety of verbal communication strategies to facilitate patient-provider relationships.

Verbal Communication Goals

Some literature on provider communication focuses primarily on goals such as persuasion, promotion, production, and marketing.[8–12] We urge caution when interpreting or applying this work. First, making persuasion a primary goal suggests that the provider's treatment objectives are more important than those of the patient, thereby undermining patient-centered care. Second, attempts at promotion and marketing may be ineffective or even counterproductive.[13,14] In a culture saturated with promotion and marketing efforts, many patients are sensitive to attempts at verbal manipulation. Such efforts may undermine the patient-provider relationship and reinforce the stereotype that dentists are greedy.

We readily acknowledge that promotion of healthy behaviors and restorative treatments usually aligns with the best interests of patients and that health marketing is a worthy field that has accomplished a great deal. Yet at the level of the patient-provider relationship, even thinking in terms such as motivating a patient and achieving patient compliance subtly prioritizes outcomes desired by the provider rather than by the patient. Rather than advocating persuasive methods per se, we believe an educational approach is most effective and most supportive of a long-term relationship with the patient. When the provider takes the time to inform the patient of his or her dental health status and the treatment options available and then gives a professional opinion about the most effective course of action, the patient will often select the recommended treatment, particularly if the provider makes the effort to address the patient's concerns related to cost, pain, scheduling, and so on.[15]

> **Q** | **Question of ethics:** Patients are prone to indulge in unhealthy behaviors, even when they have been informed of healthier options. Patients also have less understanding of oral health and dental treatments than do dental professionals, whose recommendations patients may discount or ignore. Is it ethical to withhold or distort the diagnostic or treatment information you provide to promote the best interests of the patient? Does your answer change based on context (eg, emergency treatment versus routine consultation)? Does your answer change based on the patient (eg, healthy adult versus senior with dementia)? Have you developed formal guidelines to decide these matters, or do you consider them on a case-by-case basis?

Clinical communication can be categorized primarily as task focused or emotion focused[16] (Table 5-1). The most effective provider communication includes both task- and emotion-focused messages.[17,18] Providers who help patients develop oral health knowledge and skill while encouraging patients consistently to apply that knowledge and skill will likely have more success than providers who focus on persuading patients to accept a treatment. Task- and emotion-focused providers will enhance both their patient relationships and their patients' oral health.

Table 5-1 Verbal communication goals

Goal	Appropriate	Inappropriate
Task-focused communication		
Education	"The space between your front teeth is called a diastema. We can close it, but lots of people keep it: David Letterman, Madonna, and SpongeBob Squarepants, to name a few."	"Yeah, you have a space there."
Promotion	"We've talked about the risks associated with chewing tobacco. Are you willing to try doing without it for a week?"	"Stop chewing tobacco."
Explanation	"I'm checking that filling from 2009, and it seems to be holding well."	"Another 5 minutes and I'll be done."
Emotion-focused communication		
Empathy	"I had braces when I was your age, and now I'm really glad I did."	"If you don't wear your retainer, you'll be sorry when nobody will date you."
Anxiety reduction	"I'll make this as pain-free as possible, and I promise to stop whenever you signal for me to stop, OK?"	"You're being ridiculous. There's nothing to be scared of."
Encouragement	"Stopping smoking is one of the hardest things you'll ever do, but I know you can do it and I'm here to help you."	"One way or another, everybody stops smoking!"
Trust enhancement	"I strongly recommend we try to save that tooth, but I will pull it, if that is what you really want me to do."	"Only an idiot would ask for an extraction when there's a chance you could keep the tooth."

Task-focused communication

Within verbal communication, **task-focused messages** are those that relate to the task of delivering competent dental health care. Although emotion-focused messages can indirectly promote oral health, task-focused communication directly addresses it. Although nonverbal communication can serve as a valuable supplement, task-focused communication relies mainly on verbal communication. Further, task-focused messages can be delivered to a mass audience (eg, a public health campaign), to a smaller group (eg, career day at an elementary school), or to an individual patient.[19] The goals of task-focused messages include educating patients about oral health, promoting acquisition of a behavioral skill, and explaining a diagnosis or procedure.

Providers can educate patients by providing accurate information regarding oral health care and correcting misinformation acquired from other individuals or media sources. The availability of task-focused messages on the Internet has led to an increasing number of patients who seek out information individually.[20] Such initiative can enhance patient-provider relationships by providing a task-focused topic of discussion during appointments.[21] The disadvantage of Internet information, however, is that patients may not discriminate among research, opinion, and propaganda, and they may not distinguish among noncommercial, commercial, and lay sources of information. When patients arrive for their appointments believing incorrect information, providers should praise their interest and initiative while sensitively correcting the mistaken belief:

> I'm so impressed that you took the time to research fluoride, Mrs Jackson! In large doses fluoride *is* toxic, the same way carbon dioxide is poisonous if you get too much. But the amount of fluoride in our toothpaste, mouthwash, and water is like the carbon dioxide in our air. It won't hurt you.

Worth noting is that 41.6% of dental patients would appreciate recommendations from dentists and hygienists regarding Internet sites that provide reliable oral health information.[22]

Providers can promote oral health simply by providing accurate information. A review of the research indicates that educational interventions on oral hygiene can yield significant short-term reductions in plaque levels.[23] Patients must have correct information before they can apply it. Historically, however, clinicians have not consistently adhered to good communication practices when promoting preventive treatments, and they overestimate their effectiveness.[24] The proliferation of information today can result in different and contradictory recommendations, confusing patients who may not be terribly motivated to address oral health in the first place. Dental professionals are highly credible sources of information, and face-to-face communication with patients enhances that credibility. Unless a patient indicates verbally or nonverbally that dental services should be confined to clinical treatment, providers should consider patient education a part of their job. Such education should include scientific findings but also experience-based and common-sense ways of integrating healthy dental behaviors into everyday life.[25] Evidence suggests that long-term improvement may be contingent on the level of support in patients' social environment.[26]

Another goal of task-focused messages is to explain dental procedures. Providers often neglect to do this, although research indicates that patients prefer that their dentist explain the function of instruments and procedures.[27] Each procedure should be described at least three times. First, when treatment is planned, the patient should be provided with descriptions of at least two or three options, with the recommended option identified and justified. Second, before treatment begins, the patient should be told in some detail what procedure will be undertaken: "Today we are planning to clean your teeth and check to make sure everything looks healthy." Finally, the procedure should be described or "narrated" briefly as the provider is carrying it out: "Now I'm checking for any signs of gum disease."

Emotion-focused communication

Effective teachers do not simply present information in class that could just as easily be found in a book. They also cultivate student interest in a subject by engaging the material in ways the students may not have considered it before. The same principle applies to dental professionals. As we have shown, patients' attitudes toward dentistry are emotionally charged, often with fear and suspicion. Effective dental professionals present information in a way that takes into account the emotional needs of patients. **Emotion-focused communication** can achieve four primary goals: empathy, anxiety reduction, encouragement, and trust (see Table 5-1).

First, to craft appropriate and effective emotion-focused messages, providers must have empathy for patients. Empathy is simply the capacity to share a patient's emotional state. When used in service of patient-centered care, empathy entails identifying the emotions of patients and responding appropriately. For professionals trained in Western medicine, sustaining patient empathy can be a challenge because medical training places a premium on objective analysis of symptoms.[28] In fact, evidence suggests that dental students' emotional empathy for patients declines as students are increasingly exposed to patients during the course of their schooling.[29,30] The challenge for dental professionals is to empathize with patients to a degree that allows for identification with patient feelings but avoids emotional involvement that compromises clinical judgment or job satisfaction.[31] Self-monitoring is a good practice; providers should ask themselves daily: Am I displaying appropriate empathy with my patients?

Because empathy primarily reflects emotional connection, it is often communicated via nonverbal messages, such as smiles, grimaces, furrowed brows, and comforting touch. Providers, however, should not neglect verbal means of communicating empathy. Coulehan et al[32] have provided a number of empathic statements providers can use in various contexts. Dentists believe empathic communication requires additional time, and this belief may be true, but time must be weighed against the benefits of empathy.[33] Empathy could be recommended for the sake of providers because it fosters healthy long-term relationships with patients, which ultimately make dentistry more rewarding.[34] Empathic communication also benefits patients in multiple ways by providing the relational foundation that facilitates patient-centered care. The very word *care* suggests how integral empathy is to the profession.

Second, emotion-focused messages can aim to minimize patient anxiety. Education was previously mentioned as a form of task-focused communication, but it can also serve an emotional function for anxious patients. When dental hygiene patients were asked what providers could do to decrease their anxiety, the most common answer (74%) was to explain the procedure.[35] Dentists can reduce patient anxiety by discussing the risks of procedures with them.[36] When patients know what to expect, they may feel more in control of a potentially painful experience. Based on a series of dental anxiety studies, Corah[37] asserted that promising to prevent pain is the single most effective way to reduce patient anxiety. We would caution providers to issue such promises sparingly, however, because patients have different pain thresholds and a broken promise can undermine trust in the patient-provider relationship.

Both children and adults can feel anxious about medical encounters. Fear-inducing medical encounters include simple vaccinations, anesthesia, pupil dilation, mammograms, prostate examinations, and a host of other procedures. Try to recall a time when you were anxious about a medical encounter. What was the purpose of the encounter? How old were you? Did you have time to prepare for it or worry about it? What, specifically, were you anxious about? How did your anxiety manifest? Were others aware? Did the provider acknowledge your anxiety? If so, did the provider deal with it effectively? After the encounter was over, did your anxiety about similar future encounters increase or decrease?

Unfortunately, emotion-focused messages can also increase patient anxiety, as when dental professionals try scaring patients into preventive or restorative treatments. Messages designed to induce fear are more popular than they are effective. The rationale of fear appeals is that patients will modify their behavior or elect dental procedures to avoid an outcome that frightens them: "If you keep smoking, you'll get oral cancer and we'll have to cut out your tongue."

Fear appeals can be effective, but their effectiveness depends on so many variables that researchers generally discourage their use.[38] For instance, with fear appeals, more is not always better. In a classic 1953 experiment, Janis and Feshbach[39] discovered that dental hygiene messages inducing moderate fear were more effective than low- or high-fear messages. A fear appeal should be just frightening enough to arouse patients' attention but not so gory and threatening that patients tune out. Busy dental professionals, however, have little time to determine just the right amount of fear to induce, and scaring patients is vaguely manipulative anyway. Research overwhelmingly advocates the use of positive reinforcement over negative and finds that positive reinforcement is perhaps the most common technique used to calm fearful patients, particularly children.[40–42]

Third, emotion-focused messages can encourage patients to undertake and sustain difficult behavioral changes supportive of oral health. Perhaps the most salient example is patients who are attempting smoking cessation. Even providers who have never smoked have experience in breaking a habit and can verbalize empathic messages that encourage patients to persist in their attempts to stop smoking: "I know this is difficult, but I also know you can do it." Or, "I've seen people who have failed repeatedly when they try to stop smoking, but if they keep trying they will eventually succeed." Again, positive reinforcement is a powerful tool for the dental professional. Providers should not neglect praise.[43–45]

Fourth, emotion-focused verbal messages can facilitate trust.[45–47] If dentists are to eradicate the suspicion that they are motivated by money or anything other than patients' well-being, they must express themselves in trustworthy ways. Communication that focuses exclusively on clinical information does not foster a trusting relationship, because patients have human concerns that may not be addressed by recommendations based on randomized clinical trials. Those concerns include how they are going to pay for expensive treatments, how they are going to fit treatments into their schedule, and how they are going to handle painful procedures.

Eliciting those concerns is the first step toward building trust: "Does anything concern you regarding the treatment I've recommended?" The second step is validating those concerns: "It is an expensive treatment, and I wish it did not cost so much. Our office can work out a payment plan, or we can simply continue to monitor the situation, although I'd rather take care of it sooner rather than later." Acknowledging the patient's concerns and expressing willingness to abide by the patient's decisions distinguish the trustworthy dental professional from those focused on their own objectives.

Oral Health Literacy

In recent decades, the medical establishment has grown aware of the problem of low health literacy among patients. The US Department of Education estimates that only 12% of English-speaking American adults possess sufficient health literacy skills.[48] Literacy is the ability to understand written information, but health literacy is more than the ability to understand written information about health. Healthy People 2010 defined **health literacy** as "the degree to which individuals have the capacity to obtain, process, and understand basic health information and services needed to make appropriate health decisions."[49] This conceptualization of health literacy includes written health literacy but also comprehension of spoken information and numeracy, which is the ability to understand health information involving numbers.[50]

In a health care system of increasing complexity, sufficient health literacy is necessary for patients to make appointments, fill out forms, understand the elements of consent, ask appropriate questions, evaluate oral and written sources of information, understand diagnoses and treatment options, and read and understand prescriptions, medical records, and insurance forms. Healthy People 2020 lists three objectives related to health literacy[51]:

1. Increase the proportion of persons who report that their health care provider always gave them easy-to-understand instructions about what to do to take care of their illness or health condition.
2. Increase the proportion of persons who report that their health care provider always asked them to describe how they will follow the instructions.
3. Increase the proportion of persons who report that their health care providers' office always offered help in filling out a form.

Insufficient health literacy results in poorer care and poorer health. In a recent systematic review, the Agency for Healthcare Research and Quality reported that lower health literacy is "consistently associated with increased hospitalizations, greater emergency care use...poorer ability to demonstrate taking medications appropriately, poorer ability to interpret labels and health messages, and, among seniors, poorer overall health status and higher mortality."[50] Limited health literacy is a stronger predictor of an individual's health status than age, income, employment status, education level, or racial or ethnic group.[52]

Less research has been conducted in oral health literacy than in health literacy, but the data are accumulating.[53] Jones et al[54] reported that 29% of adults have a low level of oral health literacy. As with health literacy, evidence suggests that oral health disparities are associated with oral health literacy. Regarding access to care, research indicates that those who regularly visit the dentist report higher oral health literacy than those who visit only when they are in pain.[55] Perhaps those with higher oral health literacy are more inclined to visit the dentist regularly, or maybe those who visit regularly increase their oral health literacy through provider education. Regarding oral health, results from the Carolina Oral Health Literacy Project indicate that oral health literacy is significantly associated with oral health status, although not significantly associated with dental neglect.[56]

Given the significant disparities, there have been calls to increase the public's oral health literacy.[57] Experts believe that efforts to improve the oral health literacy of children could prove particularly beneficial.[58] Lower oral health literacy scores among children's caregivers are associated with unhealthy childcare practices such as nighttime bottle use and neglect of brushing or cleaning teeth.[59] Lower oral health literacy among parents unsurprisingly is associated with poorer oral health in children.[60]

Large-scale interventions targeting children can increase oral health literacy and cultivate healthy habits before periodontal disease causes lasting damage. Dental professionals should likewise perceive patient interactions as opportunities for small-scale interventions to increase oral health literacy.[61] Patient education is, after all, a goal of verbal communication. A more immediate goal, however, is to deliver clinical information at a level patients can understand. Accomplishing this goal requires skill at assessing patients' oral health literacy.

Although dental professionals acknowledge the importance of targeting communication to a patient's literacy level, a recent study found that 62% of dental hygiene students reported that appointments do not allow enough time to assess patient comprehension of oral health concepts.[62] Further, a survey of dentists found that only 54% were confident in their ability to recognize patients with limited oral health literacy.[63] There are several ways to assess patients' oral health literacy, and they fall into two general categories: formal and informal assessments.

Formal oral health literacy assessments

The research on oral health literacy has required the development of valid and reliable measures specific to dentistry. These formal measures may be impractical for everyday use with patients, but providers should be aware of them. They could be used for specific patients if circumstances warrant. Instruments typically are one of two types: measures of word recognition or measures of comprehension.

The best known oral health literacy measures are variations of the Rapid Estimate of Adult Literacy in Dentistry (REALD), a word-recognition instrument. The REALD-30 instrument includes 30 dental terms arranged in order of increasing complexity, based on word length, number of syllables, and difficulty of sound combinations.[64] All the words were taken from the American Dental Association's (ADA's) *Glossary of Common Dental Terminology*.[65] The REALD-99 instrument includes 69 additional words chosen to represent disease etiology, anatomy, prevention, and treatment.[66]

More recently, a two-stage version has been developed, the REALD-TS.[67] The words in the first stage determine which follow-up words the participant will receive. First-stage words are *denture, abscess, restoration, fistula,* and *temporomandibular.* Performance routes the participant to follow-up words in one of three levels: low literacy (*braces, plaque, pulp,* and *extraction*); average literacy (*enamel, genetics, sealant, halitosis, cellulitis,* and *incipient*); or high literacy (*hyperemia, hypoplasia,* and *analgesia*).

The Rapid Estimate of Adult Literacy in Medicine and Dentistry (REALM-D) is an instrument that measures both general health literacy and oral health literacy by testing patients' familiarity with 84 medical and dental terms.[5] The number of terms requires more time to administer than some other measures, but it is a comprehensive measure that may be appropriate for facilities or patients requiring an integrated medical-dental measure of health literacy.

These word-recognition instruments have the advantage of being easy to administer in a clinic, but they measure only the patient's ability to recognize or pronounce words (or to correctly guess them). At least one study suggests no significant association between the ability to read dental terms and the ability to comprehend them.[68]

Three other instruments do not simply measure word recognition but instead evaluate comprehension of oral health concepts. The Test of Functional Health Literacy in Dentistry (TOFHLiD) includes one test of reading comprehension and another test of numeracy.[69] In the reading test, patients select among key words to fit omissions in three passages on instructions following application of fluoride varnish, consent for treatment, and Medicaid rights and responsibilities. The 12 numeracy questions are related to instructions on fluoride toothpaste, a pediatric dental appointment, and labels for fluoride drops and tablets.

The Oral Health Literacy Instrument (OHLI) also includes two tests.[55] The first is a 38-item measure of reading comprehension in which patients select the appropriate word to fill omissions in passages on dental caries and periodontal disease. The second is a 19-item numeracy test addressing common dental prescriptions, postextraction instructions, and dental appointments.

The Comprehensive Measure of Oral Health Knowledge (CMOHK) is a comprehension test administered via patient interview.[70] The test poses 44 multiple-choice questions in four categories: basic knowledge of oral health and prevention (20 questions) and management of dental caries (8), periodontal disease (8), and oral cancer (8).

In a general medical context, Chew et al[71] found a single question to be a valid measure of health literacy. The patient is asked, "How confident are you filling out forms by yourself?" Response choices range from 0 to 4: not at all confident, a little confident, somewhat confident, quite confident, and extremely confident. For a dental practitioner requesting the patient to fill out health history forms, asking that single question beforehand could indicate the patient's level of health literacy. For a patient with less confidence, the provider might verify the accuracy of information and might offer assistance in completing all forms.

Informal oral health literacy assessments

The societal stigma associated with illiteracy is also associated with low health literacy. Individuals often are reluctant to acknowledge that they do not know or understand information they believe they should know or understand. They can be even more reluctant to reveal a lack of understanding to health care providers. The patient-provider dynamic involves an inherent power differential that evokes that of a student and teacher. Further, patients often believe they ought to know health information because it is so personal and relevant to their physical and mental well-being. They can find themselves in a double-bind: simultaneously wanting to understand and wanting to be perceived as already understanding. Directly challenging patients on their level of health literacy is never recommended, as it would likely embarrass them and lead them to be uncommunicative. Instead, providers can rely on four informal means of determining patients' oral health literacy.

First, the provider should be aware of characteristics associated with lower oral health literacy. A study of adult participants in dental research found that marginal health literacy was associated with age, sex, and race.[72] A separate study of low-income patients reported that males and Hispanics are significantly more likely than others to have health literacy–related problems when interacting with a dental professional.[73] Another study found that economically disadvantaged patients are less likely to say that health care providers explained things so they always understood.[74] Although common sense suggests that a patient's education level should correspond with oral health literacy, at least one study does not bear that out.[55]

The provider should always remain sensitive to patients' health literacy skills, but especially so when treating older patients, the economically disadvantaged, Hispanics, or any non-native English speaker. In their research on physicians, Ferguson and Candib[75] noted that a provider must also remain aware of changes in his or her own verbal communication when treating diverse populations: "Minority patients, especially those not proficient in English, are less likely to engender empathic response from physicians, establish rapport with physicians, receive sufficient information, and be encouraged to participate in medical decision making."

Second, the provider should monitor the patients' behaviors as they process information. The chapter on listening (chapter 4) provided general guidance for monitoring patients' nonverbal expressions. When patients are reading or hearing information, specific nonverbal signals of confusion are often seen in movement of the eyes and (less often) the mouth.[76] Such movement is more often asymmetric than symmetric. Eye signals include eyebrows that are raised, lowered, or furrowed and eyes that are squinted. Mouth signals include raised lips and smiles. Of course, the blank stare can also signal confusion.

A patient with compromised basic literacy skills may show common behaviors: omitting responses on the health history form, being unable to name prescribed medications or explain what the medications are for, missing appointments, and neglecting to follow up on referrals.[77] The low-literacy patient more often asks the provider to repeat something but overall is less likely to ask questions, refer to medications by name, or request additional information or services.[78] The patient may try to hide this shortcoming with common excuses: "I forgot my glasses," "I don't have time to fill out forms right now," "My spouse handles all the paperwork," or "My handwriting is so bad someone should complete the form for me."

Third, the provider can and should periodically ask whether the patient understands the information presented. Such comprehension checks should be performed when completed forms are required or when information is provided in spoken or written form. The provider can use the words he or she is most comfortable with, but they should be some variation of, "What questions do you have about these forms?" or "Does what I just said make sense?" Written information can be very helpful, because brochures allow the patient to process information at his or her own pace and allow others at home to help the patient understand the information. However, many dental brochures are written at a difficult level for a person with low oral health literacy to understand.[79]

A fourth informal method for assessing health literacy is also a communication strategy for reinforcing information. The provider who wants a patient to understand and remember important information should present the information and ask the patient to repeat, explain, or demonstrate what was just heard or read. (RED is a useful acronym for remembering this approach.) After explaining the importance of rinsing out the mouth following consumption of sugary soft drinks, the provider might ask for a repetition: "Now, what did we discuss for you to do after you drink your afternoon Mountain Dew?" After providing instructions on postextraction socket care, the provider might ask for an explanation: "Why is it important to rinse frequently?" After showing a patient how to clean around a fixed retainer, a provider might ask for a demonstration: "Please show me how you will clean your teeth with the retainer in place."

Activity 5-2

To better appreciate how patients with limited dental health literacy experience verbal communication, read and decipher the following:

After a thorough noitanimaxe, your tsitned has determined you have a ralom that has deyaced and is in danger of noitcefni. It is dednemmocer you undergo citnododne ypareht, or what is commonly called a toor lanac. In this erudecorp, a tsitned or tsitnododne will drill a hole in the htoot and remove the htoot plup, the decayed evren eussit, and any remaining airetcab. The htoot will then be delaes. Any questions?

Verbal Communication Strategies

As we noted in the preface to this book, scripted communication does not facilitate productive patient-provider relationships. If we could generate a list of phrases for providers to match to a given circumstance, that list would be far too long to memorize. Even if providers could memorize it, relying on someone else's prepackaged words turns the providers into performers and undermines patient trust. Instead, we offer guidelines—verbal strategies that can help providers develop their own messages tailored to the patients they treat. With increased research attention focusing on health literacy, lists of recommendations are proliferating.

In the previous section, we mentioned Healthy People 2020's health literacy objectives: provide easy-to-understand instructions, ask patients to describe how they will follow instructions, and offer to help with forms.[51] These national objectives can also serve as personal objectives for health care providers in their patient interactions. Similarly, the ADA's Health Literacy in Dentistry Action Plan 2010–2015 includes the six best practices listed in Box 5-1.[80]

Box 5-1	Best practices from the ADA's Health Literacy in Dentistry Action Plan*

1. Create a respectful and "shame-free" environment and use a universal standards approach, where all patients are offered assistance to better understand and use printed and written communications.
2. Periodically assess the office/clinic for ways to improve communication.
3. Use clear and plain language in talking and writing.
4. Encourage question-asking and dialogue.
5. Use the "teach-back" or "teach-to-goal" method to check on successful communication by asking patients to repeat their interpretation of instructions and other information that has been provided.
6. Offer take-home tools designed for easy use with clear directions.

*Reprinted from the American Dental Association Council on Access, Prevention and Interprofessional Relations[80] with permission.

The National Action Plan to Improve Health Literacy proposes three criteria for all health information, noting that information should always be accurate, accessible, and actionable.[81] Those "three A's" can also serve as verbal communication guidelines.

We offer our own six strategies for crafting verbal messages, which fit into the mnemonic **SPEAKS**:

- **S**implify language.
- **P**aint an accurate picture.
- **E**xpress concerns.
- **A**llow time.
- **K**eep calm.
- **S**elf-disclose.

These strategies are particularly relevant to spoken interactions with a patient but also apply to written communication. If the provider implements these strategies after first assessing a given patient's level of oral health literacy, they should help appointments run smoothly while simultaneously facilitating patient understanding and satisfaction.

Simplify language

After assessing a patient's knowledge of oral health concepts, the provider should use language comprehensible at that level. A provider who has spent many years pursuing education and who interacts regularly with well-educated and articulate people may overestimate the reading level of the general public and of patients. The average American reads three to five grade levels below his or her last year of education.[82] Therefore, the average reading level is eighth grade, which is the level at which *USA Today* is written.[83] Experts in health literacy recommend using language below that level—at a sixth-grade reading level—and including pictures and illustrations.[84]

Table 5-2 lists some common dental terms and simpler terms that could be substituted when a provider is talking to a patient. However, the provider should occasionally introduce proper dental terms and explain what they mean to elevate the patient's oral health literacy.

Table 5-2 Dental terms versus simple terms

Dental term	Simple term
Permanent tooth	Adult tooth
Periodontitis or gingivitis	Gum disease
Amalgam restoration	Silver filling
Canine or cuspid	Eye tooth
Gingivae	Gums
Deciduous or primary tooth	Baby tooth
Restoration	Filling
Malocclusion	Uneven bite
Crown	Cap
Molars and premolars	Back teeth
Calculus	Tartar
Complete or partial denture (removable)	Plate
Incisors and canines	Front teeth
Nitrous oxide	Laughing gas

In addition to simplifying vocabulary, the provider should simplify the way he or she speaks to patients. Individuals with limited literacy skills are more likely to understand information that has short words and short sentences and that contains only essential information. The active voice ("Clean the dentures.") is more understandable than passive constructions ("Dentures need cleaning."), particularly when instructions are provided. Also, actionable instructions tend to be more specific. "Floss a couple of times a day" is not as actionable as "Floss twice a day, once when you get up and again before you go to bed." Finally, patients will vary dramatically in their oral health literacy and, if the provider is doing his or her job well, the oral health literacy levels of those patients will improve over time. The provider should not use the simplest terms uniformly with all patients, as more advanced patients may feel patronized. Assessing patient literacy levels and targeting communication to those levels is essential.

Paint an accurate picture

Accuracy is paramount in the information provided by the dental professional. The provider should resist the urge to exaggerate or selectively cite statistics, even when doing so might motivate a patient to adopt a healthy behavior. Telling a smoker that he or she faces a 90% chance of contracting lung cancer may prompt the patient to quit smoking, but it does have negative consequences for the patient-provider relationship. Patients now have access to an enormous amount of literature on oral health. If the provider disseminates incorrect information, these mistakes will be caught and could undermine the provider's credibility and the trust bestowed by patients.

The word *paint* was chosen advisedly for this strategy because it evokes visual imagery that can effectively supplement verbal messages. Whenever appropriate, the provider should rely on simile and metaphor, using everyday objects and events to translate unfamiliar dental concepts.

For instance, when telling patients what plaque is and why it must be removed regularly, we tell them it has the consistency of peanut butter. It sticks to teeth, and brushing alone will not remove all of it. If patients do not remove plaque a couple of times each day by flossing, then the plaque will remain there, just as peanut butter would. Using this simile (ie, plaque is like peanut butter), we not only teach patients a little bit about plaque but also emphasize that flossing is a fundamental component of daily oral health care.

Activity 5-3

We described our use of peanut butter to paint an accurate picture of what plaque is. Generate some of your own metaphors and similes you can use when trying to explain dental concepts to children or adults. Consider how you might explain calculus, a root canal procedure, a crown, or the damage caused by sugary drinks.

Express concerns

Patient-centered care depends on open dialogue. Research on patient preferences finds that explanation of oral health conditions is the dentist behavior most preferred by patients.[85] Such explanations are incomplete if they do not include provider concerns. All patients who are competent to grant consent for dental procedures should be privy to the dental professional's concerns regarding their oral health. Patients are not paying for the provider's silence.

Concerns should be expressed verbally and in a respectful manner. Pursed lips, "tsk tsk," rolled eyes, wagging fingers, and other nonverbal expressions of disapproval are likely ineffective in motivating a patient to accept a recommended restorative or preventive treatment. They are definitely unsupportive of the patient-provider relationship. The provider should instead explain with simple words and illustrations the problems that have been observed and the problems that are anticipated, given the practitioner's observations and knowledge of the patient's oral health behaviors.

If a patient is not in a position to consent (eg, the patient is very young or has cognitive limitations requiring a custodial caregiver), the provider should express concerns only to the extent the information will not alarm or disturb the patient. When this is not possible, concerns instead should be expressed to the caregiver in private.

Allow time

Greater amounts of time spent in patient education and information exchange are associated with better patient outcomes.[86] Building relationships with patients through effective communication requires more time than simply running from operatory to operatory performing examinations and procedures. Among health care providers, however, dental professionals hold an advantage in having long periods of time during most appointments in which they can speak uninterrupted. Although this time is not well suited to questioning and interaction, if this time is managed well, much oral health information can be imparted. In this way, the time after clinical work can be used for exploring the information provided through patient interaction and questioning. An approach in which procedures are narrated and explained has the additional advantage of providing something other than anxiety for the patient to focus on.

Although time management can streamline appointments, providers should allow adequate time to describe their observations and concerns, to question patients regarding their oral health practices, and to elicit patients' questions and concerns. Providers should bear in mind that the oral health information and terminology may be unfamiliar to patients, who may struggle to formulate articulate comments and questions. Pressuring patients to speak quickly might only make them silent or more inarticulate.

The provider should aim to allow at least 30 seconds for the patient to respond, as he or she may require time and silence to formulate replies or questions. The provider also should resist the urge to anticipate or finish a patient's thought or sentence.

Keep calm

Many patients have dental anxiety, so the provider should avoid verbal alarms. The provider can sabotage years of effort to minimize a patient's anxiety by speaking alarmingly. The anxious patient may mistake a provider's schedule-related stress for alarm over the state of the patient's oral health. For instance, a provider who cries, "Oh no!" because he or she forgot to defrost something for dinner may startle a patient into thinking the clinician has found a serious problem during the oral examination. Subsequent explanations to the contrary likely will not reverse the adrenaline unleashed by the comment. Even when the patient realizes that a provider's frenzy is unrelated to oral health, having a stressed-out medical provider hovering nearby does not inspire confidence in the patient.

In addition to avoiding verbal alarms, the provider should avoid dental terminology that can trigger panic. Patients, particularly children, often respond negatively to words such as *probe*, *drill*, *shot*, *needle*, *pain*, *tumor*, *pick*, and *hatchet*. While the provider should have a commitment to accuracy, he or she should use such trigger words only when less alarming alternatives cannot be found.

Finally, calming vocabulary can be enhanced when the provider uses two nonverbal strategies: speaking slowly and modulating the speaking tone. In a busy dental office dealing with ringing telephones and unexpected events, keeping calm can be a challenge for even the most professional oral health provider. However, patients associate a medium rate of speech with professional competence.[87] The provider can breathe deeply before speaking to patients to slow the rate of speech and modulate the tone.

Self-disclose

A final verbal strategy the provider should integrate into the patient communication repertoire is self-disclosure. Although the patient technically holds power because he or she is paying for a service, in reality the dental professional wields far more power during the time the patient is in the chair. That power relates to the provider's greater oral health knowledge, the provider's ability to inflict pain, and the provider's access to the patient's personal health information. Regarding personal health information, the provider not only has access to the patient's health records but also asks intrusive questions regarding personal habits. Moreover, during the course of an examination, the provider may discover information the patient does not yet know or understand. The unequal power in this relationship can leave the patient feeling vulnerable and exposed.

Self-disclosure by the provider can represent a small step toward equalizing the perceived power differential in the patient-provider relationship. Methods and topics for self-disclosure are addressed in more detail in chapter 7. At this point, we can simply recommend that the provider reveal a bit of personal information; this will humanize the provider in the patient's perception. Providers should carefully consider the potential impact of clinical disclosures. Providers can correct patient misperceptions about mercury poisoning from amalgam fillings or about the horrors of root canal by revealing their own or other (anonymous) patient experiences. Personal disclosures about one's own dental work, however, can be misinterpreted as a recommendation or warning, even if they are not meant as such. Providers who are unsure how a patient will interpret a disclosure should self-disclose on neutral topics: food, pets, hometowns, sports teams, traffic, etc.

There are disadvantages to self-disclosure: It may require extra time, it does not provide therapeutic value, and it risks inviting too much patient intimacy. Yet we believe these negatives are outweighed by the positives: It enhances the patient's trust and loyalty and likely enhances the provider's experiences by allowing the provider to develop a degree of mutuality in his or her patient relationships.

Chapter Checklist ✓

Verbal communication goals
- ❑ Take an educational approach to patient communication to develop an effective long-term relationship.
- ❑ Task-focused communication: Educate the patient by providing accurate information regarding oral health care.
- ❑ Task-focused communication: Praise a patient who researches oral health issues, but tactfully correct misinformation acquired from other individuals or media sources.
- ❑ Task-focused communication: Promote oral health by providing accurate information.
- ❑ Task-focused communication: Present scientific findings but also suggest experience-based and common-sense ways of integrating healthy dental behaviors into everyday life.
- ❑ Task-focused communication: Explain procedures at least three times—during treatment planning, before the treatment begins, and as the treatment is underway.
- ❑ Emotion-focused communication: Express empathy by identifying the patient's emotions and responding appropriately.
- ❑ Emotion-focused communication: Empathize to a degree that allows for identification with patient feelings but that avoids emotional involvement.
- ❑ Emotion-focused communication: Self-monitor empathy levels daily.
- ❑ Emotion-focused communication: Express empathy both verbally and nonverbally.
- ❑ Emotion-focused communication: Discuss risks of procedures as a way to minimize anxiety.
- ❑ Emotion-focused communication: Avoid promises to eliminate pain.
- ❑ Emotion-focused communication: Avoid fear appeals, relying instead on positive reinforcement.
- ❑ Emotion-focused communication: Encourage the patient through praise in his or her efforts to change poor oral health behaviors.
- ❑ Emotion-focused communication: Facilitate trust by eliciting and validating the patient's concerns.
- ❑ Emotion-focused communication: Facilitate trust by expressing a willingness to abide by a patient's decisions.

Oral health literacy
- ❑ Perceive patient interactions as opportunities for small-scale interventions to increase oral health literacy.
- ❑ Remain aware of formal measures of oral health literacy and use them when indicated: REALD, REALM-D, TOFHLiD, OHLI, and CMOHK.

- ❏ Rely on the Chew question: "How confident are you filling out forms by your-self?"
- ❏ Never directly challenge a patient's literacy.
- ❏ Informal evaluations: Remain aware of characteristics associated with lower oral health literacy, including age, sex, and race.
- ❏ Informal evaluations: Avoid adopting verbal behaviors that reduce empathic responses to the patient with limited literacy skills.
- ❏ Informal evaluations: Look for signs of confusion, particularly around the eyes and mouth.
- ❏ Informal evaluations: Look for common behaviors such as omitting answers on forms and an inability to name medications.
- ❏ Informal evaluations: Look for common excuses for not completing forms, such as a patient's claiming to have forgotten his or her eyeglasses or not to have time to fill out forms.
- ❏ Informal evaluations: Ask the patient if he or she understands information presented.
- ❏ Informal evaluations: Ask the patient to repeat, explain, or demonstrate what was heard or read.

Communication strategies promoted by organizations
- ❏ Healthy People 2020: Always give easy-to-understand instructions.
- ❏ Healthy People 2020: Always ask the patient to describe how he or she will follow instructions.
- ❏ Healthy People 2020: Always offer help in filling out forms.
- ❏ ADA Health Literacy Action Plan: Create a respectful and shame-free environment.
- ❏ ADA Health Literacy Action Plan: Periodically assess the practice for ways to improve communication.
- ❏ ADA Health Literacy Action Plan: Use clear and plain language.
- ❏ ADA Health Literacy Action Plan: Encourage questions and discussion.
- ❏ ADA Health Literacy Action Plan: Use the teach-back or teach-to-goal method.
- ❏ ADA Health Literacy Action Plan: Offer take-home tools and brochures.
- ❏ National Action Plan to Improve Health Literacy: Provide information that is accurate.
- ❏ National Action Plan to Improve Health Literacy: Provide information that is accessible.
- ❏ National Action Plan to Improve Health Literacy: Provide information that is actionable.

SPEAKS strategies
- ❏ Simplify language: Use language comprehensible at the patient's level of under-standing.
- ❏ Simplify language: Include pictures and illustrations.
- ❏ Simplify language: Occasionally use proper dental terms and explain what they mean.
- ❏ Simplify language: Use short words and sentences, active voice, and specific phrasing.
- ❏ Paint an accurate picture: Avoid the temptation to exaggerate consequences.

- ❑ Paint an accurate picture: Rely on simile and metaphor to relate dental concepts to everyday objects and events.
- ❑ Express concerns: Explain in simple words and illustrations which problems are observed and/or anticipated.
- ❑ Express concerns: If the patient is unable to give consent, do not frighten the patient but instead express concerns privately to the caregiver.
- ❑ Allow time: Permit adequate appointment time to describe observations and concerns, question the patient, and elicit questions and concerns from the patient.
- ❑ Keep calm: Avoid verbal alarms that can increase patient anxiety.
- ❑ Keep calm: Avoid dental terminology that can trigger panic.
- ❑ Keep calm: Speak slowly and modulate the speaking tone by breathing deeply before speaking.
- ❑ Self-disclose: Reveal a bit of personal information on neutral topics to lend some humanity to the patient's perception of you.

For More Information

Talking to patients
- http://www.rdhmag.com/articles/print/volume-33/issue-11/features/the-fine-art-of-patient-engagement.html
- http://www.chickmoorman.com/dentalTalk/worstThingsToSay.pdf

Oral health websites for consumers
- http://www.ada.org/en/publications/jada/jada-for-the-dental-patient
- http://www.mouthhealthy.org
- http://www.adha.org/resources
- http://www.yourdentistryguide.com
- http://www.knowyourteeth.com
- http://www.cdc.gov/OralHealth
- http://healthfinder.gov/scripts/SearchContext.asp?topic=603
- http://www.nlm.nih.gov/medlineplus/mouthandteeth.html
- http://www.cancer.gov/cancertopics/types/head-and-neck
- http://www.nidcr.nih.gov/oralhealth
- http://www.mychildrensteeth.org
- http://www.perio.org/consumer
- http://www.healthyteeth.org
- http://www.cda.org/public-resources/patient-fact-sheets
- http://oralhealthamerica.org
- http://www.simplestepsdental.com

Oral health literacy
- http://www.ahrq.gov/research/findings/final-reports/oral-health/index.html
- http://www.mchoralhealth.org/highlights/literacy.html
- http://apha.confex.com/apha/135am/webprogram/Session21729.html
- http://www.health.gov/communication/HLActionPlan/pdf/Health_Literacy_Action_Plan.pdf

References

1. Buck R, VanLear CA. Verbal and nonverbal communication: Distinguishing symbolic, spontaneous, and pseudo-spontaneous nonverbal behavior. J Commun 2002;52:522–541.
2. Earl H. Mechanics of verbal ability. Psychol Rev 1978;85:109–130.
3. Alwin DF. Family of origin and cohort differences in verbal ability. Am Sociol Rev 1991;56:625–638.
4. Sabbah W, Tsakos G, Sheiham A, Watt RG. The effects of income and education on ethnic differences in oral health: A study in US adults. J Epidemiol Community Health 2009;63:516–520.
5. Atchison KA, Gironda MW, Messadi D, Der-Martirosian C. Screening for oral health literacy in an urban dental clinic. J Public Health Dent 2010;70:269–275.
6. Centers for Disease Control and Prevention. Disparities in Oral Health. Atlanta: Centers for Disease Control and Prevention, 2009.
7. Cooper LA, Powe NR. Disparities in Patient Experiences, Health Care Processes, and Outcomes: The Role of Patient-Provider Racial, Ethnic, and Language Concordance. New York: The Commonwealth Fund, 2004.
8. Jameson C. Great Communication Equals Great Production, ed 2. Tulsa, OK: PennWell, 2002.
9. Weinstein P, Harrison R, Benton T. Motivating parents to prevent caries in their young children: One-year findings. J Am Dent Assoc 2004;135:731–738.
10. Wintersteen L. Marketing with a patient focus. J Am Dent Assoc 1997;128:1657–1659.
11. Odom JG, Odom SS, Jolly DE. Informed consent and the geriatric dental patient. Spec Care Dentist 1992;12:202–206.
12. Christensen GJ. Developing your staff into a patient education team. J Am Dent Assoc 2009;140:1536–1539.
13. Clow KE, Stevens RE, McConkey C, Loudon DL. Attitudes of dentists and dental patients toward advertising. Health Mark Q 2007;24(1–2):23–34.
14. Clow KE, Fischer AK, O'Bryan D. Patient expectations of dental services. Image affects expectations, and expectations affect perceived service quality. J Health Care Mark 1995;15(3):23–31.
15. Quill TE, Brody H. Physician recommendations and patient autonomy: Finding a balance between physician power and patient choice. Ann Intern Med 1996;125:763–769.
16. Sondell K, Soderfeldt B, Palmqvist S. Underlying dimensions of verbal communication between dentists and patients in prosthetic dentistry. Patient Educ Couns 2003;50:157–165.
17. Panagopoulou E, Montgomery A, Benos A. Health promotion as a behavioural challenge: Are we missing attitudes? Glob Health Promot 2011;18(2):54–57.
18. Roter DL, Hall JA, Merisca R, Nordstrom B, Cretin D, Svarstad B. Effectiveness of interventions to improve patient compliance: A meta-analysis. Med Care 1998;36:1138–1161.
19. Satur JG, Gussy MG, Morgan MV, Calache H, Wright C. Review of the evidence for oral health promotion effectiveness. Health Educ J 2010;69:257–266.
20. Cox JE. Oral health information on the Internet. J Consum Health Internet 2008;12:131–142.
21. Ahluwalia S, Murray E, Stevenson F, Kerr C, Burns J. 'A heartbeat moment': Qualitative study of GP views of patients bringing health information from the internet to a consultation. Br J Gen Pract 2010;60(571):88–94.
22. Harris CE, Chestnutt IG. The use of the Internet to access oral health-related information by patients attending dental hygiene clinics. Int J Dent Hyg 2005;3:70–73.
23. Watt RG, Marinho VC. Does oral health promotion improve oral hygiene and gingival health? Periodontol 2000 2005;37:35–47.

24. Weinstein P, Milgrom P, Melnick S, Beach B, Spadafora A. How effective is oral hygiene instruction? Results after 6 and 24 weeks. J Public Health Dent 1989;49:32–38.
25. Goldberg KL. The role of the dental team in implementing EBD and communicating the evidence with your patients. J Evid Based Dent Pract 2008;8:159–161.
26. Smedley BD, Syme L. Promoting Health: Intervention Strategies from Social and Behavioral Research. Washington, DC: Institute of Medicine, 2000.
27. Hamilton MA, Rouse RA, Rouse J. Dentist communication and patient utilization of dental services: Anxiety inhibition and competence enhancement effects. Health Commun 1994;6:137–158.
28. Dobie S. Viewpoint: Reflections on a well-traveled path: Self-awareness, mindful practice, and relationship-centered care as foundations for medical education. Acad Med 2007;82:422–427.
29. Sherman JJ, Cramer A. Measurement of changes in empathy during dental school. J Dent Educ 2005;69:338–345.
30. Yarascavitch C, Regehr G, Hodges B, Haas DA. Changes in dental student empathy during training. J Dent Educ 2009;73:509–517.
31. Rouse RA. A paradigm of intervention: Emotional communication in dentistry. Health Commun 1989;1:239–252.
32. Coulehan JL, Platt FW, Egener B, et al. "Let me see if I have this right...": Words that help build empathy. Ann Intern Med 2001;135:221–227.
33. Loignon C, Allison P, Landry A, Richard L, Brodeur JM, Bedos C. Providing humanistic care. J Dent Res 2010;89:991–995.
34. Stenman J, Wennström JL, Abrahamsson KH. Dental hygienists' views on communicative factors and interpersonal processes in prevention and treatment of periodontal disease. Int J Dent Hyg 2010;8:213–218.
35. Harp H, Hook E, Solberg E, Anderson D. A patient's perspective on how hygienists can decrease patient anxiety. J Dent Hyg 2000;74:322.
36. Gerbert B, Bleecker T, Saub E. Risk perception and risk communication: Benefits of dentist-patient discussions. J Am Dent Assoc 1995;126:333–339.
37. Corah NL. Dental anxiety. Assessment, reduction and increasing patient satisfaction. Dent Clin North Am 1988;32:779–790.
38. Soames Job RF. Effective and ineffective use of fear in health promotion campaigns. Am J Public Health 1988;78:163–167.
39. Janis IL, Feshbach S. Effects of fear-arousing communications. J Abnorm Soc Psychol 1953;48:78–92.
40. Marshall J, Sheller B, Mancl L, Williams BJ. Parental attitudes regarding behavior guidance of dental patients with autism. Pediatr Dent 2008;30:400–407.
41. Roberts JF, Curzon ME, Koch G, Martens LC. Review: Behaviour management techniques in paediatric dentistry. Eur Arch Paediatr Dent 2010;11:166–174.
42. Zhou Y, Cameron E, Forbes G, Humphris G. Systematic review of the effect of dental staff behaviour on child dental patient anxiety and behaviour. Patient Educ Couns 2011;85:4–13.
43. Weiner AA (ed). The Fearful Dental Patient: A Guide to Understanding and Managing. Ames, IA: Wiley-Blackwell, 2011.
44. Nash DA. Engaging children's cooperation in the dental environment through effective communication. Pediatr Dent 2006;28:455–459.
45. Kvale G, Milgrom P, Getz T, Weinstein P, Johnsen TB. Beliefs about professional ethics, dentist-patient communication, control and trust among fearful dental patients: The factor structure of the revised Dental Beliefs Survey. Acta Odontol Scand 2004;62:21–29.
46. Nash DA. Ethics, empathy, and the education of dentists. J Dent Educ 2010;74:567–578.
47. Fiscella K, Meldrum S, Franks P, et al. Patient trust: Is it related to patient-centered behavior of primary care physicians? Med Care 2004;42:1049–1055.
48. Kutner M, Greenberg E, Jin Y, Paulsen C. The health literacy of America's adults: Results from the 2003 National Assessment of Adult Literacy (NCES 2006-483). Washington, DC: US Department of Education, National Center for Education Statistics, 2006.
49. US Department of Health and Human Services. Healthy People 2010, vol 1, ed 2. Washington, DC: Government Printing Office, 2000.

50. Agency for Healthcare Research and Quality. Health Literacy Interventions and Outcomes: An Updated Systematic Review. Rockville, MD: US Department of Health and Human Services, 2011.

51. Objectives. Health Communication and Health Information Technology. US Department of Health and Human Services. Office of Disease Prevention and Health Promotion. Healthy People 2020. http://www.healthypeople.gov/2020/topics-objectives/topic/health-communication-and-health-information-technology/objectives. Accessed 6 January 2015.

52. American Medical Association Committee on Health Literacy for the Council on Scientific Affairs. Health literacy: Report of the Council on Scientific Affairs. JAMA 1999;281:552–557.

53. Schiavo JH. Oral health literacy in the dental office: The unrecognized patient risk factor. J Dent Hyg 2011;85:248–255.

54. Jones M, Lee JY, Rozier RG. Oral health literacy among adult patients seeking dental care. J Am Dent Assoc 2007;138:1199–1208.

55. Sabbahi DA, Lawrence HP, Limeback H, Rootman I. Development and evaluation of an oral health literacy instrument for adults. Community Dent Oral Epidemiol 2009;37:451–462.

56. Lee JY, Divaris K, Baker AD, Rozier RG, Vann WF Jr. The relationship of oral health literacy and self-efficacy with oral health status and dental neglect. Am J Public Health 2012;102:923–929.

57. Vargas CM, Arevalo O. How dental care can preserve and improve oral health. Dent Clin N Am 2009;53:399–420.

58. Behrens D, Lear JG. Strengthening children's oral health: Views from the field. Health Aff 2011;30:2208–2213.

59. Vann WF, Lee JY, Baker D, Divaris K. Oral health literacy among female caregivers. J Dent Res 2010;89:1395–1400.

60. Miller E, Lee JY, DeWalt DA, Vann WF Jr. Impact of caregiver literacy on children's oral health outcomes. Pediatrics 2010;126:107–114.

61. Horowitz AM, Kleinman DV. Oral health literacy: The new imperative to better oral health. Dent Clin North Am 2008;52:333–344.

62. Barron LM. Oral Health Literacy Educational Experiences of North Carolina Dental Hygiene Students: Implications for Dental Hygiene Research [thesis]. Chapel Hill, NC: University of North Carolina at Chapel Hill, 2011.

63. Sanzone L, Lee JY, Prada E, Rozier G, Zeldin L. Dentists' awareness of oral health literacy and confidence in communication. Presented at the IADR/AADR/CADR 87th General Session and Exhibition, Miami, April 2, 2009.

64. Lee JY, Rozier RG, Lee SYD, Bender D, Ruiz RE. Development of a word recognition instrument to test health literacy in dentistry: The REALD-30—A brief communication. J Public Health Dent 2007;67:94–98.

65. American Dental Association. Glossary of Common Dental Terminology. Chicago: American Dental Association, 1999.

66. Richman JA, Lee JY, Rozier RG, Gong DA, Pahel BT, Vann WF Jr. Evaluation of a word recognition instrument to test health literacy in dentistry: The REALD-99. J Public Health Dent 2007;67:99–104.

67. Stucky BD, Lee JY, Lee SYD, Rozier RG. Development of the two-stage Rapid Estimate of Adult Literacy in Dentistry. Community Dent Oral Epidemiol 2011;39:474–480.

68. Richman JA, Huebner CE, Leggott PJ, Mouradian WE, Mancl LA. Beyond word recognition: Understanding pediatric oral health literacy. Pediatr Dent 2011;33:420–425.

69. Gong DA, Lee JY, Rozier RG, Pahel BT, Richman JA, Vann WF. Development and testing of the Test of Functional Health Literacy in Dentistry (TOFHLiD). J Public Health Dent 2007;67:105–112.

70. Macek MD, Haynes D, Wells W, Bauer-Leffler S, Cotten PA, Parker RM. Measuring conceptual health knowledge in the context of oral health literacy: Preliminary results. J Public Health Dent 2010;70:197–204.

71. Chew LD, Griffin JM, Partin MR, et al. Validation of screening questions for limited health literacy in a large VA outpatient population. J Gen Intern Med 2008;23:561–566.

72. Jackson RD, Eckert GJ. Health literacy in an adult dental research population: A pilot study. J Public Health Dent 2008;68:196–200.

73. Cohen LA, Bonito AJ, Eicheldinger C, Manski RJ, Edwards RR, Khanna N. Health literacy impact on patient-provider interactions involving the treatment of dental problems. J Dent Educ 2011;75:1218–1224.

74. DeVoe JE, Wallace LS, Fryer Jr GE. Measuring patients' perceptions of communication with healthcare providers: Do differences in demographic and socioeconomic characteristics matter? Health Expect 2009;12:70–80.

75. Ferguson WJ, Candib LM. Culture, language, and the doctor-patient relationship. Fam Med 2002;34:353–361.

76. Rozin P, Cohen AB. High frequency of facial expressions corresponding to confusion, concentration, and worry in an analysis of naturally occurring facial expressions of Americans. Emotion 2003;3:68–75.

77. Weiss BD. Health Literacy and Patient Safety: Help Patients Understand: A Manual for Clinicians, ed 2. Chicago: American Medical Association Foundation, 2007.

78. Katz MG, Jacobson TA, Veledar E, Kripalani S. Patient literacy and question-asking behavior during the medical encounter: A mixed-methods analysis. J Gen Intern Med 2007;22:782–786.

79. Amini H, Casamassimo PS, Lin HL, Hayes JR. Readability of the American Academy of Pediatric Dentistry patient education materials. Pediatr Dent 2007;29:431–435.

80. American Dental Association Council on Access, Prevention and Interprofessional Relations. Health Literacy in Dentistry Action Plan 2010–2015. Chicago: American Dental Association, 2009.

81. US Department of Health and Human Services. National Action Plan to Improve Health Literacy. Rockville, MD: Office of Disease Prevention and Health Promotion, 2010.

82. Glassman P. Health Literacy. Rockville, MD: National Network of Libraries of Medicine, 2011.

83. Center for Health Care Strategies. Fact Sheet: What is Health Literacy? Lawrenceville, NJ: Center for Health Care Strategies, 2002.

84. Safeer RS, Keenan J. Health literacy: The gap between physicians and patients. Am Fam Physician 2005;72:463–468.

85. Zimmerman RS. The dental appointment and patient behavior: Differences in patient and practitioner preferences, patient satisfaction, and adherence. Med Care 1988;26:403–414.

86. Beck RS, Daughtridge R, Sloane PD. Physician-patient communication in the primary care office: A systematic review. J Am Board Fam Pract 2002;15:25–38.

87. Ray GB, Ray EB, Zahn CJ. Speech behavior and social evaluation: An examination of medical messages. Commun Q 1991;39:119–129.

6

Refining Nonverbal Communication Skills

Why Nonverbal Skills Matter

Chapter 5 mentioned two sets of communication goals. Task-focused goals include educating, promoting, and explaining. Emotion-focused goals include empathizing, reducing anxiety, encouraging, and enhancing trust. Verbal communication can accomplish both types of goals entirely without nonverbal communication. Providers can educate patients, promote oral health, and explain procedures without such nonverbal enhancements as facial expression, gestures, or interpretive dance, but they must use spoken or written language. Language is also rich in expressing messages that accomplish emotion-focused goals.

Why, then, does nonverbal communication deserve any attention? We offer two primary reasons. First, by reinforcing what is said through a different communication channel, nonverbal messages complement task-focused verbal messages. As a result, such messages are both easier to understand and easier to remember. Consider classroom experiences. Instructors who integrate images and objects into presentation of material are providing little information not already included in their lectures, but such lectures are more comprehensible than an hour of uninterrupted talking or a recorded lecture. For those with limitations in hearing, English language skills, literacy, or cognition, nonverbal communication becomes particularly important in facilitating comprehension of task-focused verbal messages.

Activity 6-1

How do you fry an egg? Instruct a colleague how to fry an egg, from cracking the shell to placing the egg on a plate. Did you notice yourself using nonverbal behaviors in addition to verbal behaviors? Do you think the nonverbal behaviors helped—or would have helped—your colleague understand? Did they help you express yourself? Would it be possible to deliver instructions without verbal messages? Try to do so by instructing a colleague on how to change a flat tire without using words.

Second, nonverbal messages are more common and persuasive than verbal messages in accomplishing emotion-focused goals.[1] Although people can articulate their emotional state (eg, "I'm happy!"), they far more often express emotions nonverbally (eg, through smiling). In many contexts, nonverbal communication delivers more information than verbal communication.[2-4]

Furthermore, nonverbal messages tend to be more reliable than verbal messages.[5,6] Consider the patient who says "I'm fine" with a flat vocal tone and a hand on her cheek. The provider would more likely believe the patient's nonverbal messages, which imply "I'm not fine." In situations similar to this example, the emotion-focused message could determine clinical outcomes. Table 6-1 reviews the different functions of verbal and nonverbal communication, providing examples of task- and emotion-focused messages.

Table 6-1 Examples of task- and emotion-focused verbal and nonverbal communication

Function	Verbal examples	Nonverbal examples
Task-focused communication		
Education	"Your tooth enamel is the hardest substance in your body."	Tap the enamel on the model teeth.
Promotion	"Try drinking your soft drinks through a straw to reduce erosion of enamel."	Make eye contact and use an authoritative tone to convey the seriousness of the suggestion.
Explanation	"A straw keeps some of the citric acid from sitting on your teeth, where it erodes the enamel."	Point through the model teeth to show how soft drinks would bypass teeth when a straw is used.
Emotion-focused communication		
Empathy	"I know how hard it is to stop drinking soft drinks."	Place your open hand on your chest to indicate personal experience.
Anxiety reduction	"This injection may pinch for just a second, but when we are finished, your tooth shouldn't bother you any more."	Hold your thumb and forefinger together when saying "just a second" to illustrate how brief the discomfort will be.
Encouragement	"Smokers often fail on the first few quitting attempts, so don't grow discouraged about your slip."	Smile to indicate that you remain positive about the long-term prospects your patient will quit smoking.
Trust enhancement	"When you ask me to stop, I'll stop, and we can take a break."	Slow your rate of speech to indicate that you take the patient's wishes seriously.

A growing body of research reveals the linkages between providers' nonverbal communication skills and patient satisfaction. Patient satisfaction and treatment adherence are more closely tied to providers' interpersonal skills than to the quantity of instruction providers supply.[7] The nonverbal behavior component of interpersonal skills is significantly associated with patient satisfaction across a variety of clinical encounters.[8–10] Researching verbal and nonverbal behaviors, Corah[11] found that the dentist behaviors most closely associated with satisfaction "were those portraying empathy, friendliness, and a calm, competent image to the patient." Such behaviors are largely nonverbal. In a 2002 study, Aruguete and Roberts[12] found that the nonverbal communication style of physicians was associated with patient preferences. Specifically, "Nonverbal concern was associated with highest satisfaction, trust, self-disclosure, recall of information, likelihood of recommending the physician, and intent to comply with the physician's recommendations." Providers who demonstrate more sensitive nonverbal communication are liked more by patients, and those patients are more engaged and less distressed.[13]

Nonverbal Communication and Fear

Previous chapters discussed the prevalence of dental fear and anxiety, ways to identify anxious patients, and verbal communication strategies to minimize dental anxiety. This chapter returns to the topic of dental anxiety for two reasons. First, a substantial proportion of the population is apprehensive of dental treatment, and the more anxious or fearful often avoid treatment entirely.[24–27] For such patients, dental anxiety can influence aspects of daily life beyond oral health care.[28] Further, the patient-provider relationship may be more salient for anxious patients than for those without anxiety.[29] Therefore, the phenomenon of dental anxiety warrants examination from multiple perspectives.

Second, apprehension, anxiety, and fear are emotions and therefore are more responsive to emotion-focused communication, which is the primary domain of nonverbal communication. Dental anxiety can be rational: Accidents happen. Yet verbal persuasion often fails to alter negative emotions such as fear. Careful use of vocabulary and language can help providers to avoid triggering or aggravating fearful responses in anxious patients, but attention to nonverbal cues may be more effective in making dental encounters a positive experience.

Research indicates that the attitude of providers partly determines the anxiety experienced by patients.[30] Corah[11] concluded that anxious patients are most satisfied when dentists portray empathy, friendliness, and competence. These behaviors are no different than those used with nonanxious patients and are addressed later in the chapter. However, in addition to these behavioral goals, providers should consider sensory stimuli that may aggravate or mitigate dental fear (Table 6-2).

In addition to the five senses, some patients identify **fear of fear** as a problem. In other words, patients are fearful that they will express fear and therefore embarrass themselves. One study found that 66% of such patients were embarrassed by their fear and their inability to control it.[31] Fear of a panic attack or of shaking or crying may make those outcomes more likely. Similarly, some patients fear that the anesthesia will not work, they fear radiographs, or they fear infection. Although patients must overcome such fears to arrive in the dental chair, they may yet fear that they will be unable to suppress these fears for the duration of the appointment.

Table 6-2 Nonverbal stimuli associated with dental fear

Stimulus	Remedies
Sounds	
Dental handpiece and instruments	Play background music
Moaning patients	Use white noise machine
Crying children	Allow patient to use MP3 player or earplugs Shut operatory doors
Sights	
Probe, pliers, and syringe	Remove instruments from sight
Bright lights	Adjust light; provide sunglasses
Problem area shown in mirror	Show patient only if he or she requests that you do so
Scrubs	Wear less traditionally medical clothes
Mask	Remove mask frequently
Sensations	
Dental probe, handpiece, and syringe	Narrate procedures
Choking or gag reflex	Explore and manipulate gently
Gritty consistency of toothpaste	Allow frequent rinsing
Blast of air on sensitive teeth	Warn patient; start air outside the mouth
Numbness of anesthesia	Offer alternatives to topical anesthesia
Smells	
Eugenol	Use chemicals with less aroma
Methyl methacrylate	Ventilate and open windows
Tooth preparation smells	Use scented candles or air freshener
Tastes	
Blood	Rinse frequently
Latex or nitrile gloves	Select vinyl and/or gloves with little or no odor
Nitrous oxide	Consider prescription medication for anxiety as an alternative to nitrous oxide

The following sections present published research on diagnosis of dental anxiety and findings on the most common and most forceful nonverbal fear stimuli. Treatment of anxious and fearful dental patients, however, is a subfield of its own, and an exhaustive exploration of the subject is beyond the scope of this book. Others have written books devoted entirely to the subject.[32,33] Further, suggestions here are limited to basic communication strategies for alleviating anxiety. Training in formal treatment modalities that have proven effective in reducing dental anxiety is also beyond the scope of this book. Interested providers should explore the research on behavioral treatments, drug treatments, and treatment by hypnosis.[34–37]

Diagnosis of dental anxiety

Chapter 4 suggested observational ways to identify anxious patients. In addition, survey instruments are available for diagnosing fearful patients in the waiting room or operatory.[38] In the four-item Dental Anxiety Scale, patients identify their level of anxiety at four stages: making the appointment, sitting in the waiting room, waiting for tooth preparation to begin, and waiting for cleaning to begin.[39,40] The 20-item Dental Fear Survey requires patients to indicate the frequency with which they experience 7 fear responses related to dental care and then to indicate the degree to which they experience fear when confronted with 13 stimuli.[26,41] A 2009 Finnish study found that providers rarely use these instruments in practice, so the researchers developed a single question to identify fearful patients: The Short Dental Fear Question[42] (see Table 2-1).

Management of frightening stimuli

Sounds

Research has established that the sounds in a dental office can stimulate a fearful response in patients.[43] The anxiety-triggering sound mentioned repeatedly in the research is that of hand instruments, particularly the handpiece.[25,44,45] One study found that 17.2% of high-fear subjects, compared with only 8.3% of low-fear subjects, reported the sound of the handpiece as aversive.[46] Sounds other than the handpiece are rarely mentioned. However, one study of noise exposure in pediatric dentistry has shown that the sound of crying children is louder than the sound of dental instruments.[47] Crying children are stressful for health care providers, so they likely are stressful for waiting patients as well.[48–51] Likewise, patients who cry out or moan in pain may elevate stress in other patients, particularly the anxious ones.[52,53]

   The provider's communication option while treating a moaning adult or crying child entails asking the patient for notification before he or she vocalizes so that the provider can make adjustments or take a break. The hand-over-mouth technique was once popular for management of the crying child, but it is now not widely recommended.[54,55] The provider may also find that inviting a patient's parent, family member, or caregiver into the operatory may quiet a patient. To mitigate the stress of instrument and handpiece sounds, the provider can play music over office speakers or use white noise machines.[56,57] In a survey, 89% of anxious dental patients indicated that background music helps.[58] The provider can also allow the patient to use an MP3 player (such as an iPod or smartphone) or earplugs as a means of distraction or to cover ambient noise.[59–61] The patient, however, should remain able to hear what the provider says. Finally, unless a dental practice has an open floor plan, operatory doors should be closed or left slightly ajar, as suggested in chapter 2, if the provider wishes to reduce the potential for sexual misperceptions. A closed or partially closed door reduces the amount of stress-inducing noise the patient hears, minimizes distractions, and enhances privacy.

Question of ethics: Some dentists still use the hand-over-mouth technique to work on uncooperative patients who are young or cognitively challenged. How do you feel about using this technique? What are the alternatives? Are there situations in which its use is preferable to no care?

Sights

Like the sound of dental instruments, the sight of dental instruments can evoke fear in anxious patients. Seeing the handpiece can induce anxiety, just as hearing it can.[42] Yet relatively silent instruments such as the dental probe, pliers, and syringe can also induce anxiety when they are seen.[62,63] Krochak and Friedman[64] found that 90% of patients acknowledge at least mild anxiety about receiving injections. In rating fears associated with 12 dental situations, Stouthard and Hoogstraten[65] found that both high- and low-anxiety patients ranked the sight of providers laying out instruments as fourth in terms of anxiety production, behind tooth preparation, being told they had bad teeth, and injections. Other visual stimuli that less consistently may induce anxiety across patients include the light directed into their eyes, the sight of scrubs and masks worn by providers, and the sight of problems such as carious teeth, sometimes glimpsed in the reflection of providers' safety glasses.

The remedies suggested to minimize these stressful stimuli are fairly straightforward but require attention by the dental team. The handpiece may be fairly stationary, but syringes, probes, pliers, and other instruments should be kept out of the patient's line of sight for as long as possible. Syringe preparation should take place where the patient cannot see (eg, behind the chair). The dental provider should always direct the light away from the patient's eyes or provide sunglasses.

Patients vary in their preferences for information on their oral health problems. Oral health problems can appear gruesome to most patients. Problem areas should not be shown to an anxious patient who may be further alarmed by them. A verbal description of the diagnosis will suffice in these cases.

Patients likewise vary in their attitude toward traditional medical attire. The provider should wear clothing that is comfortable and professional but remain aware that traditional scrubs may trigger stress in some patients. The mask may do likewise and is particularly stressful because it obscures the provider's facial expressions. The mask should be pulled down or removed whenever its use is not required.

Sensations

Although anxious patients also report fear of receiving bad news, losing their teeth, embarrassing themselves, or fainting in the chair, the most commonly cited dental fear is fear of pain.[66] Physical pain is necessarily associated with the sense of touch, and just as the sight and sound of dental instruments can evoke anxiety, so too can the sensation of the dental instruments. Particularly in mouths of patients unaccustomed to invasive exploration or with sensitivity related to gingivitis or periodontitis, the slightest touch of the probe, handpiece, or syringe can trigger pain. Even when touch does not cause pain, anticipation of pain can lead to distress.[67,68] Aside from pain, some patients fear that the procedure will cause them to choke or gag.[28,69–71]

In addition, some patients become anxious about injections of local anesthetic. Morse and Chow[72] concluded that "local anesthetic injection is the most anxiety producing aspect of endodontic treatment." Anesthetic anxiety can relate to fear of injections, fear of allergic reaction, fear that the anesthetic will not anesthetize the area, or fear of the ensuing loss of feeling.

The fear of experiencing pain, the fear of choking or gagging, and the fear of anesthesia are rational fears. As a result of the provider's touch, the patient sometimes feels pain, chokes or gags, or experiences negative outcomes from anesthesia. The provider may reduce the patient's anxiety by acknowledging fears and assuring that he or she will perform procedures gently.

The patient's vulnerability and loss of control are central to all these fears, so the provider should enhance the agency of the patient as much as possible. One way to do so is to narrate procedures and notify the patient about what is about to occur. Surprising the patient with a brief but excruciating poke or pull may accomplish the clinical goal, but it completely undermines the trust central to future treatment. Patients tend to respond better to adequate, time-sensitive warnings such as, "You are about to feel a small pinch, but it will last for less than 2 seconds." Agency can also be enhanced by allowing the patient to signal when he or she needs a break.

A final way to help the patient experience more control is to allow the patient to choose from alternatives whenever possible. For minor procedures, the patient may choose to forego local anesthesia; for longer or more complex procedures, the patient may wish to use nitrous oxide, or if appropriate, the practitioner may suggest conscious sedation (eg, for the extraction of impacted wisdom teeth). Even the patient who does opt to receive local anesthesia should feel less vulnerable because he or she made the choice.

Smells

The sense of smell is particularly adept at evoking emotions, both positive and negative. Scents that are otherwise not offensive can become associated through experience with negative emotional states. The smell of antiseptic, for instance, holds negative associations for many hospital patients and visitors. A pair of studies in the 1990s examined smells common to the dental operatory and their association with dental fear. One study found that menthol was rated as pleasant by both fearful and nonfearful patients, whereas methyl methacrylate was rated as unpleasant by both types of patient.[73] Interestingly, the smell of eugenol was rated as unpleasant by fearful patients but pleasant by nonfearful ones.[74]

Other smells that patients sometimes mention as unpleasant or stressful are associated with the preparation of the tooth for a restoration. Caries removal is sometimes associated with an odor that some patients may find objectionable. Even when this is not the case, any trace of what is often described as a "burning smell" emerging from the mouth can be off-putting.[46] Occasionally, patients react negatively to the smell of gloves, and some patients are hypersensitive to perfume.[75,76]

The primary remedy for unpleasant olfactory stimuli is to stop the smell at its source. Dental offices and adjacent laboratories should use low-odor or no-odor chemicals when possible. The provider should offer an alternative to latex gloves—either mint-scented latex gloves or latex-free gloves.

The use of ceiling fans or air cleaners to facilitate airflow in the office may reduce stress-inducing odors. Air fresheners, particularly those that neutralize odors, may help. Essential oils used in aromatherapy may simultaneously mask stressful smells while contributing an anxiety-reducing benefit for the patient.[77] Studies have found that the scent of lavender and the scent of orange significantly reduce anxiety in dental patients.[78,79] However, many patients find air fresheners and essential oils to have cloying smells, so they should be used sparingly. The provider should avoid or minimize the use of perfume and use fragrance-free personal products.

> **Activity 6-3**
>
> Discuss with your colleagues the significance of smell as a form of nonverbal communication. What smells do you associate with these public places: a hair salon, a gym, a parking garage, a bar, a hospital, and a funeral parlor? Do you find any of these smells offensive? Do you have negative emotional associations with any of them? Would efforts to reduce or mask these signature smells improve the environment, or do those smells seem to belong to the place? What do you think of efforts to minimize or mask the smells in a dental practice?

Tastes

Certain tastes can increase anxiety among patients. Whether in or out of a dental operatory, the taste of blood holds negative associations, even if people are expecting it. Further, dental phobia and phobia associated with blood seem to be related and share many of the same characteristics.[80–82] Like the smell, the taste of gloves can trigger anxious responses in some patients. Other patients associate anxiety with the taste of nitrous oxide.[83]

Each of the following remedies shifts some control back to the patient, making him or her feel less vulnerable to painful or embarrassing stimuli. To minimize the taste of blood, there should be frequent rinsing and suctioning of the mouth, and the patient should be allowed to indicate a need to rinse and suction during the procedure. The importance of frequent rinsing cannot be overemphasized. Also, providers have called on glove manufacturers to consider taste when developing products.[84] Some individuals express a taste preference for either latex or nitrile gloves.[85] Such preferences should be accommodated and noted in the patient record for subsequent visits.

The patient who associates fear with nitrous oxide can prove challenging, because nitrous oxide is sometimes used to reduce anxiety. The best approach is to discuss the fear and offer an alternative anesthetic if one is available.

Place and Time as Forms of Nonverbal Communication

This manual focuses on patient-provider interaction. Yet, as previous discussions on nonverbal communication and dental anxiety have shown, patients can attach meaning to environmental stimuli (such as operatory smells) as well as provider behaviors. These messages can influence or eclipse the messages providers intend to send, so providers should consider what their spatial and temporal environment might communicate about them. Preemptively addressing potential place- and time-related barriers to communication facilitates effective patient-provider communication. This section considers four environmental contexts: waiting room, operatory, scheduling, and time spent on interaction.

Waiting room

The dental operatory should be a sterile environment for obvious reasons, but the waiting area also should be immaculately clean because it is the first visual representation of a practice that the patient encounters. The patient also may spend several minutes in the waiting area with little else to do but examine the furnishings, floors, walls, and ceiling. Any sign that these areas are unclean might increase a patient's anxiety.

A practice that treats pediatric patients should provide books, toys, or videos for children and make arrangements to clean the waiting area quickly when a child creates a mess. The availability of sanitizing wipes may be of some comfort to parents, particularly during the cold and flu season.

When asked, patients state a strong preference for comfortable furniture in the waiting area, and comfortable furniture is likely to reduce anxiety.[86] A significant majority of anxious patients prefer adorned walls, a cooler temperature, background music, and magazines.[58]

Corah[11] found that relaxation (eg, through relaxation recordings) and distraction (eg, through video games) are the two most reliable methods of reducing dental anxiety. Increasingly, the patient is likely to be carrying a smartphone or tablet computer that makes obsolete the copies of old magazines that traditionally litter waiting areas. The provider might offer suggestions for games or relaxation techniques that the patient can access through electronic devices. Online sources for relaxation and meditation apps are listed at the end of this chapter.

> **Activity 6-4**
>
> Take a field trip to one or more nearby dental practices and observe the waiting area. How are waiting patients spending their time? Does the room provide distraction or relaxation that could help the anxious patient? Is it inviting for children? Do you notice any smells or sounds? What would you change if the space were part of your practice?

Operatory

Seeing and hearing are crucial aspects of effective communication. Lighting in a dental operatory differs from lighting in other types of medical environments, so care must be taken to illuminate the workspace without directing light into the reclining patient's eyes.[87]

Regarding noise, one in five Americans now has hearing loss severe enough to compromise communication.[88] One study found that the surgical mask does not significantly impair patients' understanding of provider speech, but dental office noise does negatively affect understanding in both hearing-impaired patients and patients with good hearing.[89] In addition, as previously noted, sounds (eg, crying children) can induce stress in anxious patients. Therefore, we reiterate that the provider should reduce ambient noise by closing doors when possible and silencing equipment that is not in use.

Andrus[86] found that patients prefer that the operatory be well equipped, presumably so that the provider will not need to leave it repeatedly to retrieve supplies or forms. When the provider must leave the operatory, he or she should always tell the patient why and for how long: "I'm afraid I must take this phone call. I'll return within 5 minutes."

By law, operatories should be compliant with the Americans with Disabilities Act.[90] The provider should anticipate a patient's characteristics (eg, age or obesity) and consider ways to address them.[91]

For noise and privacy reasons, patients seem to prefer closed operatories to open-layout plans, but the former can be much more expensive. The provider should consult the literature on dental office design when organizing an operatory.[92–94]

Perhaps the most significant physical change to the dental operatory in the last 50 years has been the introduction of technology to the environment. Hardware, particularly monitors and keyboards, have not always been integrated well into the operatory environment.[95] These devices are sometimes placed behind the dental chair, so the provider is forced in the interview either to call out questions from behind the patient or to wheel between the patient and the keyboard to ask the questions face to face. If a keyboard and monitor are used, they should be situated so that the provider can face the patient while asking questions and entering responses. As technology advances, more portable tablets may solve this problem entirely. The provider should keep abreast of developments in information technology to take advantage of advances.[96]

Scheduling

Although the scheduling of a patient is not explicitly a domain of patient-provider communication, the timing of an appointment can profoundly affect the way the patient perceives and interacts with the provider and even the amount of information a patient can recall afterward. One communication strategy is to schedule morning appointments for the patient with a cognitive or physical disability. A patient with a disability (eg, Down syndrome, Alzheimer disease, or Parkinson disease) may be more cooperative or alert in the morning, and the patient's caregiver may be better able to assist at that time.[97,98] Skipped appointments may also be a symptom of dental anxiety, so morning appointments may allow the anxious patient less time in the day to worry about the appointment.

A patient with a physical or mental disability may respond better to several shorter appointments, but the caregiver might prefer fewer longer appointments to minimize the challenge of transportation. Scheduling should therefore be a matter jointly decided in consultation with the patient and the caregiver. Worth noting is that a tight recall schedule can enhance adherence to a treatment plan.[99]

> **Q** **Question of ethics:** A problem that patients persistently complain about is delays. Appointments may start late for various reasons. Once an appointment starts, the provider may be called to address another patient's needs before completing examination or treatment of the original patient. As a patient, do you see such delays in ethical terms, that the provider does not value your time as much as another patient's? As a provider, do you have a different perspective on delays? How can communication, and communication technology, reconcile patient impatience and provider delays?

Time spent on interaction

When the patient is in the operatory, the timing of communication should also be considered. Research has shown that spending 40 seconds engaging in compassionate (emotion-focused) communication with the patient can result in significantly reduced anxiety and more positive ratings of the provider.[100]

The timing of interactions can also affect recall. Patient recall is notoriously poor, so the provider should take every opportunity to enhance it. A 2008 study found that patients were unable to correctly classify more than half of the dental statements made by the dental provider, and the percentage of correct answers dropped below 40% for those in a high-stress condition just prior to oral surgery.[101] The implication of this finding is that important treatment information should be given during a time of lower stress. In addition, information and instruction should be reinforced—by repetition, by providing it in written form (eg, brochure or follow-up email), and by including a friend or family member in the conversation, in compliance with Health Insurance Portability and Accountability Act (HIPAA) regulations regarding release of patient information.

Presentation Aids

Anyone who has sat through a lecture knows that presentation aids can facilitate audience understanding. Anyone who has designed a presentation knows that presentation aids can facilitate delivery. In short, presentation aids help the audience and the speaker by accomplishing a number of task-focused goals.[102] They provide clarity to spoken messages, they generate interest in the spoken message, and they enhance retention of the spoken message by reproducing it through another medium.

A 1986 study on public speaking found that those who use presentation aids can increase the persuasiveness of their message by more than 40%.[103] The speakers also are perceived as more credible, professional, and dynamic. Since the time of that study, the advance and proliferation of digital and media technology have altered audience expectations. Even personal conversations now are often complemented by photographs, video, and multimedia websites available on personal electronic devices.

Box 6-1 categorizes seven types of easy and accessible presentation aids that the dental provider can use to enhance educational messages and provides examples of each type:

Box 6-1	Types and examples of presentation aids

Provider and patient
- Point to a tooth.
- Use a fist to illustrate a root canal.

Objects and models
- Use a pen to represent a dental handpiece.
- Use model teeth to indicate how periodontal disease spreads.

Photographs and illustrations
- Show before-and-after photographs.
- Use a diagram to illustrate a procedure.
- Display illustrations on a flip chart.

Radiographs and imaging
- Use a radiograph to indicate an area of concern.

Graphs and charts
- Point out the current level of water fluoridation on a graph.
- Show the decrease in smoking rates over time.

Video and multimedia
- Play an instructional video on a computer monitor, tablet computer, or smartphone.

Brochures and samples
- Provide instructions to take home.
- Give a complimentary ("free") toothbrush.

Traditionally, these have been called **visual aids**, but the term **presentation aids** is more accurate because audio aids (such as digital readers for the visually impaired) and product samples do not require visual attention. Nor are these presentation aids strictly nonverbal, as they can include written and spoken information.

This offered list of presentation aids is not exhaustive. In discussing the dental team's tools for patient education, Christensen[104] also included diagnostic casts, intra-oral video, books, and patient testimonials delivered over the telephone. We suggest that the provider first integrate the standard presentation aids into patient interactions before including these more advanced tools.

Provider and patient

The most accessible presentation aid is the human body. No additional tools are needed when the provider uses his or her own mouth or the patient's mouth to indicate where a problem is located or how it might be treated. A mirror can help the patient see problem areas in his or her mouth; the provider should keep a larger hand mirror available because the patient may have difficulty seeing or fail to wear corrective lenses when in the dental chair.

Demonstration is also a core communication skill. Showing a patient how to perform an oral health–related task (such as flossing teeth) is another way to use the body as a presentation aid.

Finally, the provider can use other body parts, such as his or her hands, to mime or illustrate oral health processes or treatment. For instance, the provider can close or splay his or her fingers to represent spaces between teeth or can rub his or her fists together to illustrate grinding or abrasion. Such visual representations might help the patient with later recall of what was said during the appointment.

Objects and models

The dental professional can also use actual objects to show the patient what the provider is speaking about. Most offices have available the following objects that can be helpful in educating patients: toothbrushes, floss, toothpaste, dentures and partial prostheses, and dental instruments. Models are simply manufactured representations of objects and can be used for the same purpose. They include model teeth, an oversized toothbrush, a model skull or jaw, and various healthy and diseased model teeth in cross section.

The dental professional should begin collecting objects and models early and continue adding to the collection during the course of his or her career. Objects and models are portable, but equipping every operatory with its own collection facilitates their use and saves time.

Photographs and illustrations

Digital photography has greatly expanded the use of photographs in multiple domains, including dentistry. The patient may be unable to simultaneously hold open his or her mouth and maneuver a mirror to see a problem area or restoration, but a digital image can be taken in an instant and magnified for clarity. Photographs representative of the problem or treatment can also be used, as long as they are published photographs and not depicting patients for whom the regulations of HIPAA apply.[105]

In the United States, before-and-after photographs are now ubiquitous, and many patients will expect to see the anticipated treatment outcomes before deciding whether to proceed with treatment. Such photographs are available in books, brochures, and on the Internet. Such images are easy to find online by describing the desired image (eg, "dental implant before and after") in a search engine like Google or Bing and then clicking "Images."

Illustrations of teeth and gingivae are also useful for many of the same purposes as photographs. With more defined lines and colors, drawings and paintings often provide greater clarity than do photographs. Illustration books and wall posters are extremely effective in conveying educational information. Illustrations are especially useful for helping patients understand more abstract concepts such as pulp chambers, incipient lesions, and implants.

Radiographs and imaging

Like patient photographs, a patient's digital images are nearly instant and easy to understand. Furthermore, digital images are replicable and portable, allowing the patient to take copies home for review.

In an exploration of the influence of information technology on the patient-provider relationship, Kirshner[106] identified digital imaging as influencing four aspects of relationship quality: communication, interpersonal treatment, contextual knowledge, and trust. He went on to say that, among technologic developments, "digital imaging may have the most profound effect on the dentist-patient relationship, due to its immediacy and ease of understanding through recognizable visualizations." Christensen[104] recommended the use of periapical, panoramic, and tomographic or cone beam digital radiography. The provider can use software to manipulate digital radiographs for more accurate diagnosis and utilize imaging software programs to show anticipated outcomes of esthetic treatment.

Graphs and charts

Given the limited literacy and numeracy of many dental patients, the recitation of numeric data can be counterproductive and confusing. Yet numeric information is an important component of treatment decisions, because the patient ought to know, for instance, the prevalence of the diagnosed problem, the cost of treatment, or the average time restorations last. A highly literate patient may comprehend and retain such numbers when they are delivered verbally, but the typical patient appreciates simplified presentations.

Graphs are visual representations of numeric data that make certain data easier to understand. Pie graphs relate parts to a whole and can be used to show prevalence. Bar graphs show comparisons between two or more alternatives, such as various treatment success rates. Line graphs show trends and are useful for illustrating replacement rates over time. Charts are typically tables with column and row categories and numeric data in the cells. Charts should be reserved for the patient with advanced understanding of numeric data.

Charts and graphs are available in books and journal articles, on the Internet, and in dental brochures. Useful charts and graphs should be kept in printed form in operatories or in digital form on a tablet computer.

Video and multimedia

Dental products and dental practices now are advertised regularly on television and online. In fact, video and multimedia are two of the most common ways patients learn about dental services outside the operatory, so these media also should be used within the operatory when they can help illustrate problems and procedures.

As in other realms, videotapes and DVDs are giving way to downloadable video files and PowerPoint presentations that can be viewed on computer monitors, tablets, MP3 players, and even smartphones. The provider should become acquainted with online video files, apps, and other Internet resources in order to guide the patient to sources of accurate information that can be consulted repeatedly after the patient has left the operatory. For example, many free dental videos are available online. The end of this chapter lists online sources for videos, such as the American Dental Association's (ADA's) website (www.ada.org/en), YouTube (www.youtube.com), and other sites. The ADA's 60-second videos address a wide variety of topics, including mouthguards, tooth whitening, and the parts of a tooth. Smartphone apps are also available to illustrate procedures (GC Restorative Dentistry Guides, Dental Aid, and DentalNavi), educate the patient who is receiving braces (iBraces Help), and show radiographs (RVG Mobile).

Brochures and samples

The provider should continue to use dental brochures and samples as presentation aids, despite their lack of technology. A patient may be unable to download recommended files or have no access to the Internet at all. Even a patient who can access links to video and multimedia can easily misplace digital files and links. Hard copies of information and instruction are more difficult to lose and serve as reminders to follow up.

For this reason, at the end of every appointment, the provider should write the date and time of the follow-up appointment on an informational brochure or card. Such brochures are available at low cost from commercial vendors, the ADA, and the American Academy of Pediatric Dentistry. The creative provider who wishes to draft his or her own brochures can find templates online. Finally, newsletters, which can include education information and descriptions of treatment, can be distributed or mailed to patients. Software is available to draft newsletters, and there are commercial services that provide a standard letter that can be customized to a particular practice.

Samples are such a staple of dental practices that patients would likely be disappointed to leave their recall appointments without the requisite "freebies": the toothbrush, floss, toothpaste, or samples of other useful hygiene aids. Such items can be used for demonstration purposes and then dispensed to the patient at the conclusion of the appointment. These inexpensive giveaways may seem trivial, but patients frequently mention to us that it is one of the most appealing parts of the dental visit. The appeal of giveaways is universal among children, who also appreciate stickers, pencils, sugarless gum, and sugarless candy. Many other items are available, and many of them can be customized with the name of the practice. These items subsequently remind the patient to follow up on oral health care, and they engender goodwill toward the provider.

> **Activity 6-5**
>
> Decide which one or two presentation aids would best help you explain the following procedures: dental implants, gingival disease, crowns, impressions, and veneers. Find your chosen presentation aids and present your explanation to a colleague using only nonverbal behavior. Ask for feedback.

Nonverbal Skills in Interaction: SMILES Approach

In order for nonverbal communication to support verbal communication effectively, the two forms of communication often must occur simultaneously. Fortunately, nonverbal communication is the more natural of the two forms, and many people are skilled at it without realizing they have developed proficiency over years of interaction with others. Even skilled communicators, however, may be challenged to adapt their nonverbal behaviors to a practice serving patients of diverse cultures, ages, and states of health. Furthermore, the nervousness and stress associated with providing clinical care can lead providers to neglect appropriate nonverbal behaviors. Therefore, a careful review of effective nonverbal provider behaviors can identify those that are working well and those that should be integrated or refined in practice.

In 2010, Crane and Crane[107] published a review of nonverbal communication research, identifying the best practices for physicians (Table 6-3). Although physicians were the research subjects in that study, no evidence suggests that the effectiveness and appeal of these skills would not also apply to oral health care professionals. The dozen best practices identified are not exhaustive, because research in this area continues, and they may be difficult to remember and perform as the provider is attempting to simultaneously talk to the patient and perform clinical duties. For practical reasons, we further distilled the most important skills into the mnemonic **SMILES**: **s**mile, **m**ake contact, **i**ncline toward the patient, **l**ower hands, **e**ye contact, and **s**it.

On encountering a patient, the provider generally can perform these behaviors sequentially. We suggest that the provider who is attempting to improve patient-provider communication attend to two or three skills in each encounter, until the behaviors come naturally, and then move on to other skills. If the details of the behaviors are forgotten, the provider should remember that all the actions focus attention on the patient and coordinate communication with the patient.

Table 6-3 Nonverbal communication best practices*

Nonverbal cue	Best practice	Worst practice
Facial expression	Smile	Frown
Gaze orientation	Equal eye contact while listening and talking	No eye contact or constant eye contact
Head nodding	More affirmative head nodding	Little or no head nodding
Body orientation	Open body, oriented toward patient	Closed body, oriented 45 or 90 degrees away from patient
	Forward lean	Backward lean
	Three feet away during personal conversation	Too close or too far
Vocal characteristics	Varied tone	Monotone
	Adjusted pace	Too slow or too fast
	Correct pausing	No pauses or too many pauses
	Varied volume	Too loud, too low
	Synchronized with patient	Unsynchronized with patient
	Use of nontechnical language	Use of technical jargon
Handshake	Firm and confident	Weak or bone-crushing

*Adapted from Crane and Crane[107] with permission.

Smile

Provider friendliness is associated with patient satisfaction.[108] In fact, friendliness is one of the top three characteristics mentioned by patients in describing an ideal dentist.[109] In addition, 93% of anxious dental patients prefer a provider to be friendly, and friendliness is associated with reduction in anxiety.[58,110] One study found that practicing dentists are even more likely than patients to identify the friendliness of the dental team as important.[111] Roter and Hall's theory of reciprocal exchange[112] holds that provider friendliness will elicit friendliness and inspire satisfaction in the patient.

Friendliness is expressed through a variety of nonverbal behaviors, but perhaps the single most important behavior is the smile, which is universally associated with friendliness.[113] The dental provider should smile frequently and always smile when greeting a patient.[114,115] Not only does a smile express friendliness, but it also displays the potential outcomes from dental care, serving as an advertisement of services.

The provider should also be aware that humans are adept at identifying a false smile (sometimes known as a Pan Am smile). A genuine and sincere smile (known as a **Duchenne smile**) includes the upper face and eyes in addition to the mouth.

Make contact

The norms for physical touch in the United States vary based on—among other things—the context of the encounter (professional versus personal), the sex of the communicators, and the intimacy between them. Given the nature of dentistry, patients arrive with an expectation that providers will touch them in order to conduct clinical duties. Nonclinical touch is also important but should be restricted to three touch behaviors. First, when greeting the patient, the provider should shake hands.[116] In each hand, the web between forefinger and thumb should touch, and the grip should be firm but not crushing. A 2007 survey found that 78.1% of patients want physicians to shake their hand.[117] Although a handshake is perceived as an "ideal dentist" behavior expressing friendliness and establishing trust, one study found that dentists shake patients' hands less than 20% of the time.[118]

Second, the provider should engage in appropriate nonclinical touch when comforting a patient. A touch can convey compassion and calm a patient suffering from anxiety or physical or emotional distress, and nonreciprocal (one-way) touch is associated with warmth and expressiveness.[119,120] One study found that 7- to 10-year-old children fidgeted significantly less when touched twice on the shoulder or arm during a dental consultation.[121]

Third, the provider may touch the patient when presenting a treatment plan. Research shows that touch is associated with compliance, so the patient may be more receptive to treatment if the presentation is accompanied by a touch.[122] Touch should be confined to the arm or shoulder, and the provider should always avoid touching the reclining patient's torso, legs, or feet.

Incline toward the patient

To communicate interest and involvement, the provider should tilt his or her head forward or lean toward the patient rather than lean against a wall or recline in a chair or on a stool. A 2002 review of physician behaviors found an association between forward lean and positive patient outcomes.[123] Furthermore, the forward lean should include an orientation facing the patient. Patients give higher ratings to providers who face them directly.[9,124]

The open-and-forward posture is part of a constellation of immediacy behaviors that patients—or any communication partners—find appealing. One study found that patients more often expect such immediacy behaviors from female providers than from male providers.[125] Female dental providers should remain aware of this gender role expectation and of patients' potential disapproval when it is violated (ie, when female providers appear less interested and involved).

> **Q** **Question of ethics:** Patients have different expectations of male and female dental professionals. Female dentists who are less friendly and more focused on clinical tasks are judged more severely than men who act similarly. How do you feel about this? Should providers accept this double standard, or should they play some role in trying to change patient expectations?

Lower hands

The provider should lower his or her hands while standing and place them in his or her lap while sitting.[126] Lowering the hands during initial rapport building prevents the provider from excessive gesturing that might make the patient nervous. Excessive gesticulations undermine the sense of calmness patients prefer from their providers.[110] During the clinical portion of the appointment, the hands will necessarily be occupied with dental instruments and tools, and during these periods the provider should also refrain from gesticulating with sharp instruments.

Open arm positions and arm symmetry are rated more positively by patients than crossed arms or arms akimbo (hands on hips, elbows turned out).[123,124] In medical encounters, providers' uncrossed arms and arm symmetry are actually associated with positive patient outcomes.[123]

Eye contact

Gaze aversion is consistently associated with negative perceptions of attraction, credibility, and relational communication.[127] Eye contact establishes and sustains trust between the patient and provider and is associated with patient satisfaction.[128,129] Similar to physical touch, eye contact is also associated with compliance with requests, suggesting that eye contact is particularly important in treatment plan presentation.[130]

Use of a computer during the patient interview is negatively associated with both eye contact and the amount of information that the provider conveys to the patient.[131] A 2007 study of electronic medical records observed that physicians who took short breaks from data entry to make eye contact and converse with a patient used more nonverbal communication than physicians who continuously worked on the computer.[132] Such breaks risk creating long pauses in the conversation, but those pauses may actually enhance communication by providing time for both the patient and provider to process information.

Activity 6-6

Locate an online video of a dental professional speaking to the camera or to a patient. Turn off the sound and observe the nonverbal aspect of the presentation or explanation. Pay close attention to facial expressions, posture, proximity, and hand gestures. What nonverbal messages are you receiving? Does the provider project friendliness? Confidence? Boredom? Nervousness?

Sit

Sitting while interacting with a patient physically represents the reduction in patient-provider power differential that the provider seeks to achieve. The standing provider towers over the patient who is sitting or reclining in a dental chair. Given the personal nature of interview questions, a standing provider can seem intimidating or condescending, even to confident patients.[128] A provider who is standing might only increase the fear of those contending with dental anxiety. The provider may occasionally need to stand during some examinations and procedures, but especially during rapport building, the information-gathering interview, and the treatment plan presentation, the provider should sit facing the patient and as close to his or her eye level as possible.

There are other, less obvious reasons for the provider to sit rather than stand. Patients tend to perceive that sitting providers spend more time with them than standing providers.[133] A recent study of provider follow-up visits to hospitalized patients confirmed that finding and also found that patients perceived that sitting providers understood their condition better than standing providers.[134]

Chapter Checklist ☑

Nonverbal communication and fear
- ❑ Portray empathy, friendliness, and competence to increase the satisfaction of the anxious patient.
- ❑ Use survey instruments, such as the Dental Anxiety Scale, Dental Fear Survey, or Short Dental Fear Question, to diagnose dental fear.
- ❑ Sounds: Understand anxiety triggers such as the sound of instruments, the dental handpiece, crying children, and patients who moan or cry out.
- ❑ Sounds: Ask the patient for notification before he or she vocalizes.
- ❑ Sounds: Invite a parent, family member, or caregiver into the operatory.
- ❑ Sounds: Play music or white noise, encourage use of MP3 players or earplugs, and close doors or leave them slightly ajar.
- ❑ Sights: Understand anxiety triggers such as the sight of instruments, direct light, scrubs and masks, and dental diagnoses.
- ❑ Sights: Keep instruments and syringes out of the patient's sight.
- ❑ Sights: Direct light away from the patient's eyes or provide sunglasses.
- ❑ Sights: Avoid showing problem areas in the mouth if the patient seems anxious.
- ❑ Sights: Pull down your mask when its use is not required.
- ❑ Sensations: Understand anxiety triggers such as the sensation of pain or dental instruments, anticipation of choking or gagging, and injections of anesthetic.
- ❑ Sensations: Acknowledge fears and assure the patient that caution and care will be taken.
- ❑ Sensations: Narrate procedures and notify the patient about what will occur.
- ❑ Sensations: Allow the patient to signal for breaks and to choose from alternatives whenever possible.
- ❑ Smells: Understand anxiety triggers such as the smell of methyl methacrylate, eugenol, carious teeth, handpiece burning, gloves, and perfume.
- ❑ Smells: Use low-odor chemicals, improve airflow, and (sparingly) use air fresheners and essential oils.

❑ Smells: Avoid wearing perfumes, use fragrance-free products whenever possible, and select gloves based on scent and taste.
❑ Tastes: Understand anxiety triggers such as the taste of blood, gloves, and nitrous oxide.
❑ Tastes: Rinse and suction the patient's mouth frequently during a procedure, and allow a means for the patient to signal when additional rinsing and suctioning are needed.
❑ Tastes: Look for signs of the patient's distaste for latex gloves and nitrous oxide, and offer alternatives (eg, nitrile gloves and anti-anxiety medications).

Place and time as nonverbal communication
❑ Consider what the spatial and temporal environment of the practice communicates about you.
❑ Waiting area: Keep the waiting area clean.
❑ Waiting area: Provide books, toys, or videos for children and arrange to clean up after them.
❑ Waiting area: Keep the waiting area cool and provide comfortable furniture, adorned walls, background music, and magazines.
❑ Waiting area: Suggest games or relaxation apps for the patient to download to a smartphone or tablet device.
❑ Operatory: Illuminate the workspace without directing light into the patient's eyes.
❑ Operatory: Reduce ambient noise by closing doors (or leaving them slightly ajar) and silencing equipment.
❑ Operatory: Fully stock and equip each operatory to minimize the transportation of supplies and equipment during treatment.
❑ Operatory: Notify patients why you must leave the operatory during the appointment and how long the delay might be.
❑ Operatory: Place keyboards and monitors so that you and the patient can maintain eye contact.
❑ Scheduling: Consider scheduling morning appointments if a patient has a disability or is anxious.
❑ Scheduling: Consider scheduling several shorter appointments, and pursue a tight recall schedule if a patient has a disability.
❑ Scheduling: Consider the caregiver's preferences, and schedule appointments in consultation with both the patient and caregiver.
❑ Interacting: Aim to spend 40 seconds in initial compassionate communication.
❑ Interacting: Give important treatment information during a time of low stress.
❑ Interacting: Reinforce information by saying it repeatedly, providing it in written form, and (within the guidelines mandated by HIPAA) including a friend or family member in the conversation.

Presentation aids
❑ Self and patient: Keep large hand mirrors available.
❑ Self and patient: Show the patient how to perform oral health tasks by miming and using other body parts such as the hands.
❑ Objects and models: Begin collecting objects and models early and supply each operatory with its own collection.
❑ Objects: Demonstrate the use of toothbrushes and floss as well as proper cleaning of full and removable partial dentures.

❑ Models: Demonstrate with model teeth, an oversized toothbrush, model skulls and jaws, and cross sections of healthy and diseased teeth.

❑ Photographs: Use digital photography, representative photographs, or before-and-after photographs to discuss problems, treatments, and potential outcomes.

❑ Illustrations: Use drawings and paintings to provide clearer renderings of problem areas and treatment options.

❑ Radiographs and imaging: Use periapical, panoramic, and tomographic or cone beam digital radiography.

❑ Radiographs and imaging: Consider using photography software to manipulate images in order to forecast results.

❑ Graphs and charts: Keep copies of graphs and charts in each operatory or in digital form on tablet computers.

❑ Graphs: Use pie graphs to relate parts to a whole.

❑ Graphs: Use bar graphs to compare two or more alternatives.

❑ Graphs: Use line graphs to show trends.

❑ Charts: Use charts sparingly, primarily with the patient who has advanced understanding of numeric data.

❑ Video and multimedia: Use video and PowerPoint presentations viewable on monitors, tablet computers, MP3 players, and smartphones.

❑ Video and multimedia: Access free dental videos online and download smartphone apps.

❑ Brochures and samples: Rely on brochures and samples to reinforce oral health messages.

❑ Brochures: Remind the patient of return appointments by using reminder cards or writing the appointment date and time on an informational brochure.

❑ Brochures: Consider distributing periodic practice newsletters.

❑ Samples: Provide a toothbrush, floss, toothpaste, or other giveaways to the patient at the end of the appointment.

❑ Samples: Provide the child patient with stickers, pencils, sugarless gum, or sugarless candy to create a positive regard for dental visits.

❑ Samples: Consider personalizing giveaways with the name of the practice or provider.

SMILES approach

❑ Focus attention on the patient and coordinate communication with the patient.

❑ Smile: Smile frequently and always smile when greeting a patient.

❑ Make contact: Touch the patient on the arm or hand when greeting the patient (handshake), when comforting the patient, and when presenting a treatment plan to the patient.

❑ Make contact: Avoid touching the reclining patient's torso, legs, or feet.

❑ Incline toward the patient: Lean forward or tilt your head forward.

❑ Incline toward the patient: Face the patient.

❑ Lower hands: Drop your hands when standing and place your hands in your lap when sitting.

❑ Lower hands: Keep your arms open and symmetric.

❑ Lower hands: Avoid gesticulating, particularly with instruments in hand.

❑ Eye contact: Regularly make eye contact when entering health history data.

❑ Eye contact: Sustain eye contact when presenting treatment plans.

❑ Sit: Sit facing the patient as close to eye level as possible during rapport building, the interview, and the treatment plan presentation.

21. Hennenlotter A, Dresel C, Castrop F, Ceballos-Baumann AO, Wohlschläger AM, Haslinger B. The link between facial feedback and neural activity within central circuitries of emotion—New insights from botulinum toxin-induced denervation of frown muscles. Cereb Cortex 2009;19: 537–542.

22. Soussignan R. Duchenne smile, emotional experience, and autonomic reactivity: A test of the facial feedback hypothesis. Emotion 2002;2:52–74.

23. Dimberg U, Söderkvist S. The voluntary facial action technique: A method to test the facial feedback hypothesis. J Nonverbal Behav 2011;35:17–33.

24. Olav V. Anxiety, pain and discomfort associated with dental treatment. Behav Res Ther 1993;31:659–666.

25. Eitner S, Wichmann M, Paulsen A, Holst S. Dental anxiety: An epidemiological study on its clinical correlation and effects on oral health. J Oral Rehabil 2006;33:588–593.

26. Kleinknecht RA, Thorndike RM, McGlynn FD, Harkavy J. Factor analysis of the Dental Fear Survey with cross-validation. J Am Dent Assoc 1984;108:59–61.

27. Heaton LJ, Carlson CR, Smith TA, Baer RA, de Leeuw R. Predicting anxiety during dental treatment using patients' self-reports: Less is more. J Am Dent Assoc 2007;138:188–195.

28. Cohen SM, Fiske J, Newton JT. Behavioural dentistry: The impact of dental anxiety on daily living. Br Dent J 2000;189:385–390.

29. Dempster L, Locker D. The role of dentist/patient interactions in dental anxiety. Presented at the IADR/AADR/CADR 87th General Session and Exhibition, Miami, April 2, 2009.

30. Gale EN. Fears of the dental situation. J Dent Res 1972;51:964–966.

31. Moore R, Brødsgaard I, Birn H. Manifestations, acquisition and diagnostic categories of dental fear in a self-referred population. Behav Res Ther 1991;29:51–60.

32. Weiner AA (ed). The Fearful Dental Patient: A Guide to Understanding and Managing. Ames, IA: Wiley-Blackwell, 2011.

33. Milgrom P, Weinstein P, Getz T. Treating Fearful Dental Patients: A Patient Management Handbook, ed 2. Seattle: University of Washington, 1995.

34. Mostofsky DI, Forgione AG, Giddon DB (eds). Behavioral Dentistry. Ames, IA: Wiley-Blackwell, 2006.

35. Peltier B. Psychological treatment of fearful and phobic special needs patients. Spec Care Dentist 2009;29:51–57.

36. Milgrom P, Heaton LJ. Enhancing sedation treatment for the long-term: Pre-treatment behavioural exposure. SAAD Dig 2007;23:29–34.

37. Forgione AG. Hypnosis in the treatment of dental fear and phobia. Dent Clin North Am 1988;32:745–761.

38. Schuurs AHB, Hoogstraten J. Appraisal of dental anxiety and fear questionnaires: A review. Community Dent Oral Epidemiol 1993;21:329–339.

39. Corah NL. Development of a dental anxiety scale. J Dent Res 1969;48:596.

40. Corah NL, Gale EN, Illig SJ. Assessment of a dental anxiety scale. J Am Dent Assoc 1978;97: 816–819.

41. Milgrom P, Kleinknecht RA, Elliott J, Liu HH, Teo CS. A cross-cultural cross validation of the Dental Fear Survey in South East Asia. Behav Res Ther 1990;28:227–233.

42. Jaakkola S, Rautava P, Alanen P, et al. Dental fear: One single clinical question for measurement. Open Dent J 2009;3:161–166.

43. Stouthard MEA, Hoogstraten J, Mellenbergh GJ. A study on the convergent and discriminant validity of the Dental Anxiety Inventory. Behav Res Ther 1995;33:589–595.

44. Smyth JS. Some problems of dental treatment. 1. Patient anxiety: Some correlates and sex differences. Aust Dent J 1993;38:354–359.

45. De Jongh A, Stouthard MEA. Anxiety about dental hygienist treatment. Community Dent Oral Epidemiol 1993;21:91–95.

46. Bernstein DA, Kleinknecht RA, Alexander LD. Antecedents of dental fear. J Public Health Dent 1979;39:113–124.

47. Jadid K, Klein U, Meinke D. Assessment of noise exposures in a pediatric dentistry residency clinic. Pediatr Dent 2011;33:343–348.

48. Zlotogorski Z, Zadik D, Evron D. The relationship between learned resourcefulness and coping with crying in pediatric dentistry: A pilot study. Pediatr Dent 1994;16:371–372.

49. Johnson JB, Pinkham JR, Kerber PE. Stress reactions of various judging groups to the child dental patient. J Dent Res 1979;58:1664–1671.

50. Elsbach HG. Crying as a diagnostic tool. J Dent Child 1963;30:13–16.

51. Trocinski DR, Pearigen PD. The crying infant. Emerg Med Clin North Am 1998;16:895–910.

52. So HM, Chan DSK. Perception of stressors by patients and nurses of critical care units in Hong Kong. Int J Nurs Stud 2004;41:77–84.

53. Bobey MJ, Davidson PO. Psychological factors affecting pain tolerance. J Psychosom Res 1970;14:371–376.

54. Newton JT, Patel H, Shah S, Sturmey P. Paediatric dental surgery: Attitudes towards the use of hand over mouth (HOM) and physical restraint amongst paediatric specialist practitioners in the UK. Br Dent J 2004;197:117–117.

55. Sotto JJ, Azari AF, Riley J, Bimstein E. First-year students' perceptions about pediatric dental behavior guidance techniques: The effect of education. J Dent Educ 2008;72:1029–1041.

56. Anderson RA, Baron R, Logan H. Distraction, control, and dental stress. J Appl Soc Psychol 1991;21:156–171.

57. Vernet-Maury E, Robin O, Vinard H. Analgesic property of white noise: An experimental study. Funct Neurol 1988;3:157–166.

58. Bare LC, Dundes L. Strategies for combating dental anxiety. J Dent Educ 2004;68:1172–1177.

59. Harp H, Hook E, Solberg E, Anderson D. A patient's perspective on how hygienists can decrease patient anxiety. J Dent Hyg 2000;74:322.

60. Chang JR, Cheng HK, Lee SY, Bai MR, Lean RI. A novel earplug system for filtering out dental noise. J Mar Sci Technol (Taiwan) 2003;11:179–188.

61. Filcheck HA, Allen KD, Ogren H, Darby JB, Holstein B, Hupp S. The use of choice-based distraction to decrease the distress of children at the dentist. Child Fam Behav Ther 2005;26(4):59–68.

62. Schmid-Leuz B, Elsesser K, Lohrmann T, Jöhren P, Sartory G. Attention focusing versus distraction during exposure in dental phobia. Behav Res Ther 2007;45:2691–2703.

63. Rubin JG, Kaplan AS. Development of a hospital-based dental phobia clinic. Spec Care Dentist 1988;8:25–27.

64. Krochak M, Friedman N. Using a precision-metered injection system to minimize dental injection anxiety. Compend Contin Educ Dent 1998;19:137–150.

65. Stouthard MEA, Hoogstraten J. Ratings of fears associated with twelve dental situations. J Dent Res 1987;66:1175–1178.

66. Hmud R, Walsh LJ. Dental anxiety: Causes, complications and management approaches. J Minim Interv Dent 2009;2:67–78.

67. Getka EJ, Glass CR. Behavioral and cognitive-behavioral approaches to the reduction of dental anxiety. Behav Ther 1992;23:433–448.

68. Weiner AA, Sheehan DV, Jones KJ. Dental anxiety—The development of a measurement model. Acta Psychiatr Scand 1986;73:559–565.

69. Armfield JM. Towards a better understanding of dental anxiety and fear: Cognitions vs. experiences. Eur J Oral Sci 2010;118:259–264.

70. Raadal M, Milgrom P, Weinstein P, Mancl L, Cauce AM. The prevalence of dental anxiety in children from low-income families and its relationship to personality traits. J Dent Res 1995;74:1439–1443.

71. Moore R, Brødsgaard I, Rosenberg N. The contribution of embarrassment to phobic dental anxiety: A qualitative research study. BMC Psychiatry 2004;4:10.

72. Morse DR, Chow E. The effect of the Relaxodont brain wave synchronizer on endodontic anxiety: Evaluation by galvanic skin resistance, pulse rate, physical reactions, and questionnaire responses. Int J Psychosom 1993;40:68–76.

73. Robin O, Alaoui-Ismaili O, Dittmar A, Vernet-Maury E. Emotional responses evoked by dental odors: An evaluation from autonomic parameters. J Dent Res 1998;77:1638–1646.

74. Robin O, Alaoui-Ismaili O, Dittmar A, Vernet-Maury E. Basic emotions evoked by eugenol odor differ according to the dental experience. A neurovegetative analysis. Chem Senses 1999;24:327–335.

75. Lahti S, Tuutti H, Hausen H, Kaariainen R. Dentist and patient opinions about the ideal dentist and patient: Developing a compact questionnaire. Community Dent Oral Epidemiol 1992;20: 229–234.
76. Christensen GJ. Operating gloves: The good and the bad. J Am Dent Assoc 2001;132: 1455–1457.
77. Harlan K, Wancour S. An overview of pain management. RDH 2008;28(12):50–53.
78. Kritsidima M, Newton T, Asimakopoulou K. The effects of lavender scent on dental patient anxiety levels: A cluster randomised-controlled trial. Community Dent Oral Epidemiol 2010;38: 83–87.
79. Lehrner J, Eckersberger C, Walla P, Pötsch G, Deecke L. Ambient odor of orange in a dental office reduces anxiety and improves mood in female patients. Physiol Behav 2000;71:83–86.
80. Locker D, Shapiro D, Liddell A. Overlap between dental anxiety and blood-injury fears: Psychological characteristics and response to dental treatment. Behav Res Ther 1997;35:583–590.
81. Öst LG, Hugdahl K. Acquisition of blood and dental phobia and anxiety response patterns in clinical patients. Behav Res Ther 1985;23:27–34.
82. De Jongh A, Bongaarts G, Vermeule I, Visser K, De Vos P, Makkes P. Blood–injury–injection phobia and dental phobia. Behav Res Ther 1998;36:971–982.
83. Faulks D, Hennequin M, Albecker-Grappe S, et al. Sedation with 50% nitrous oxide/oxygen for outpatient dental treatment in individuals with intellectual disability. Dev Med Child Neurol 2007;49:621–625.
84. Burke FJT. Use of non-sterile gloves in clinical practice. J Dent 1990;18:79–89.
85. Bahr D. Nobody Ever Told Me (or My Mother) That! Everything from Bottles and Breathing to Healthy Speech Development. Arlington, TX: Sensory World, 2010.
86. Andrus D. Office atmospherics and dental service satisfaction. J Prof Serv Market 1986;1(4): 77–85.
87. Preston JD, Ward LC, Bobrick M. Light and lighting in the dental office. Dent Clin North Am 1978;22:431–451.
88. Lin FR, Niparko JK, Ferrucci L. Hearing loss prevalence in the United States. Arch Intern Med 2011;171:1851–1852.
89. Mendel LL, Gardino JA, Atcherson SR. Speech understanding using surgical masks: A problem in health care? J Am Acad Audiol 2008;19:686–695.
90. Americans with Disabilities Act of 1990, Pub L No. 101-336, 104 Stat 328 (1990).
91. Ettinger R, Beck J, Glenn R. Eliminating office architectural barriers to dental care of the elderly and handicapped. J Am Dent Assoc 1979;98:398–401.
92. Malkin J. Medical and Dental Space Planning: A Comprehensive Guide to Design, Equipment, and Clinical Procedures, ed 3. New York: Wiley, 2002.
93. Demaree HL. Dental office design. Curr Opin Dent 1991;1:672–676.
94. Goldstep F. Designing the esthetic dental environment. Dent Clin North Am 1998;42:643–651.
95. Schleyer TKL. Why integration is key for dental office technology. J Am Dent Assoc 2004;135(suppl 1):4S–9S.
96. Schleyer TKL, Spallek H, Bartling WC, Corby P. The technologically well-equipped dental office. J Am Dent Assoc 2003;134:30–41.
97. Pilcher ES. Treating the patient with Down syndrome. J Contemp Dent Pract 2001;2(4):58.
98. Pilcher ES. Dental care for the patient with Down syndrome. Down Syndr Res Pract 1998;5:111–116.
99. Witt E, Bartsch A. Effects of information-giving and communication during orthodontic consultation and treatment. 3. Optimized orthodontist-patient communication. J Orofac Orthop 1996;57:154–167.
100. Fogarty LA, Curbow BA, Wingard JR, McDonnell K, Somerfield MR. Can 40 seconds of compassion reduce patient anxiety? J Clin Oncol 1999;17:371–379.
101. Eli I, Schwartz-Arad D, Bartal Y. Anxiety and ability to recognize clinical Information in dentistry. J Dent Res 2008;87:65–68.
102. Lucas SE. The Art of Public Speaking, ed 9. New York: McGraw-Hill, 2007.
103. Vogel DR, Dickson GW, Lehman JA. Persuasion and the role of visual presentation support: The UM/3M study. Minneapolis, MN: Management Information Systems Research Center, University of Minnesota School of Management, 1986.

104. Christensen GJ. Developing your staff into a patient education team. J Am Dent Assoc 2009;140:1536–1539.
105. Health Insurance Portability and Accountability Act of 1996, Pub L No. 104-191, 110 Stat 1936 (1996). http://www.gpo.gov/fdsys/pkg/PLAW-104publ191/html/PLAW-104publ191.htm. Accessed 12 January 2015.
106. Kirshner M. The role of information technology and informatics research in the dentist-patient relationship. Adv Dent Res 2003;17:77–81.
107. Crane J, Crane FG. Optimal nonverbal communications strategies physicians should engage in to promote positive clinical outcomes. Health Mark Q 2010;27:262–274.
108. Comstock LM, Hooper EM, Goodwin JM, Goodwin JS. Physician behaviors that correlate with patient satisfaction. J Med Educ 1982;57:105–112.
109. Van Groenestijn MA, Maas-de Waal CJ, Mileman PA, Swallow JN. The ideal dentist. Soc Sci Med 1980;14A:533–540.
110. Corah N, O'Shea R, Bissell G, Thines T, Mendola P. The dentist-patient relationship: Perceived dentist behaviors that reduce patient anxiety and increase satisfaction. J Am Dent Assoc 1988;116:73–76.
111. Woelber JP, Deimling D, Langenbach D, Ratka-Krüger P. The importance of teaching communication in dental education. A survey amongst dentists, students and patients. Eur J Dent Educ 2012;16:e200–e204.
112. Roter DL, Hall JA. Health education theory: An application to the process of patient-provider communication. Health Educ Res 1991;6:185–193.
113. Ekman P, Keltner D. Universal facial expressions of emotion: An old controversy and new findings. In: Segerstrale U, Molnar P (eds). Nonverbal communication: Where nature meets culture. Mahwah, NJ: Lawrence Erlbaum, 1997:27–46.
114. Levin RP. Interpersonal communication. J Am Dent Assoc 2006;137:239–240.
115. Lill MM, Wilkinson TJ. Judging a book by its cover: Descriptive survey of patients' preferences for doctors' appearance and mode of address. BMJ 2005;331:1524–1527.
116. Levin RP. The interpersonal factor. J Am Dent Assoc 2008;139:986–987.
117. Makoul G, Zick A, Green M. An evidence-based perspective on greetings in medical encounters. Arch Intern Med 2007;167:1172–1176.
118. Lahti S, Tuuti H, Hausen H, Kaariainen R. Comparison of ideal and actual behavior of patients and dentists during dental treatment. Community Dent Oral Epidemiol 1995;23:374–378.
119. Terézhalmy GT, Huber MA, Jones AC. Physical evaluation in dental practice. Ames, IA: Wiley-Blackwell, 2009.
120. Major B, Heslin R. Perceptions of cross-sex and same-sex nonreciprocal touch: It is better to give than to receive. J Nonverbal Behav 1982;6:148–162.
121. Greenbaum PE, Lumley MA, Turner C, Melamed BG. Dentist's reassuring touch: Effects on children's behavior. Pediatr Dent 1993;15:20–24.
122. Willis FN, Hamm HK. The use of interpersonal touch in securing compliance. J Nonverbal Behav 1980;5:49–55.
123. Beck RS, Daughtridge R, Sloane PD. Physician-patient communication in the primary care office: A systematic review. J Am Board Fam Pract 2002;15:25–38.
124. Harrigan JA, Rosenthal R. Physicians' head and body positions as determinants of perceived rapport. J Appl Soc Psychol 1983;13:496–509.
125. Mast MS, Hall JA, Köckner C, Choi E. Physician gender affects how physician nonverbal behavior is related to patient satisfaction. Med Care 2008;46:1212–1218.
126. Harrigan JA, Rosenthal R. Nonverbal aspects of empathy and rapport in physician-patient interaction. In: Blanck PD, Buck R, Rosenthal R (eds). Nonverbal Communication in the Clinical Context. University Park, PA: Pennsylvania State University Press, 1986:36–73.
127. Burgoon JK, Coker DA, Coker RA. Communicative effects of gaze behavior. Hum Commun Res 1986;12:495–524.
128. Levin RP. Body language speaks volumes. J Am Dent Assoc 2008;139:1262–1263.
129. Mast MS. On the importance of nonverbal communication in the physician-patient interaction. Patient Educ Couns 2007;67:315–318.

130. Guéguen N, Jacob C. Direct look versus evasive glance and compliance with a request. J Soc Psychol 2002;142:393–396.
131. Noordman J, Verhaak P, van Beljouw I, van Dulmen S. Consulting room computers and their effect on general practitioner-patient communication. Fam Pract 2010;27:644–651.
132. McGrath JM, Arar NH, Pugh JA. The influence of electronic medical record usage on nonverbal communication in the medical interview. Health Informatics J 2007;13:105–118.
133. Johnson RL, Sadosty AT, Weaver AL, Goyal DG. To sit or not to sit? Ann Emerg Med 2008;51: 188–193.
134. Swayden KJ, Anderson KK, Connelly LM, Moran JS, McMahon JK, Arnold PM. Effect of sitting vs. standing on perception of provider time at bedside: A pilot study. Patient Educ Couns 2012;86:166–167.

Part III

Communication During the Appointment

Up to this point, discussion has focused separately on the key components of communication: listening, verbal communication, and nonverbal communication. In life, and in the dental operatory, providers do not engage in those behaviors in isolation. Some researchers suggest, therefore, that the components not be studied in isolation.* This section presents an integration of those skills, discussing ways to communicate with patients during three phases of a typical dental appointment: initiating and interviewing (chapter 7), interacting during and after procedures (chapter 8), and presenting treatment plans (chapter 9). Although providers should maintain basic patient-centered behaviors throughout their interactions with patients, the specific skills used will vary in each context.

*Jones SE, LeBaron CD. Research on the relationship between verbal and nonverbal communication: Emerging integrations. J Commun 2002;52:499–521.

7

Initiating and Interviewing

Why Initiating and Interviewing Skills Matter

Accurate information regarding a patient's health status and history is crucial to clinical encounters. Effective consultation, examination, diagnosis, and treatment planning depend on the clinician's knowledge of a patient's background, former treatments, risk factors, and health behaviors. This is the case for both the traditional (disease-centered) and the patient-centered health care delivery models, although the latter requires that the provider also determine the patient's capabilities and preferences. Moreover, this large amount of information is required at the beginning of the patient-provider relationship, and updates are required at the beginning of each appointment. This characteristic, more than any other, distinguishes the patient-provider relationship from other types of social and professional relationships: It inverts the normal course of relational self-disclosure.

Not only is the disclosure primarily one way (from patient to provider), but also the most intimate personal and physical details must be divulged before strong relational ties are established.

Initiating relationships with patients matters because providers must establish professional intimacy quickly if they are to perform their clinical duties effectively. In a personal relationship, two individuals might share a meal or a movie and divulge superficial information (eg, likes and dislikes) for months or years before learning some of the more intimate details asked in the health history: allergies, infectious diseases, prescriptions, and so on.[1,2] Dental professionals do not have the luxury of so much time. Within minutes of meeting patients for the first time, providers must explore their patients' physical and behavioral problems.

Such an accelerated timetable can be disconcerting for patients, so providers must become skilled at eliciting disclosures in a way that does not offend patients or lead them to withhold information. Achievement of these goals can be challenging with patients who arrive with negative expectations based on cultural stereotypes or negative personal experiences with dental professionals. Patients' first impressions of their dental providers are therefore extremely important.[3] The first impression affects both comfort and anxiety level during the appointment.[4] The first impression may also determine whether patients return and the quality of the subsequent relationship—including loyalty, trust, and treatment adherence.[5]

Soon after the greeting and initial exchanges, providers begin the health history interview. For returning patients, a briefer health history update may be conducted, but for new patients a more thorough interview is necessary. The questions asked often duplicate the questions patients answered on the health history form they previously completed. This redundancy can lead to frustration, irritation, and embarrassment for many patients, including those who have limited literacy skills, who cannot recall the answers to certain questions, who are disclosing information on stigmatized conditions or behaviors, or who do not understand the relevance of the questions to oral health. Defusing these negative attitudes and eliciting correct and thorough information quickly are also necessary communication skills.[6]

Interviewing skills matter because these are intimate questions and patients are justifiably concerned about their privacy. From a clinical perspective, skilled questioning facilitates accurate diagnosis. Evidence also suggests that patient-centered interviewing is associated with treatment adherence.[7]

This chapter begins broadly and narrows to specific sequential skills that dental providers must master. The first section addresses communication from a legal perspective, outlining the parameters of the Privacy Rule of the Health Insurance Portability and Accountability Act (HIPAA) and identifying aspects of the law that might facilitate trust and patient disclosure. The second section discusses professional consensus recommendations, identifying essential elements of patient-physician communication and detailing lists of patient interview processes. The third section discusses the impact and goals of the initial dental consultation. The final section describes specific practical skills to implement in dental practice.

People we do not know personally often ask for information we would otherwise keep confidential. Retailers sometimes want telephone numbers or addresses. Charities sometimes ask for email addresses. Insurance companies sometimes require Social Security numbers. Can you think of other individuals or organizations that routinely ask for information that seems disconnected from their mission? How do you respond to these requests? Does it depend on the organization or individual who is asking, or do you have a blanket policy regarding information requests? Discuss your responses and response options with your colleagues. Also discuss whether patients perceive requests from health care providers differently than they perceive these other requests.

HIPAA Privacy Rule

The Health Insurance Portability and Accountability Act became federal law in 1996.[8] For many years, health care organizations, the insurance industry, and government bureaucracies had failed to draft and implement standards for information sharing among various entities. HIPAA pursued four objectives: curtailing fraud and abuse, enforcing health information standards, guaranteeing information privacy and security, and assuring insurance portability.[9] HIPAA resulted in much confusion and frustration as its provisions were implemented, interpreted, and revised over the years. In an age when medical record keeping has transitioned from paper to digital formats, however, HIPAA has successfully introduced standardization that permits the sharing of information among a patient's various providers and has successfully introduced standards that safeguard that information.

HIPAA compliance is a practice-management concern that exceeds the scope of this manual on patient-provider communication. Numerous articles have been written to guide compliance by practitioners.[10–13] Yet one element of HIPAA, the **Privacy Rule**, does merit attention here because it relates to communication in two ways. First, it prescribes the parameters and legal requirements for discussing, documenting, and distributing patients' protected health information. Second, HIPAA has changed patients' expectations regarding privacy and ownership of their medical information. Ultimately, these changes in rules and expectations support patient-centered care and therefore are positive developments. Providers should acquaint themselves with, and even embrace, the provisions of the Privacy Rule.

Legal requirements

In general, the Privacy Rule restricts the type of patient information that can be shared and with whom it can be shared.[14,15] Protected health information includes patients' medical history, diagnostic tests and results, dental treatments, prescriptions, and other health data. However, protected health information also includes data that are not directly related to a patients' health, such as email addresses[14] (Box 7-1). Further, this information is covered by the Privacy Rule whether it is in oral, written, or electronic form.

Box 7-1	**Nonmedical information protected by the HIPAA Privacy Rule***
• Names	• Birth dates
• Addresses (all elements)	• Account numbers
• Telephone numbers	• Credit card information
• Fax numbers	• Certificate numbers
• Email addresses	• Social Security numbers
• License numbers	• Full-face photographs

*This list provides examples of protected information and is not comprehensive.

The Privacy Rule allows providers to share patients' information with specific others to the degree necessary to accomplish a specific purpose: coordination of care, arrangement of insurance payments, and so on. In all cases, providers should minimize the amount of protected health information that they share (ie, minimum necessary disclosure), limit the number of people with whom the information is shared, and document everything.

Box 7-2 summarizes key provisions of the Privacy Rule. These are fairly straightforward, and providers are granted some discretion in the way the provisions are implemented in practice. In exercising that discretion, providers should keep in mind several caveats. First, many patients have low literacy levels, so privacy notices should be written at a level that patients can understand. A 2007 study of the privacy notices used by all 56 US dental schools found that they were written in language significantly more complex than "plain language."[16] Efforts to notify patients of a practice's privacy efforts are useless if patients cannot understand them.

Second, as mentioned previously, some dental offices are better configured for privacy than others are. Providers can attempt to minimize exposure of others to protected information by shutting a door or lowering their voice. Such efforts not only are appreciated by patients but also provide evidence of providers' intention to comply with HIPAA regulations.

Third, many patients (particularly the very young or old) are accompanied by companions, and providers are rightly concerned about disclosing protected information within companions' hearing.[17] Under HIPAA, providers are generally allowed to exercise professional judgment in disclosing information in the presence of family members or companions. The exception is when patients expressly request that information be disclosed confidentially. In these cases, patients' wishes should be honored.

Box 7-2	Key provisions of the Privacy Rule

- The patient has the right to access his or her personal health information, obtain copies of medical records, request correction of errors, and restrict use of protected health information.
- The patient has the right to file a complaint with the practice or the federal Office for Civil Rights in the event of a privacy violation.
- The provider must give the patient a written disclosure of privacy rights under HIPAA and the provider's use and disclosure practices regarding protected health information. This disclosure must be provided during the patient's first visit.
- The practice must post a copy of privacy rights and practices in each dental office and on any practice website.
- The practice must implement HIPAA privacy and security measures.
- The practice must designate a privacy officer—a staff member responsible for compliance.
- The provider must undergo training in HIPAA privacy and security measures.
- The provider must identify and contract with specific business associates who will have access to patient data.
- The provider must develop patient consent forms that document each patient's preferences regarding use of protected health information.

Patient expectations

Although several states had previously done so, the Privacy Rule is the first attempt by the federal government to protect patients' health information.[18] Since its implementation on April 14, 2001, patients have been provided oral and written notices of their rights to view and challenge the collection and distribution of their health information. Although HIPAA regulates only those practices that transmit electronic patient data, all practices would do well to adhere to its privacy standards, as patients have come to expect a certain level of privacy regarding their treatment that they may not have expected previously.

Patients may be less likely to request copies of their health records in a dental setting than in a medical practice. Even so, dental professionals must expect such requests, and similar privacy-related requests, and be prepared to explain their practice's security measures to ensure privacy (eg, encryption, passwords, and restricted physical access to terminals). Patients have a right to make such requests, so the information should be available and provided cheerfully.

> **Question of ethics:** HIPAA's Privacy Rule clarifies that disclosing patient information to others uninvolved in patient care is illegal and unethical. Yet discussion of cases—formally at conferences or informally among colleagues—has a long tradition in medicine. Such discussions can confirm diagnoses and generate treatment ideas. If you are not directly consulting a dental professional, is it ethical to discuss a case with colleagues? What if you conceal the patient's identity? Is it ethical to discuss a case if you are not sharing or seeking professional expertise but rather sharing a humorous or unusual experience? Does your answer change if your audience is a friend or family member rather than a dental professional?

Guidelines for Communication

As organizations and practices increasingly adopted the patient-centered model of health care, professionals increasingly acknowledged the centrality of provider communication to the effective integration of patient-centered care.[19] Recognition of a gap between best practices and the abilities and skills of many providers led to calls for more and better training, particularly of physicians.[20] Much as HIPAA attempted to standardize health information, the communication initiatives and resulting reports sought to standardize the communication curricula offered in medical schools. Two of those initiatives were the Kalamazoo Consensus Statement[21,22] in the United States and the Calgary-Cambridge Guide to the Medical Interview[23,24] in Canada. Although they focus primarily on patient-physician communication, they are presented here because their recommendations apply equally to the oral health context and because they identify communication goals and practices that dental professionals should keep in mind, particularly as they initiate relationships and appointments.

Kalamazoo Consensus Statement

A 1999 conference sought to develop a set of essential communication elements to guide curriculum development for medical education on the subject of patient-provider communication. The result was a synthesis of five communication models, articulated as the Kalamazoo Consensus Statement.[21] The statement comprises seven essential elements of patient-provider communication, which generally approximate the steps in a primary care consultation: *(1)* establishing rapport, *(2)* opening discussion, *(3)* gathering information, *(4)* understanding the patient's perspective, *(5)* sharing information, *(6)* reaching agreement on problems and plans, and *(7)* providing closure. Each of the elements includes specific objectives to be met. Therefore, the statement lends itself to checklist format. Indeed, the Kalamazoo Essential Elements Communication Components have been validated and used in medical school communication curricula.[22]

The Kalamazoo Consensus Statement is based on the best available evidence, and its elements should guide dental professionals as well as family practice physicians. Some of these recommendations, however, may be more challenging to implement in a dental consultation than in a primary medical care setting. For instance, the "sharing information" goal of "checks for understanding" is fairly easy for the medical provider to accomplish by simply asking the primary care patient. The dental professional, on the other hand, must plan ahead and check for understanding before beginning work on a patient's mouth or arrange for signals from the patient to indicate understanding during examination or treatment. The eight-step health history interview we propose later in this chapter incorporates principles of the Kalamazoo statement and adapts them to dentistry.

Calgary-Cambridge Guide

About the time the Kalamazoo Consensus Statement was issued in the United States, Canadian researchers were developing and publishing the Calgary-Cambridge Guide to the Medical Interview.[23,24] Their work was also evidence based. The research focused on communication as a skill set comprising three domains: content, process, and perceptual skills. In other words, providers should refine what they say, how they say it, and what they think and feel about it.

To help providers accomplish those goals, the Calgary-Cambridge Guide structures the medical interview in seven steps and indicates the goals to be achieved in each: (1) initiating the session, (2) gathering information, (3) providing structure, (4) building the relationship, (5) explaining and planning, (6) closing the session, and (7) opting for alternatives in explanation and planning. In turn, those goals can be accomplished by 71 specific behaviors (which can be reviewed online; resources are listed at the end of the chapter). For instance, the goal "attending to flow" involves (21) structuring the interview in logical sequence and (22) attending to timing and keeping the interview on task.[25]

The authors of the Calgary-Cambridge Guide acknowledge that the specificity of 71 objectives can intimidate skill-seeking providers, but they emphasize that not all objectives must be used in every patient encounter.[25] Guides such as the Kalamazoo Consensus Statement and the Calgary-Cambridge Guide are most useful when they are integrated into providers' natural communication patterns. Some providers will do this by committing those 71 objectives to memory and applying them in every patient encounter. Providers unfamiliar with US culture and those who struggle with English may need to take a more rigorous approach. Others with long experience as patients in the United States and with good communication skills may need only to remember the basic elements of a successful clinical interview. The Common Ground Instrument integrates the Kalamazoo and Calgary skills into an assessment measure that can serve as a simpler guide to exemplary communication (Box 7-3).

Box 7-3	**Exemplary interview skills from the Common Ground Global Rating Guide***

1. **Rapport building:** Demonstrates rapport-building skills such that most patients would subsequently go out of their way to tell friends or family about this interviewer with extraordinary interpersonal skills. Usually includes two or more elements of "positive speak" and expressions of nonverbal interest that are exceptionally warm.

2. **Agenda setting:** Explores complete agenda at the beginning until the point that the patient says, "Nothing else." If there are several agenda items, prioritizes among them. Explores for additional agenda at end.

3. **Information management:** Begins interview with open-ended question and non-directed facilitation. Continues in this mode (with occasional closed-ended points of clarification) until most/all of the patient's information about the condition has been expressed. Performs appropriate summary. Asks appropriate focused (closed) questions toward the end.

4. **Active listening to understand the patient's perspective on illness:** Very effective at identifying the patient's perspective on illness (PPI) (ie, what the patient thinks may be going on, the greatest concern about the problem, and the expectation for the visit). The PPI is repeatedly explored using active listening to understand the meaning behind the patient's "clues." Once the PPI is disclosed, these elements are acknowledged, normalized, and used as part of a plan to address the diagnosis and the PPI.

5. **Addressing feelings:** Responds to all opportunities to address feelings. When the patient expresses a feeling, these are acknowledged, normalized, or legitimized and are addressed with a follow-up, which at least explores how the patient would like these feelings to be addressed. Also seeks out the "potential feelings" when situations with high likelihood of feelings surface in the interview.

6. **Reaching common ground:** Works very effectively at bridging differences between the interviewer and the patient. Requires a full exploration of the PPI and use of the PPI to reach common ground. Uses a number of the more effective skills in reaching common ground (eg, full exploration of the PPI, decision analysis, reframing, patient-centered suggestions, criteria setting, brainstorming, compromise). Avoids less effective methods (eg, use of authority, personal appeal, repetition of serious complications). Would likely facilitate a desirable change in behavior toward health.

7. **Overall global rating criteria:** At the level of an experienced clinician who is expert in using all communication skills effectively. Skills demonstrated such that a patient would likely note such skills to friends and family.

*Adapted from Lang et al[26] with permission.

Our experience suggests that providers initially overestimate their ability to effectively communicate during the initiation and interview stages of a consultation. Perhaps they assume that the interaction is a simple conversation, and they never had to study how to carry on a conversation. This is true, but social conversations do not require the same level of attention and goal attainment as patient-provider interviews. The best providers make these exchanges seem like conversations, but their ease with communication has emerged from an early focus on integrating the details into their communication repertoire.

The beginning of a consultation is a period of cognitive overload, as providers complete an appointment with one patient, prepare for another, and attend to clinical details while trying to put patients at ease and elicit necessary information. It is more difficult than it looks. Providers will not consult a checklist when engaging their patients, so at the very least **providers should commit to memory the steps of the process and have a thorough understanding of what to say and do in each step**.

Projecting Professionalism

First impressions presumably matter no less in professional encounters than in personal ones, but little research has been conducted on the significance of the initial encounter with a patient. As discussed in chapter 2, individuals hold various preconceptions and stereotypes regarding dentists. Dental professionals can assume that adults who arrive at a dental office have positive expectations that eclipse the negative ones. A selection bias operates to keep the anti-dentistry individuals away—at least until their pain is more intense than their fear or dislike of dentistry. (Children are a different story, as they are usually compelled to visit the dentist.) The selection bias works in favor of dental professionals. Patients arrive with the positive expectation that dentistry and dental providers can help them. From a communication perspective, the primary task of the initial encounter is simple: Do nothing that will undermine patients' initial positive regard toward providers.[27]

Whether providers are meeting patients for the first time or greeting returning patients, the key to sustaining patients' positive regard is professionalism. Professionalism is a concept increasingly attracting the attention of both boards and researchers in the health community.[28,29] The concept has also drawn attention within the dental field of medicine, including both discussions and disputes over what constitutes professionalism.[30–33] Masella,[34] for instance, perceived an American focus on profit as undermining professionalism in dental education and dentistry. Profit and professionalism should not conflict; the former should be a consequence of the latter.

Brosky et al[4] examined patient perceptions of professionalism in dentistry and defined **professionalism** as "an image that will promote a successful relationship with the patient." That image is expressed through communication, including both the appearance and behavior of health care providers. Initial patient encounters profoundly influence the patient-provider relationship and determine patient responses in four interrelated areas: trust, anxiety, adherence, and loyalty.

Patient trust

Trust in the health care provider may be more important in predicting use of services than satisfaction with the provider.[35] Initial patient trust may be affected more by the way dental professionals act than the way they dress. A 2005 randomized experiment found that pharmacists' communication performance was the most important determinant of patients' trust in a pharmacist.[36] Somewhat surprisingly, trust was unrelated to the pharmacists' dress (casual, business casual, or formal) or the presence of a white coat. Whether these findings hold for dental professionals has not been reported, but they suggest that dental professionals' communication behavior should project credibility from the very first encounter.

Credibility suggests the level of trust a patient places in the provider. Although providers cannot directly manipulate patients' trust, they can monitor their own expression of three characteristics that elicit trust: competence, charisma, and character.[37,38] Competence is a significant predictor of attraction in interpersonal relationships and is expressed both verbally and nonverbally.[39] Diplomas and other credentials on an operatory wall enhance perceptions of competence, but providers also express competence by projecting clinical confidence—that is, they act like they know what they are doing. Competent providers avoid surprises by preparing for the appointment. They know where their equipment and implements are, scan the patient file before meeting patients, and speak with authority, in both what they say and how they say it. Charisma encompasses enthusiasm and likeability and is largely expressed nonverbally. Expressive and extroverted providers are more attractive to patients.[40] Character comprises patients' perceptions of provider honesty and impartiality.[41,42] In a dental context, character is primarily a function of message content: Providers should avoid saying anything that suggests they have any motive other than the well-being of patients.

Activity 7-2

Speaking authoritatively takes practice. Have a group or an individual give you a topic you know little about (eg, growing roses or cleaning a carburetor). Try speaking authoritatively on the subject for 2 minutes. You and your audience should judge how authoritatively you spoke. Consider content performance: the number of times you said "uh," "I think...," or "I've heard...." Consider nonverbal performance: what you did with your hands and eyes and the tone of your voice. Try the activity again, speaking on a dental topic you know well. Is it easier to project authority when you are familiar with the topic? Can you fake it when you are unfamiliar with the topic? Should you?

Patient anxiety

Even if patient trust is unrelated to provider dress, what providers wear may be related to other patient responses. The anxiety level of some patients may be affected by the attire of dental providers.[4] A 2007 study of British patients found that they prefer that dentists dress more formally and wear white laboratory coats or tunics.[43] A majority also endorsed the wearing of safety glasses and face masks, which older American patients may remember as once being optional. Shulman and Brehm[44] found that a majority of American patients have similar preferences and also strongly prefer the use of plastic barriers for infection control. Such obvious infection-control measures likely reduce patient anxiety.

Both studies[43,44] also reported that patients prefer that providers wear name tags. All patients—and especially anxious patients—are processing unfamiliar information during a dental visit, and they may easily forget the names of various providers. Name tags fix this problem.

Name tags might also clarify the jobs of different providers. Clarifying the various jobs of individuals on the dental team is important to patients and may alleviate anxiety. Years ago, nearly all dentists were male and nearly all hygienists were female, so patients knew who did what. Fortunately, gender no longer determines job assignment, but patients therefore need help knowing who is who. A 2010 study found that 67% of patients prefer that dentists wear white coats, and 63% of those with that preference believe that the coat aids in identification of the dentist.[45] The researchers found, however, that the preference for a white coat is much more prevalent in older patients than in younger ones.

As patient cohorts age in coming decades, preferences for dress may change. Dental professionals should continually assess issues of patient satisfaction in their practice, including perceptions of professional attire, and exceed in formality the preferences of a majority of patients. The reason is simple: Patients with lower expectations are unlikely to be offended by more formal dress, but those with higher expectations are more likely to be offended by casual dress. Some patients may also attach infection-control significance to the white coat (or any other protective clinic gown), so the coat must be kept clean. One study found that 15.7% of coats worn by dentists were dirty, and a dirty coat does nothing to alleviate patient anxiety.[46] The use of disposable clinic coats is becoming an increasingly used substitute for the white coat and facilitates the usage of clean clinic apparel.

What hygienists and dental assistants should wear is less clear. A study of patients' first impressions of nurses indicates that patients prefer the white pant uniform with stethoscope—a uniform that simultaneously reinforces clinical competency while distinguishing the nurse from the physician.[47] We recommend that hygienists wear scrubs to likewise project an image of competency while avoiding patient confusion about their role. Hurley-Trailor,[48] however, disagrees about distinguishing dental roles through dress. She recommends a dental office dress code in which everyone wears scrubs or everyone wears coats. To project professionalism, she says professionals should avoid scrubs in red and unflattering pastels and scrubs that sport animal or cartoon characters. Juvenile imagery on scrubs might be appropriate in a pediatric dentistry practice but might increase anxiety among adult patients.

Patient adherence

In keeping with the patient-centered health care model, **patient compliance** is now called **patient adherence** to better reflect the shift from provider-ordered treatment to a treatment plan developed together by the patient and provider. As in any collaboration, communication matters. Although communication during the treatment plan presentation is particularly salient to adherence (and is addressed in a later chapter), the evidence suggests that provider communication earlier in the appointment might also affect patient adherence.[49] For instance, the patient-provider working alliance is significantly and positively associated with patient adherence.[50] Such alliances do not begin after the examination but rather begin (or falter) when the provider and patient first meet.

Among patients who are members of racial and ethnic minorities, being treated with dignity is significantly associated with adherence.[51] Treating patients with dignity involves a patient-centered approach that acknowledges patients' concerns, respects their time and intelligence, and defers to their treatment decisions. In addition, a 2008 study filtered out the content of providers' speech to determine the impact of the tone of voice.[52] Those researchers determined that patient adherence is significantly associated with vocal affect—speaking in a tone expressing empathy, concern, or humor, as appropriate to the context.

Perhaps due to the importance of patient behaviors between appointments, much of the adherence research focuses on orthodontics.[53] A 1996 study found that patient adherence is significantly associated with two orthodontist behaviors. Adherence is positively related to provider politeness and negatively related to provider criticism of patients' teeth or oral health habits.[54] In short, establishing a positive patient-provider relationship from the beginning can positively influence clinical outcomes by enhancing patient adherence.

Question of ethics: Patients do not like to be criticized by their dental providers. This is unsurprising, since most people do not appreciate negative comments about their behavior, practices, or character. A provider who minimizes criticism will be better liked and achieve better treatment adherence from patients. Yet the oral health practices and habits of some patients are egregious. Consider the teenager who wants a large tongue stud or the parent who fills a child's sippy cup with sugary soda. Is it ethical not to criticize such behaviors? What are the alternatives to criticism? In such cases, would these alternatives be more effective than criticism?

Patient loyalty

New patients never become loyal patients if the initial consultation goes so poorly that they never return. Establishing new relationships involves effort from both patients and providers. Patients prefer long-term relationships. Returning to the same dental provider reduces uncertainty, reduces paperwork, and reduces embarrassment and effort in disclosing personal health history information. Patients select providers they believe offer prospects for a long-term relationship, and patients want to be loyal. This is the good news for providers: Patients want to like their dentist.

To cultivate patient fondness, providers should act likeable and approachable. A study of patient loyalty by Holt and McHugh[55] suggested specific ways to do that. Pain control and safety consciousness are "very important" determinants of loyalty, but the most important is expression of care and attention (reported by 90% of respondents). Another very important determinant is putting the patient at ease.

The verbal and nonverbal behaviors prescribed in earlier chapters are means of expressing care and attention, and they tend to put the patient at ease. The importance of engaging in such behaviors from the very beginning cannot be overstated. Research indicates that communication performance determines patient satisfaction, which in turn influences loyalty.[56] In short, if, through their clinical and communication skills, providers are able to achieve patient loyalty, they should find themselves treating satisfied patients.

Health History Communication Strategies

The twin goals of the first phase of every routine dental consultation are to initiate the encounter on a positive footing and to gather a comprehensive and accurate health history. This phase corresponds to the first four of the Kalamazoo Consensus Statement's seven steps: establishing rapport, opening discussion, gathering information, and understanding the patient's perspective of illness. The Calgary-Cambridge Guide prescribes seven steps for conducting the medical interview. Using these evidence-based guides, we have developed an eight-step framework for the oral health interview (Box 7-4).

Our framework could be elaborated with very detailed instructions regarding what to say and how to say it for every moment of the encounter, but we have instead attempted a more practical guide. We have reduced the instructions to essential steps, with two or three strategies for each step. Providers should be able to recall the framework from memory until it becomes habitual. Providers who feel they need more detailed guidance, however, should consult the Calgary-Cambridge Guide and the resources listed at the end of this chapter.

Box 7-4	Eight steps of the initial patient interview

Step 1: Greet the patient
- Smile.
- Shake hands and make eye contact.
- Exchange names using proper pronunciation and title.

Step 2: Establish rapport
- Introduce neutral topics.
- Listen more than you speak.
- Contribute appropriate personal disclosures.

Step 3: Structure the appointment
- State the purpose of the appointment.
- Preview the phases of the appointment.
- Confirm patient expectations for the appointment.

Step 4: Provide rationale and review
- Preview the type of questions you will ask.
- Explain why you need accurate answers.
- Solicit corrections, questions, and clarifications from the patient.

Step 5: Ask key health history update questions
- Ask first about the chief complaint.
- Ask the eight key update questions (see Box 7-7).
- Follow up answers that trigger concern.
- Verify and update any other health conditions documented in the patient's comprehensive health history that are not included in the eight health history update questions.

Step 6: Check patient understanding
- Ask if the patient has any questions or needs explanation.
- Observe the patient's verbal and nonverbal signals.

Step 7: Summarize health history findings
- Briefly review answers to key questions.
- Close with, "Is that correct?" and "Do you have any questions?"

Step 8: Structure the next step of the appointment
- State what will happen next with transition words.
- Avoid initiating words such as *start* or *begin*.

Step 1: Greet the patient

Depending on the procedures adopted in the specific practice, the provider may greet the patient in the waiting room or in the operatory. If greeting a patient in the waiting room, the provider should first determine which patient has the appointment (if the patient is not recognized) and then face the patient when greeting. Calling out a patient's name across a waiting room is disrespectful, and hard-of-hearing patients may not hear it. After the waiting room greeting, the provider should escort the patient to the operatory, walking side by side if possible, and invite the patient to sit in the chair.

Whether in the waiting room or the operatory, the provider should always enter the room with a smile.[57] Smiling will not come naturally during all points of a busy day, and some patients may inspire dread rather than enthusiasm, but a provider's smile will improve the chances that the ensuing consultation will be a positive experience for both provider and patient.[58]

In keeping with the SMILES approach (see chapter 6), the provider should always shake hands and establish eye contact with the patient. A brief verbal greeting (eg, "Hello" or "Good morning") is also appropriate. A 2007 study found that 78.1% of patients want the provider to shake their hand in greeting.[59] Older patients expect it as a sign of courtesy.[60] Younger patients appreciate it as a sign of respect. Anxious patients may be comforted by the contact.[61] The handshake, moreover, is a nonverbal expression of the mutuality and collaboration to which patient-centered health care aspires.

Any physical contact, of course, is an infection risk. Therefore, the provider should wash his or her hands in view of the patient at some point before putting on gloves. Although gloves offer protection, witnessing hand washing reassures the patient that infection control is a priority. Increasingly, the use of hand sanitizer is accepted as a substitute for hand washing, and it should also be used in view of the patient.

The final communication strategy involved in the greeting is the exchange of names. The provider should introduce himself or herself when meeting a patient for the first time and on return visits for a patient with memory deficits (eg, Alzheimer disease or dementia). Most patients want providers to introduce themselves using first and last names.[59] We suggest that the provider include a job title and any preference about how he or she is addressed by the patient. These preferences may vary based on the patient's age. For instance, the provider might say, "I'm Jack Milton, your hygienist. You can call me Jack." For a young patient, the provider might say, "I'm Sally Washington, your dentist. You can call me Dr Sally." However, some patients prefer to use *Doctor* rather than call dentists by their first name.[62]

What are the advantages of being on a given-name basis with patients? What are the advantages of having patients call you by your title and last name? Develop a policy for what patients should call you. Your policy should accommodate your preferences, patient preferences, and demographic or cultural differences. For instance, younger dentists may decide to use *Doctor* to emphasize their clinical competence. Compare your policy with the policies developed by your colleagues.

Patients prefer that doctors call them by their given name, although the preference is not a strong one.[63–65] The given name is typically the first name, but many patients prefer diminutives (Johnny for John or Terry for Teresa), and many patients use their middle name rather than their first name. In the first meeting, the provider should clarify what the patient prefers to be called. Otherwise, the provider might call a patient "Sam" for years before learning everyone else calls him "George." (People may be too intimidated to correct those in authority, such as dentists and teachers.)

Traditionally, all adults were called by their title and surname. Adults granted permission to use their first name only after a close long-term relationship had been established. People are far less formal today, but no research addresses what other members of the dental team should call patients. We suggest that the hygienist or assistant use a title for a patient who is significantly (20 or more years) older than the staff member. The patient may then request use of his or her given name, which should be respected. A patient in the provider's age range or younger should be called by the given name.

Step 2: Establish rapport

In the rapport-building step, the provider should implement the remaining SMILES strategies (see chapter 6): inclining toward the patient, lowering the hands, maintaining eye contact, and sitting. Patient-provider rapport entails three components: mutual attentiveness, positivity, and coordination.[66] The relative importance of these components shifts over the course of the relationship; positivity and attentiveness are more important in newer relationships, and coordination and attentiveness are more important to long-standing relationships.

A study of physician consultations indicated that patient satisfaction is associated with rapport during the interview phase but not during the actual examination phase of the appointment.[67] In addition, rapport is encouraged by a focus on social themes—neutral topics—rather than on clinical information.[68] Such findings suggest that patients expect an initial conversation with providers to touch on neutral topics before switching to the medical topics that constitute the purpose of the appointment.[69] Skipping the neutral topics may save time, but it also may leave patients feeling like specimens or experimental subjects, of interest only for the information and insurance payments they can provide.

The provider can initiate rapport by introducing a neutral topic with a new patient or returning to a neutral topic discussed with a returning patient. Neutral topics are simply those that do not invite strong opinions; in other words, small talk.[70] The weather is the prototypical neutral topic, and it is a reliable topic when nothing is known about a patient, because everyone has experience with weather. Other neutral topics can be introduced to test whether they are relevant to the specific patient: hometowns, pets, sports teams, cooking or food, traffic or road construction, parking challenges at the dental office, and plans for upcoming holidays. The provider should develop a short mental list of neutral topics that fit the interest of the provider and most patients. The provider should not, for instance, ask about a favorite sports team if he or she does not follow sports. The ensuing conversation would be brief.

When reestablishing rapport with a returning patient, a good practice is to note a topic or question for the ensuing visit in the patient's record. For instance, following a routine examination, the provider might note, "Ask pt abt Nov trip to Cozumel." Keeping track of a single personal detail like this is easy, and the patient will be enormously appreciative of the effort.

For rapport to succeed, it must contain an element of the personal. During rapport building, the provider should listen more than talk. Doing so will help build trust and balance the relationship, because the provider will do nearly all the talking during the clinical examination or procedure. The provider should introduce topics, actively listen to responses, and contribute appropriate personal disclosures, such as, "You are from Metropolis? I have an aunt who lives there."

A study on provider disclosure found that only 34% of encounters with new patients involve provider disclosures.[71] In disclosing information, the provider should carefully consider the implications of the disclosure. Acknowledgment by the provider that he or she underwent a specific dental procedure, for instance, could be interpreted by the patient as evidence that it is a superior treatment choice. Disclosure that the provider just bought an expensive car could confirm the stereotype that dentists are greedy.

The rapport-building step need not go on for long. One study found that 40 seconds is adequate to reduce patient anxiety, so 1 or 2 minutes of small talk should be sufficient to cultivate a relationship.[72]

Activity 7-4

Interview someone whose job entails meeting new patients or clients. Health care professionals, hair stylists, insurance agents, and massage therapists are common examples. Ask them how they establish rapport. What do they talk about? How do they handle those who talk very little? Do they ever struggle to maintain boundaries between the professional and the personal? Do they have stories of conversations that went horribly wrong? What advice do they have for you?

Step 3: Structure the appointment

The third step of the oral health history phase consists of only one or two sentences that indicate the purpose of the appointment and how it will proceed. At this point we should emphasize the function of redundancy in communicating with the dental patient. Providers often overestimate how much information their patients understand and retain for later recall. Along with providing written information, repeating information is a very effective way to ensure patients understand what services will be or have been provided. The amount of unfamiliar information coupled with patient anxiety is a recipe for misunderstanding and forgetting, two unfortunate outcomes with significant ramifications for informed consent, treatment planning, treatment adherence, and payment. Therefore, the advice offered to students in public speaking courses can be adapted for dental professionals as well: Tell patients what you are going to say, say it, and then tell them what you said. This much repetition will seem unnatural to most providers, who find the information routine and the repetition tedious. Nevertheless, it is crucial to patient understanding and satisfaction.

When 1 or 2 minutes of rapport building have taken place, the provider should transition to the clinical topic by stating the purpose of the appointment: "Well, today you are here for an amalgam filling in one of your back teeth. Is that what you were expecting for today's appointment?" On occasion, such a brief statement will bring to light errors in scheduling when the provider discovers that the patient is there for an altogether different procedure.

The opening statement should be followed by a brief overview of the stages of the appointment: "First we'll verify your health history, then we'll apply the anesthesia and complete the filling, and then we'll schedule your follow-up." Although such information seems routine for the dentist, and although a returning patient may understand how appointments are structured, previewing what will happen is a way to alleviate the patient's anxiety and make the patient feel a part of the dental team. If this step is omitted, the patient can feel like a mouth to be worked on rather than a person involved in his or her own oral health care.

Step 4: Provide rationale and review

The patient's health history involves three types of self-report communication. The first is the health history form, which patients (or their literate companions) usually complete in the waiting room or online before arriving at the dental office. The second is the health history interview, which involves a comprehensive questioning of new patients to establish a patient record. The third is a health history update, which is an abbreviated interview administered to returning patients to ensure that the record reflects the patient's current health status, prescription medications, and so on.

Self-reports of health behaviors and treatments are subject to faulty memory and misrepresentation, so a great deal of attention has been focused on enhancing the reliability and validity of oral health history forms and interviews.[73–77] Comprehensive health histories include questions on sensitive subjects that patients may perceive as incriminating or irrelevant to dentistry. For instance, one study found that the health history form correctly identified only 57.4% of adolescents who smoke daily.[78]

The portability of health records promised by HIPAA may enhance the accuracy of health history information, but self-reports will remain the primary source of information. Providing a rationale to the patient for collecting such health data can reduce misrepresentation, even if it does not correct poor memory. The rationale includes standard components, so the provider should develop wording that sounds natural and rehearse delivering it in a conversational manner (Box 7-5). To incorporate redundancy, the provider should begin by stating that the health history questions are coming up. Next, a rationale should explain why seemingly irrelevant information is necessary and why questions duplicate what the patient reported on the health history form. Without such a rationale, the patient may feel that his or her health history form was completely ignored, so the provider should explicitly state that the same questions that the patient answered in writing will be asked again in order to be absolutely sure the information is correct. If the provider neglects to provide this rationale, the patient may become frustrated or suspicious of provider competency.

The final three components seek patient input. First, the patient should be allowed to ask questions regarding the health history and to receive truthful answers. Second, the patient should be encouraged to alter or add information on the health history form. If the patient changes any answers, the provider must refrain from criticism or reprimand. Disclosing sensitive health information is deeply personal, and the patient may legitimately fear social disapproval, canceled insurance policies, or legal action if he or she answers truthfully. The patient must be assured that in the medical context of the dental practice, his or her information will not be misused. Third, the patient should be asked to clarify positive responses on the health history form. Such forms often lack nuance and often use medical language a patient does not understand. Talking through positive responses is a way to clear up misunderstandings on the part of the patient or provider and to gain more accurate information.

| Box 7-5 | Steps of rationale and review for the health history |

1. State what you are going to do.
"I am going to ask you some questions about your general health."

2. State why it is important.
"This information is important to us as we provide dental care for you. Many patients are not aware that their general health status can affect their oral health and some oral conditions are indicative of general health problems. In addition, some medications we routinely use may interact with drugs you are currently taking. This includes any over-the-counter drugs or drugs prescribed for you or others. Do the best you can at remembering the names of the drugs and how much you take."

3. Ask for questions or concerns.
"What questions can I answer for you?"

4. Allow the patient to review the health history.
"Please look over your health history form and make any adjustments or additions to give the most accurate report on your health."

5. Clarify positive responses on the health history form.
"You indicated you have high blood pressure and hepatitis C. Now do you simply carry the hepatitis C virus, or do you actually have acute hepatitis C with symptoms?"

[Note: Diabetes, asthma, seizure disorders, and other chronic health conditions are not included in the eight recommended health history update questions but are important to verfiy, and appropriate follow-up questions are essential.]

Step 5: Ask key health history update questions

The number and nature of questions asked during the health history interview and health history update may vary depending on the reason for the visit, the amount and type of information already collected in the patient's records, and the patient's responses on the health history form. The initial health history interview of a new patient should be more comprehensive than the health history update for a returning patient. The interview closely tracks whatever health history form the practice uses. The health history update, on the other hand, focuses mainly on changes in the patient's health and medications since the previous visit and verfies important health information that ensures patient safety during and after treatment.

If the appointment is anything other than a routine cleaning and examination, the chief complaint was likely stated in the purpose for the appointment (step 3). If not, the provider should first confirm the patient's chief complaint or presenting problem. The provider should determine answers to questions on complaints, pain, and soreness, if those answers are not already known (Box 7-6).

Box 7-6	Questions about complaints, pain, and soreness

- Could you tell me more about what's been happening?
- Do you associate the [name symptom] with anything you were doing when you first noticed it?
- Is the [name symptom] getting better, worse, or staying the same?
- Has the [name symptom] changed?
- Has anything made it better?
- How has this affected your daily routine? Your leisure hours? Your sleep?
- Who have you seen about this condition?
- Have you ever had an injury to your head or neck?
- Have you ever been in a motor vehicle accident?
- Where does it hurt? Is it localized or does it spread? Where does it spread to?
- What is the character of the pain? Sharp, shooting, dull, burning, pressure, stabbing, throbbing?
- When does it hurt? All the time or episodically? Time of day? How long does it hurt?
- What seems to bring on the pain? What makes it worse or makes it better?
- What have you done to try to relieve the pain?

When all details regarding the chief complaint are documented, the provider should then address the eight health history update questions (Box 7-7). Research documents a strong relationship between encouraging communication behaviors, such as signals of active listening, and patient participation in the exchange (eg, quantity of speech and length of answers).[79] Therefore, the provider should attend to the nonverbal signals he or she is giving while asking questions, such as engaging in eye contact, nodding, and affirming backchannels.[80] The provider should avoid nonverbal expressions of doubt, surprise, or disapproval and instead aim for a tone of clinical interest. All verbal and nonverbal messages sent by the provider should aim to encourage the patient to provide accurate and thorough answers.

Box 7-7	Eight key questions in the health history update

1. Have there been any changes in your health or medical history since [date of last update]?
2. When did you last see a physician?
3. Have you been treated at a hospital or same-day surgery center since your last visit here on [date of last update]?
4. Are you currently taking any prescribed or over-the-counter medication? Over-the-counter medication includes items such as pain medications, vitamins, and herbal remedies.
5. Do you regularly or occasionally use tobacco products? Do you regularly or occasionally use alcohol? Do you regularly or occasionally use recreational drugs?
6. Are you aware of any medications that you are allergic to or are unable to take?
7. Has a physician ever told you that you have any problems with your heart?
8. Is there anything else about your health that we have not discussed?

Regarding question content, question 2 asks for a numeric response and the other seven key questions require a *yes* or *no* response. The wording of the key questions should remain consistent to enhance accuracy (ie, validity and reliability). Patients often provide inaccurate self-reports. One study compared patient self-reports of wearing orthodontic headgear with accurate electronic recordings of wear.[81] For nearly one-third of patients, the accuracy of self-report was less than 59%.

Methods for enhancing the accuracy of self-reports are listed in Box 7-8. The provider should be careful to avoid double-barreled questions. For instance, "Do you brush and floss every day?" invites a *yes* or *no* response, but a *no* response could have multiple meanings: The patient does one, or the other, or both but not every day. Similarly, accuracy can be undermined through leading questions. The patient perceives the provider as having both power and authority, so leading questions can cause the patient to agree in order to please the provider. For instance, "You don't chew tobacco, do you?" nudges the patient to provide a negative response. The patient may feel that a positive response to such a leading question would contradict the provider.

Box 7-8	Strategies to enhance interview accuracy

- Ask every patient the same questions.
- Use scripted key questions.
- Ensure that questions mean the same thing to every patient.
- Maintain complete wording.
- Avoid multiple or double-barreled questions.
- Avoid leading questions.
- Vary the interview with closed and open follow-up questions.

The key update questions are gateway questions. Questions the patient responds "yes" to will require follow-up questions. If the patient indicates that he or she has visited a physician, hospital, or surgery center, the provider will want to know who the patient saw, why the patient went, what the diagnosis was, and what treatment was prescribed and/or implemented.

The provider should also ask about usage of tobacco products, alcohol, and recreational drugs and ask a question about each separately. Screening for alcohol use is inconsistent on oral health history forms, even though moderate alcohol use significantly increases the risk of oral and pharyngeal cancer and even though the majority of patients do not mind the screening questions.[82–84] The provider should also remain aware that the distinction between prescription and illicit drugs is an ambiguous one, as the former can be more addictive than the latter. Further, a patient who has experience with addiction or recovery may view addiction as an illness and therefore may be less sensitive to these questions than the provider might assume.

Regardless of the number and type of follow-up questions that the key update questions trigger, the final question should always be, "Is there anything else about your health that we have not discussed?" Barrier et al[85] suggested that the two words that can instantly improve patient-provider communication are, "Anything else?" The authors correctly noted that the three purposes of the health history phase of the appointment are information gathering, relationship building, and patient education. The "anything else" question ostensibly aims at information gathering, but it likewise builds the relationship by showing that the provider is interested in the patient's input.

The question also educates the patient by indicating the importance of health information to clinical practice and may jog the patient's memory about health information that may not have been directly addressed in the health history update.

Step 6: Check patient understanding

After the health history form has been updated and confirmed and after all the interview or update questions have been asked, the provider should ask whether the patient would like to pose any questions: "I want to be sure that we understand things in the same way. Is there anything I could clarify for you? Is there anything additional that you want to ask me?" The provider can adapt the phrasing as long as the patient understands that he or she now has an opportunity to elicit information and can reduce patient reluctance to ask questions by indicating that questions are expected.

When the patient responds, the provider should observe the patient's verbal and nonverbal signals for indications of misunderstanding or reluctance to question. If the patient says that he or she understands and has no further questions, but tone and expression suggest that the patient may be holding back, the provider should gently press for elaboration: "I'm getting the sense you are a little unsure about something. Are you sure I can't clear anything up for you?"

Step 7: Summarize health history findings

The interview or update should conclude with a summary of the information collected. The provider should begin with a redundant preview of the summary: "I am going to summarize all of the health history information to make sure I have correctly interpreted all that we have discussed." Then, the provider should summarize the indicators of good health before listing the conditions and medications disclosed on the health history form. Even if the patient is healthy, the provider should summarize answers to the eight key questions:

> After updating your medical history and asking about how you are currently feeling, it appears you are in good health. As I understand, there have been no changes in your health. You are not under the care of a physician. You are not taking any medications. You have not been treated in a same-day surgery center, and you are not allergic to any medication.

It is most important that the provider strive for accuracy, as the patient may interpret an inaccurate summary as evidence that a provider is not listening.[86] The provider should conclude this step with another request for confirmation: "Is that correct? Do you have any questions?" Such statements provide closure and allow for a smooth transition to the final step.

Step 8: Structure the next step of the appointment

The final step is, by now, a familiar one. The provider should tell the patient what is going to happen next. Typically, this will entail a description of the next procedures. The provider should use transition words and phrases such as, "We will continue with your care by administering the anesthesia," and avoid initiating words such as *start* or *begin*. If the provider says, "Now we will begin," the effect is to diminish or negate the importance of the conversation and health history efforts that have already taken place. The health history phase is an integral part of treatment; the provider must appreciate this fact and hone his or her initiating and interviewing skills if the patient is to fully appreciate how important open and accurate communication is to effective oral health care.

Chapter Checklist ✓

HIPAA Privacy Rule
- ❏ Understand that the Privacy Rule prescribes the parameters and legal requirements for discussing, documenting, and distributing the protected health information of patients.
- ❏ Understand that the Privacy Rule has changed patients' expectations regarding privacy and access to their health information.
- ❏ Minimize the amount of protected health information shared.
- ❏ Minimize the number of people with whom protected information is shared.
- ❏ Document everything that is shared and with whom.
- ❏ Know what information is considered protected health information.
- ❏ Caveat: Write privacy notices at a level the patient can understand.
- ❏ Caveat: Minimize exposure of others to protected information (eg, by lowering your voice and closing doors).
- ❏ Caveat: Use professional judgment when disclosing information in the presence of others.
- ❏ Provision: Understand that the patient has a right to access to, to obtain copies of, to request corrections to, and to restrict use of his or her protected health information.
- ❏ Provision: Acknowledge that the patient has a right to file a complaint for Privacy Rule violations.
- ❏ Provision: Give the patient written disclosure of privacy rights.
- ❏ Provision: Post a copy of privacy rights and practices in every office and on any website.
- ❏ Provision: Implement HIPAA privacy and security measures.
- ❏ Provision: Designate a privacy officer.
- ❏ Provision: Undergo training in HIPAA privacy and security measures.
- ❏ Provision: Identify and contract with specific business associates who will have access to patient data.
- ❏ Provision: Develop consent forms documenting patient preferences regarding use of protected health information, and ask if the patient wishes to authorize release of his or her health information to anyone else, such as a spouse or other family members.
- ❏ Patient expectations: Prepare to explain security measures to the patient.
- ❏ Patient expectations: Provide information cheerfully.

Common Ground exemplary interview skills
❑ Rapport building: Use positive verbal communication.
❑ Rapport building: Use warm expressions of nonverbal interest.
❑ Agenda setting: Explore the patient's agenda until the patient says "Nothing else."
❑ Agenda setting: Prioritize agenda items.
❑ Agenda setting: Explore for additional agenda items at the end of the agenda-setting phase.
❑ Information management: Begin with open-ended questions and nondirected facilitation.
❑ Information management: Continue (with occasional closed-ended questions for clarification) until all information about the condition has been expressed.
❑ Information management: Appropriately summarize.
❑ Information management: Ask focused closed-ended questions toward the end.
❑ Active listening to the patient's perspective on illness: Identify what the patient thinks is going on, the patient's greatest concern, and the patient's expectations for the visit.
❑ Active listening to the patient's perspective on illness: Explore the patient's perspective on illness using active listening.
❑ Active listening to the patient's perspective on illness: Acknowledge, normalize, and use the patient's perspective on illness as part of a plan to address the medical diagnosis.
❑ Addressing feelings: Acknowledge, normalize, and legitimize the patient's expressed feelings.
❑ Addressing feelings: Address feelings with a follow-up, which may explore how the patient wants feelings to be addressed.
❑ Addressing feelings: Seek out potential feelings when they are likely to surface in the interview.
❑ Reaching common ground: Work to bridge differences with the patient.
❑ Reaching common ground: Fully explore the patient's perspective on illness and use it to reach common ground.
❑ Reaching common ground: Use effective skills like decision analysis, reframing, patient-centered suggestions, criteria setting, brainstorming, and compromise.
❑ Reaching common ground: Avoid ineffective skills like use of authority, personal appeal, and repetition of serious complications.

Professionalism
❑ Do nothing to undermine the patient's initial positive regard.
❑ Trust: Communicate credibility from the first encounter.
❑ Trust: Express competence by projecting clinical confidence.
❑ Trust: Enhance attractiveness by being expressive and extroverted.
❑ Trust: Avoid saying anything suggesting that you have any motive other than patient well-being.
❑ Anxiety: The dentist should dress more formally and wear a clinic coat or gown.
❑ Anxiety: The hygienist should wear scrubs of a solid color.
❑ Anxiety: Communicate infection control by wearing safety glasses, face masks, and plastic barriers and by daily cleaning or disposing of clinic coats.
❑ Anxiety: Wear a name tag.
❑ Adherence: Treat the patient with dignity and respect.
❑ Adherence: Speak in a tone expressing empathy, concern, or humor.
❑ Adherence: Be polite and avoid criticism.

❑ Adherence: Express care and attention.
❑ Adherence: Communicate concern about pain control and safety consciousness.
❑ Loyalty: Put the patient at ease.

Health history communication strategies
❑ Greet the patient: Face the patient and smile.
❑ Greet the patient: Shake hands and make eye contact.
❑ Greet the patient: Exchange greetings, offer your first and last name, and explain your role in the patient's care.
❑ Greet the patient: Address the patient by first and last name, using a title when appropriate, and verify the correct pronunciation and how the patient prefers to be addressed.
❑ Greet the patient: Escort the patient to the operatory.
❑ Greet the patient: Wash hands or use sanitizer in view of the patient.
❑ Establish rapport: Incline toward the patient, lower your hands, maintain eye contact, and sit.
❑ Establish rapport: Introduce neutral topics or revisit a topic discussed previously.
❑ Establish rapport: Listen more than you speak.
❑ Establish rapport: Contribute appropriate personal disclosures.
❑ Establish rapport: Note a topic or question for the ensuing visit in the patient's record.
❑ Establish rapport: Maintain rapport for 1 or 2 minutes.
❑ Structure the appointment: State the purpose of the appointment.
❑ Structure the appointment: Preview the phases of the appointment.
❑ Provide rationale and review: State what you are going to do and preview the type of questions you will ask.
❑ Provide rationale and review: Explain why you need accurate answers.
❑ Provide rationale and review: Solicit questions or concerns from the patient.
❑ Provide rationale and review: Allow the patient to review and correct the health history form.
❑ Provide rationale and review: Clarify positive responses on the health history form.
❑ Ask key update questions: Ask first about the chief complaint, if any.
❑ Ask key update questions: Ask the eight key questions.
❑ Key update question 1: Have there been any changes in your health or medical history since [date of last update]?
❑ Key update question 2: When did you last see a physician?
❑ Key update question 3: Have you been treated at a hospital or same-day surgery center since your last visit here on [date of last update]?
❑ Key update question 4: Are you currently taking any prescribed or over-the-counter medications? Over-the-counter includes items such as pain medications, vitamins, and herbal remedies.
❑ Key update question 5: Do you regularly or occasionally use tobacco products? Do you regularly or occasionally use alcohol? Do you regularly or occasionally use recreational drugs?
❑ Key update question 6: Are you aware of any medications that you are allergic to or are unable to take?
❑ Key update question 7: Has a physician ever told you that you have any problems with your heart?

❑ Key update question 8: Is there anything else about your health that we have not discussed?
❑ Ask key update questions: Maintain consistent wording of questions.
❑ Ask key update questions: Attend to nonverbal signals.
❑ Ask key update questions: Maintain a tone of clinical interest.
❑ Ask key update questions: Follow up on answers that trigger concern.
❑ Check patient understanding: Ask if the patient has any questions or needs explanation.
❑ Check patient understanding: Observe the patient's verbal and nonverbal signals.
❑ Summarize health history: Tell the patient that you are going to summarize his or her health status.
❑ Summarize health history: Briefly review the indicators of good health followed by conditions and/or medications disclosed or verified.
❑ Summarize health history: Close with, "Is that correct?" and "What questions do you have for me?"
❑ Structure the next step: State what will happen next with transition words.
❑ Structure the next step: Avoid words such as *start* or *begin*, which may diminish the importance of the interview in the patient's mind.

For More Information

HIPAA
- http://www.hhs.gov/ocr/privacy/hipaa/administrative/privacyrule/index.html
- http://www.aspe.hhs.gov/admnsimp/final/pvcguide1.htm
- http://www.adha.org/resources-docs/7267_HIPAA_Implications_for_Dental_Hygiene.pdf
- http://www.hhs.gov/ocr/privacy/hipaa/understanding/coveredentities/index.html
- http://www.ama-assn.org/ama/pub/physician-resources/solutions-managing-your-practice/coding-billing-insurance/hipaahealth-insurance-portability-accountability-act/hipaa-compliance-resources.page?

Professionalism
- http://acd.org/ethicshandbook.htm
- http://www.adea.org/Pages/Professionalism.aspx
- http://www.jdentaled.org/content/67/8/909.full.pdf
- http://www.pierce.ctc.edu/dept/denthyg/ref/files/dh-competencies.pdf

Kalamazoo Consensus Statement and Calgary-Cambridge Guide
- http://ipepweb.org/wp-content/uploads/2013/10/Essential-elements-communication-Kalamazoo-Consensus.pdf
- http://www.shockmd.com/2009/04/07/cinemeducation-improves-communication-skills-of-residents

- http://www.gp-training.net/training/communication_skills/calgary/guide.htm
- http://www.skillscascade.com/handouts.htm

Establishing rapport
- http://www.nursetogether.com/creating-a-partnership-building-rapport-wit
- http://www.dentalnursenetwork.com/news/dental-nursing-news/235-good-patient-communication-and-rapport-building-skills.html
- http://www.rdhmag.com/index/display/article-display/373065/articles/rdh/volume-30/issue-2/feature/small-talk-big-business.html
- http://www.dentaleconomics.com/articles/print/volume-99/issue-8/columns/comprehensive-case-acceptance/develop-rapport-with-patients.html

Initial consultations
- http://www.dentistryiq.com/articles/2013/06/three-best-practice-management-tips-for-the-new-dental-patient.html
- http://www.mdanderson.org/education-and-research/resources-for-professionals/professional-educational-resources/i-care/complete-library-of-communication-videos/basic-principles.html

Health history
- http://bphc.hrsa.gov/technicalassistance/resourcecenter/clinicalservices/designatedrecordssetprotocol.pdf
- http://dental.pacific.edu/Documents/dental_prof/intrv_sheet.pdf
- http://www.peterjacobsen.com/handouts/index.htm
- http://clinicalskills.machealth.ca/index.php/content/table1
- http://www.dentaleconomics.com/articles/print/volume-100/issue-11/features/preparing-for-the-transition-to-electronic-medical-records.html

References

1. Knapp M. Interpersonal Communication and Human Relationships. Boston: Allyn and Bacon, 1984.
2. Altman I, Taylor D. Social Penetration: The Development of Interpersonal Relationships. New York: Holt, 1973.
3. Marston J. The first five minutes; making the most of a first impression. J Ala Dent Assoc 1993;77(4):40–41.
4. Brosky M, Keefer O, Hodges J, Pesun I, Cook G. Patient perceptions of professionalism in dentistry. J Dent Educ 2003;67:909–915.
5. Price B. First impressions: Paradigms for patient assessment. J Adv Nurs 1987;12:699–705.
6. Gafaranga J, Britten N. "Fire away": The opening sequence in general practice consultations. Fam Pract 2003;20:242–247.
7. Stewart MA. What is a successful doctor-patient interview? A study of interactions and outcomes. Soc Sci Med 1984;19:167–175.
8. Health Insurance Portability and Accountability Act of 1996, Pub L No. 104-191, 110 Stat 1936 (1996). http://www.gpo.gov/fdsys/pkg/PLAW-104publ191/html/PLAW-104publ191.htm. Accessed 12 January 2015.

9. Pai SS, Zimmerman JL. Health Insurance Portability and Accountability Act (HIPAA). Implications for dental practice. Dent Today 2002;21(10):106–111.

10. McLellan TS. Understanding HIPAA: The Health Insurance Portability and Accountability Act. J Mich Dent Assoc 2002;84(3):38–42.

11. Rossi MS. Are you ready for HIPAA? A regulatory primer for dentists. N Y State Dent J 2002;68(7):6–9.

12. Rossi MS. A five-step program for attaining HIPAA compliance. N Y State Dent J 2003;69(2):5–7.

13. Wun C, Dym H. How to implement a HIPAA compliance plan into a practice. Dent Clin North Am 2008;52:669–682.

14. Standards for Privacy of Individually Identifiable Health Information; Final Rule. Fed Regist 2002;67(157):53181–53273. Codified at 45 CFR parts 160 and 164.

15. US Department of Health and Human Services, Office for Civil Rights. HIPAA Administrative Simplification: Regulation Text. Codified at 45 CFR Parts 160, 162, and 164. Washington, DC: US Department of Health and Human Services, 2013.

16. Ha AT, Gansky SA. HIPAA notice of privacy practices used in U.S. dental schools: Factors related to readability or lack thereof. J Dent Educ 2007;71:419–429.

17. Rosland AM, Piette JD, Choi H, Heisler M. Family and friend participation in primary care visits of patients with diabetes or heart failure: Patient and physician determinants and experiences. Med Care 2011;49:37–45.

18. Walker R. The Health Insurance Portability and Accountability Act: Implications for the dental profession. Dent Clin North Am 2002;46:553–563.

19. Simpson M, Buckman R, Stewart M, et al. Doctor-patient communication: The Toronto consensus statement. BMJ 1991;303:1385–1387.

20. Buyck D, Lang F. Teaching medical communication skills: A call for greater uniformity. Fam Med 2002;34:337–343.

21. Makoul G. Essential elements of communication in medical encounters: The Kalamazoo Consensus Statement. Acad Med 2001;76:390–393.

22. Joyce BL, Steenbergh T, Scher E. Use of the Kalamazoo Essential Elements Communication Checklist (Adapted) in an institutional interpersonal and communication skills curriculum. J Grad Med Educ 2010;2:165–169.

23. Kurtz S, Silverman J, Draper J. Teaching and Learning Communication Skills in Medicine, ed 2. Abingdon, England: Radcliffe Medical Press, 2004.

24. Kurtz SM. Doctor-patient communication: Principles and practices. Can J Neurol Sci 2002;29(suppl 2):S23–S29.

25. Kurtz S, Silverman J, Benson J, Draper J. Marrying content and process in clinical method teaching: Enhancing the Calgary-Cambridge guides. Acad Med 2003;78:802–809.

26. Lang F, McCord R, Harvill L, Anderson D. Communication assessment using the Common Ground Instrument: Psychometric properties. Fam Med 2004;36:189–198.

27. Newsome PRH, Wright GH. Qualitative techniques to investigate how patients evaluate dentists: A pilot study. Community Dent Oral Epidemiol 2000;28:257–266.

28. Arnold L. Assessing professional behavior: Yesterday, today, and tomorrow. Acad Med 2002;77:502–515.

29. Wynia MK. The short history and tenuous future of medical professionalism: The erosion of medicine's social contract. Perspect Biol Med 2008;51:565–578.

30. Fricker JP, Kiley M, Townsend G, Trevitt C. Professionalism: What is it, why should we have it and how can we achieve it? Aust Dent J 2011;56:92–96.

31. Shaw D. Ethics, professionalism and fitness to practise: Three concepts, not one. Br Dent J 2009;207:59–62.

32. Zijlstra-Shaw S, Robinson PG, Roberts T. Assessing professionalism within dental education; the need for a definition. Eur J Dent Educ 2012;16:e128–e136.

33. Trathen A, Gallagher JE. Dental professionalism: Definitions and debate. Br Dent J 2009;206:249–253.

34. Masella RS. Renewing professionalism in dental education: Overcoming the market environment. J Dent Educ 2007;71:205–216.

35. Thom DH, Hall MA, Pawlson LG. Measuring patients' trust In physicians when assessing quality of care. Health Affairs (Millwood) 2004;23:124–132.
36. Bentley JP, Stroup LJ, Wilkin NE, Bouldin AS. Patient evaluations of pharmacist performance with variations in attire and communication levels. J Am Pharm Assoc 2005;45:600–607.
37. DeVito JA. The Communication Handbook: A Dictionary. New York: Harper & Row, 1986.
38. DeVito JA. Messages: Building Interpersonal Skills, ed 6. Boston: Pearson Education, 2005.
39. Sprecher S. Insiders' perspectives on reasons for attraction to a close other. Soc Psychol Q 1998;61:287–300.
40. Friedman HS, Riggio RE, Casella DF. Nonverbal skill, personal charisma, and initial attraction. Pers Soc Psychol Bull 1988;14:203–211.
41. Adler RB, Rodman G, Hutchinson CC. Understanding Human Communication, ed 11. New York: Oxford University Press, 2011.
42. Paunonen SV. You are honest, therefore I like you and find you attractive. J Res Pers 2006;40: 237–249.
43. McKenna G, Lillywhite GRR, Maini N. Patient preferences for dental clinical attire: A cross-sectional survey in a dental hospital. Br Dent J 2007;203:681–685.
44. Shulman ER, Brehm WT. Dental clinical attire and infection-control procedures: Patients' attitudes. J Am Dent Assoc 2001;132:508–516.
45. Tibdewal H, Sharma S, Tadakamadla J, Duraiswamy P, Kulkarni S. Should dentist wear white coat? A cross-sectional study. J Oral Health Res 2010;1:76–81.
46. Priya H, Acharya S, Bhat M, Ballal M. Microbial contamination of the white coats of dental staff in the clinical setting. J Dent Res Dent Clin Dent Prospects 2010;3:136–140.
47. Mangum S, Garrison C, Lind C, Hilton HG. First impressions of the nurse and nursing care. J Nurs Care Qual 1997;11(5):39–47.
48. Hurley-Trailor J. The office dress code. RDH 2011;31(10):20.
49. Alexander SC, Sleath B, Golin CE, Kalinowski CT. Provider-patient communication and treatment adherence. In: Bosworth HB, Oddone EZ, Weinberger M (eds). Patient Treatment Adherence: Concepts Interventions and Measurement. Mahwah, NJ: Lawrence Erlbaum, 2008:329–372.
50. Fuertes JN, Mislowack A, Bennett J, et al. The physician–patient working alliance. Patient Educ Couns 2007;66:29–36.
51. Beach MC, Sugarman J, Johnson RL, Arbelaez JJ, Duggan PS, Cooper LA. Do patients treated with dignity report higher satisfaction, adherence, and receipt of preventive care? Ann Fam Med 2005;3:331–338.
52. Haskard K, Williams S, DiMatteo M, Heritage J, Rosenthal R. The provider's voice: Patient satisfaction and the content-filtered speech of nurses and physicians in primary medical care. J Nonverbal Behav 2008;32:1–20.
53. Sergl HG, Zentner A. Predicting patient compliance in orthodontic treatment. Semin Orthod 2000;6:231–236.
54. Sinha PK, Nanda RS, McNeil DW. Perceived orthodontist behaviors that predict patient satisfaction, orthodontist-patient relationship, and patient adherence in orthodontic treatment. Am J Orthod Dentofacial Orthop 1996;110:370–377.
55. Holt V, McHugh K. Factors influencing patient loyalty to dentist and dental practice. Br Dent J 1997;183:365–370.
56. Ford WSZ. Communication practices of professional service providers: Predicting customer satisfaction and loyalty. J Appl Commun Res 2003;31:189–211.
57. Lill MM, Wilkinson TJ. Judging a book by its cover: Descriptive survey of patients' preferences for doctors' appearance and mode of address. BMJ 2005;331:1524–1527.
58. Levin RP. The interpersonal factor. J Am Dent Assoc 2008;139:986–987.
59. Makoul G, Zick A, Green M. An evidence-based perspective on greetings in medical encounters. Arch Intern Med 2007;167:1172–1176.
60. Kahn MW. Etiquette-based medicine. New Engl J Med 2008;358:1988–1989.
61. Levin RP. Body language speaks volumes. J Am Dent Assoc 2008;139:1262–1263.
62. McKinstry B. Should general practitioners call patients by their first names? BMJ 1990;301: 795–796.

63. Bergman JJ, Eggertsen SC, Phillips WR, Cherkin DC, Schultz JK. How patients and physicians address each other in the office. J Fam Pract 1988;27:399–402.
64. Gallagher J, Waldron Lynch F, Stack J, Barragry J. Dress and address: Patient preferences regarding doctor's style of dress and patient interaction. Ir Med J 2008;101:211–213.
65. Gillette RD, Filak A, Thorne C. First name or last name: Which do patients prefer? J Am Board Fam Pract 1992;5:517–522.
66. Tickle-Degnen L, Rosenthal R. The nature of rapport and its nonverbal correlates. Psychol Inq 1990;1:285–293.
67. Eide H, Graugaard P, Holgersen K, Finset A. Physician communication in different phases of a consultation at an oncology outpatient clinic related to patient satisfaction. Patient Educ Couns 2003;51:259–266.
68. Bain DJ. Doctor-patient communication in general practice consultations. Med Educ 1976;10:125–131.
69. Liang ZY. Classification of Dentists' Types of Talk and Their Application in Doctor-Patient Conversation: In the Case of Pediatric Dental Treatment [thesis]. Tainan, Taiwan: National Cheng Kung University, 2008.
70. Handelman SL, Stege PM, Baric JM, Espeland MA, Saunders RH. Dentists' verbal communication leads during an interview with geriatric patients. Spec Care Dent 1986;6:253–257.
71. McDaniel SH, Beckman HB, Morse DS, Silberman J, Seaburn DB, Epstein RM. Physician self-disclosure in primary care visits: Enough about you, what about me? Arch Intern Med 2007;167:1321–1326.
72. Fogarty LA, Curbow BA, Wingard JR, McDonnell K, Somerfield MR. Can 40 seconds of compassion reduce patient anxiety? J Clin Oncol 1999;17:371–379.
73. Brady W, Martinoff J. Validity of health history data collected from dental patients and patient perception of health status. J Am Dent Assoc 1980;101:642–645.
74. Jolly DE. Interpreting the medical history. J Calif Dent Assoc 1995;23(10):19–28.
75. Minden NJ, Fast TB. The patient's health history form: How healthy is it? J Am Dent Assoc 1993;124:95–101.
76. Minden NJ, Fast TB. Evaluation of health history forms used in U.S. dental schools. Oral Surg Oral Med Oral Pathol 1994;77:105–109.
77. Thibodeau EA, Rossomando KJ. Survey of the medical history questionnaire. Oral Surg Oral Med Oral Pathol 1992;74:400–403.
78. Hennrikus D, Rindal DB, Boyle RG, Stafne E, Lazovich D, Lando H. How well does the health history form identify adolescent smokers? J Am Dent Assoc 2005;136:1113–1120.
79. Klages U, Sergl HG, Burucker I. Relations between verbal behavior of the orthodontist and communicative cooperation of the patient in regular orthodontic visits. Am J Orthod Dentofacial Orthop 1992;102:265–269.
80. Platt FW, Gaspar DL, Coulehan JL, et al. "Tell me about yourself": The patient-centered interview. Ann Intern Med 2001;134:1079–1085.
81. Cole WA. Accuracy of patient reporting as an indication of headgear compliance. Am J Orthod Dentofacial Orthop 2002;121:419–423.
82. Miller PM, Ravenel MC, Shealy AE, Thomas S. Alcohol screening in dental patients: The prevalence of hazardous drinking and patients' attitudes about screening and advice. J Am Dent Assoc 2006;137:1692–1698.
83. Tramacere I, Negri E, Bagnardi V, et al. A meta-analysis of alcohol drinking and oral and pharyngeal cancers. 1. Overall results and dose-risk relation. Oral Oncol 2010;46:497–503.
84. Yellowitz J, Goodman H, Horowitz A, al-Tannir M. Assessment of alcohol and tobacco use in dental schools' health history forms. J Dent Educ 1995;59:1091–1096.
85. Barrier PA, Li JT, Jensen NM. Two words to improve physician-patient communication: What else? Mayo Clin Proc 2003;78:211–214.
86. Quilligan S, Silverman J. The skill of summary in clinician-patient communication: A case study. Patient Educ Couns 2012;86:354–359.

Interacting During and After Procedures

Why Interacting During and After Procedures Matters

For both patients and providers, treatment planning too often is the focal point of the entire consultation. As a result, the interview, procedure, and diagnosis are neglected or completed too rapidly. In chapter 7, we emphasized the importance of conducting a thorough health history. Just as important is the communication that takes place during the examination or procedure. Whether patients are undergoing cleaning, extraction, root canal treatment, or something more extensive, providers should build on the positive foundations established during the initiating and interviewing phase.

Providers must resist the temptation to begin treating patients as a mouth as soon as the chair reclines. This temptation to objectify patients is strong because providers are performing clinical work, so clinical skills of observation and objectivity are needed, and because patients have limited ability to respond. Providers should remain aware that patient-centered care requires them to treat patients as people at all times. Further, the effectiveness of any treatment plan hinges on both clinical and relational communication. Clinically, an accurate diagnosis and the patient's capacity and willingness to implement treatment determine its effectiveness.[1] Relationally, providers' attitudes of sympathy and their establishment of informal relationships with patients are associated with oral hygiene adherence.[2]

Effective communication during the procedure and diagnosis is therefore crucial to the treatment planning that follows. It may also save time, as examinations and procedures usually provide dental professionals extended lengths of time in which to present information to dental patients who have little else to do but pay attention. Too often, this time is wasted by providers who either remain silent throughout the procedure or engage in a lengthy monologue unrelated to the task at hand. Neither approach facilitates patient-centered care, and both may actually undermine it by making patients nervous or fearful. In this chapter, we propose an alternative approach for communicating with patients during examinations and procedures and for discussing findings afterward.

Communication During Procedures

An appointment's initiating and interviewing phase ends when the provider says something like this: "If you have no more questions, let's move on to your examination [or procedure]." The purpose of the appointment will dictate the precise actions that follow. Providers should remain aware that communication is taking place even if they are not speaking or listening. Patients are watching and responding, and these behaviors constitute communication. At a minimum, providers should make sure that patients see them wash their hands (or use hand sanitizer) and don gloves. They should also notify patients before they recline the chair or adjust head rests or arm rests: "I'm going to recline the chair so I can get a better view of your mouth. Please let me know how I can make you more comfortable." As providers begin an examination or procedure, silence often prevails, and silence can enhance the clinical proceedings by fostering concentration. Yet during procedures, verbal and nonverbal forms of communication (aside from silence) are necessary and beneficial, serving six interrelated functions: coordinating, instructing, calming, monitoring, narrating, and educating (Box 8-1).

Box 8-1	Communication functions and strategies during procedures

Coordinating
- Practice smooth patient handoffs from one practitioner to another.
- Treat the patient as a member of the dental team.
- Minimize interruptions.

Instructing
- Evaluate the patient's control preferences.
- Tell the patient what you expect of him or her.
- Politely instruct the patient how to facilitate the procedure.

Calming
- Project calmness and confidence during the procedure.
- Avoid negative comments during the procedure.
- Provide encouragement and benchmarks.

Monitoring
- Observe the patient's nonverbal behavior for signs of distress.
- Take breaks when needed.
- Periodically ask how the patient is doing.

Narrating
- Describe what you are doing as you do it.
- Describe what you are observing, unless it will cause distress.
- Offer praise and compliments when appropriate.

Educating
- Describe the etiology and risk factors of any observed problem.
- Explain the consequences if no treatment is undertaken.
- Mention preventive and/or restorative treatment options.

Coordinating

Communication can become complicated during examinations and other dental procedures because often more than two participants are involved. When a dentist speaks, for instance, the message may be meant for the patient, for the hygienist, for a dental assistant, or for all three. Over time, dental teams develop patterns of communication that serve their purposes, but they should keep in mind that patients may be unfamiliar with those patterns. For instance, if a dentist says, "Please move your arm," the hygienist may understand who the comment is directed to, but the patient may not. We recommend three particular strategies for coordinating patient care during an examination or procedure.

First, the team should practice smooth patient handoffs. Often, the hygienist cleans the patient's teeth, and the dentist arrives later for the health history, examination, or procedure. The professional who cleans the teeth gains significant information that the dentist should know regarding a patient's oral health practices and concerns. Failure to disclose this information is an error.

If the patient's oral health practices are poor, the hygienist may be tempted to disclose this information to the dentist outside the patient's hearing or to use a code that rates the patient's (poor) oral health in a way the patient may not understand. Instead, the provider should disclose the patient's oral health status clearly and in the presence of the patient.[3] The dentist should deliberately mark a time when the hygienist will provide the information, and the patient should be able to hear it and offer any clarifications: "Jane, did you find out anything I should know about Mr Brady's oral health?"

Any disclosures should be made discreetly, preserving the privacy of the patient. Disclosure should also be done without judgment. The person who conducted the tooth cleaning should confine remarks to what was observed and not speculate about the patient's motivations or character, remembering that many reasons could account for poor oral health.

Second, the provider should treat the patient as a member of the dental team. The patient likely possesses less dental knowledge and skill, but he or she makes the treatment decision and lives with the consequences and therefore is entitled to the same respect other members of the dental team receive.[4] The patient should be enlisted to assist others on the dental team in accomplishing the tasks at hand.[5,6] However, the provider should avoid overuse of the first person plural, which patients do not like: "What flavor toothpaste do we want today?"[7]

For the patient, the "specimen" position of reclining while the provider works hovering above can seem depersonalizing. Depersonalization is increased when the members of the dental team ignore the patient's presence.[8] We have heard reports of remarkably unprofessional conversations among dental providers unaware or unconcerned that the patient they were working on could hear them. Even if a patient is sedated, the provider should say nothing in a patient's presence that would alarm or offend and should periodically acknowledge the patient's presence. Because the mask obscures facial expression and the hands are often occupied, the provider should use eye contact to indicate for whom the message is intended.

Third, the provider should minimize interruptions. A recent observational study of comprehensive dental examinations in the United States found frequent workflow interruptions, most of which were related to technology interfering with workflow.[9] The result was duplication of work and an increase in the number of steps involved to complete tasks. We can assume that the patient will be frustrated or distressed by such delays and lack of coordination among the dental team members. The provider should keep track of interruptions and find solutions when specific types of interruption recur frequently.

Instructing

A second function of communication during procedures is to instruct a patient what to do so that the clinical work can be completed. First, the provider should determine a patient's preferences for control. As with other types of communication, the messages should be adapted to the patient, and patients vary in the level of control they prefer. Patients with a higher need for control may experience more stress and even pain if they perceive that the procedure renders them helpless.[10,11]

Attending to the patient's verbal and nonverbal responses to instructions should indicate the level of control the patient desires. The provider can politely direct a patient with lower control preferences. The provider should more often check on the comfort of a patient with higher control preferences and indicate an obvious willingness to take a break when asked.

Second, the provider should tell the patient what is expected of him or her. Patients prefer knowing what will happen and what is expected of them.[4,12] Satisfaction is a function of patient expectations, so providing realistic expectations for what will take place should enhance patient satisfaction.[13] The provider should give the patient a brief summary of expectations: "We'll mostly need you to keep your mouth open and let us know when you need a break or a rinse."

For dental providers, the structure of appointments is so routine that they may not realize that patients do not always know what they are supposed to do. This is especially true of younger patients, patients new to the practice, or patients who have avoided or neglected dental care. These are precisely the patients who need guidance so they are not taken by surprise or left feeling embarrassed. For such patients, specific expectations should be clarified. For instance, if a new patient who was loyal to an older dentist has only used a cuspidor and is unaware how to use suction, some embarrassment would be avoided for the patient if, on the first visit, the hygienist asks: "Are you familiar with the use of a suction device?" A hesitation or a "no" reply would offer an opportunity to instruct the patient in the proper use of suction.

Third, the provider should politely instruct the patient on how to facilitate clinical work. Politeness toward the patient should be expected, but the majority of respondents in a 2008 study agreed that "dentists sometimes act rude to their patients."[14] This was the case even though a study of 25 communication behaviors performed by orthodontists found that politeness is the one behavior most predictive of satisfaction, accounting for nearly 61% of the variance in patient satisfaction.[15] In addition, politeness is one of two communication behaviors significantly associated with adherence.

Because the initiating and interviewing phase involves social interaction and the treatment presentation phase involves persuasion, clinical interaction during the procedure may be the time the provider is most likely to forget manners. Patients generally do not expect to be asked nicely every time a provider requires something of them, but they also do not expect to be ordered. The provider should avoid single-word commands: *Open! Spit! Move! Rinse!* The patient will be satisfied if the provider simply softens the tone and adds *please* to instructions. Politeness may also benefit the provider.[16–18] In recent years, research has suggested that providers who apologize for errors and mistakes may avert patient legal action.[19,20] At the very least, the provider should apologize when he or she causes pain.

> **Activity 8-1**
>
> Describe a time when a medical or service provider was rude to you or when you witnessed a provider being rude to another patient or client. Was the rudeness triggered by something? What was the patient's or client's response? Was there an apology that defused the situation or did it escalate? What was the long-term consequence of the rudeness for the patient or client?

Calming

A third function of communication during dental procedures and examinations is to reduce patient anxiety. Because fear of the unknown fosters anxiety, coordinating care and providing instructions may have a calming effect.[21] The provider can also implement three deliberate strategies to calm a patient during a procedure. First, the provider should project calmness and confidence. Feelings of calmness and confidence are insufficient if the provider does not communicate them to the patient; the provider therefore should minimize habits that can be interpreted as nervousness: jerky hand and eye movements, distractedness, and constant chattering.

Emotions, like viruses, are contagious.[22] The provider should be careful not to "infect" the patient with anxiety and at the same time should avoid becoming "infected" by a patient's preexisting anxiety. Emotional contagion can also play a role when a parent or caregiver is in the operatory. Research indicates that children tend to reflect the anxiety of a present parent (especially mothers).[23,24] Unlike viruses, emotional contagion can benefit the patient, as is the case when the provider taps into a patient's anxiety in order to empathize or boosts the confidence of the patient by modeling confidence.[25,26]

Second, the provider should avoid negative comments during the procedure. For a patient, few things are more alarming during an examination or procedure than to hear a provider saying, "Oh no!" or "This is bad." Negative comments significantly predict patient anxiety, which may in turn increase pain.[27–29] On hearing negative comments, the patient's thoughts likely turn toward negative outcomes: short- or long-term pain, loss of teeth, expensive treatments, and so on. The patient may even begin deciding what treatment he or she can accept and afford before the provider completes the examination and offers a diagnosis and prognosis.

Negative comments may also be interpreted as criticism of oral health status or practices, and this interpretation can make anxiety worse.[30,31] Even patients who are not dentally anxious dislike criticism, so the provider should also avoid critical comments (eg, "I can tell you haven't been flossing").[32–34]

Third, the provider should communicate encouragement and provide benchmarks. When a patient known to be anxious is treated, encouraging commentary can be very soothing: "You are doing great"; "I don't think we are going to have any trouble today"; or "You are a trooper." Benchmarks can help the patient feel less vulnerable by providing information about the progress of the procedure. The provider should narrate the procedure anyway, but an anxious patient may also be helped with time-relevant comments: "We are already halfway finished"; or "After this I'm going to pack in some gauze and you'll be on your way." The provider should remember that the patient cannot see what is happening, and an anxious patient's sense of time may be distorted, so regular progress reports can be tremendously reassuring.

Monitoring

All patients—but especially anxious patients—should be monitored for signs of distress. Vigilance on this front is warranted. Dental providers' field of vision may be narrowed or restricted due to the use of loupes. Or they can become so clinically focused that they ignore indications that patients are in emotional or physical distress.

Three communication strategies can facilitate monitoring of the patient's status. First, the provider should observe the patient's nonverbal behavior for signs of distress. Human beings can intuitively identify distress signals such as moaning, interjections, rapid breathing, and tensed muscles. In addition, a patient may occasionally engage in annoying behaviors such as grabbing the provider's hand or—a verbal behavior—unduly criticizing the provider. These expressions of hostility can also be signs of anxiety.[35] If more than one member of the dental team is involved in the procedure, one provider should be tasked with tracking the patient's responses.

Second, the provider should take breaks when needed by either the patient or the provider. Occasional breaks offer the opportunity to focus on the patient's emotional state. These breaks also offer the opportunity to de-stress from both mental and physical strain.[36,37] Both performing and undergoing dental procedures can induce stress, and the tendency toward emotional contagion suggests that when one person experiences emotional intensity, others nearby may do the same. The provider should designate a hand signal, such as a raised hand, to provide the patient a sense of control. More than half of dental hygiene patients indicate that using hand signals to request breaks is effective in reducing their anxiety.[38]

The patient-provider power dynamic, however, may lead some patients to endure pain rather than ask for some relief.[39,40] Whenever the emotional climate becomes intense, the provider should either ask the patient if he or she would like a short break or simply find an excuse to allow some time before resuming, such as allowing the patient to rinse, asking the patient a question, or retrieving an instrument or supplies. After 20 seconds or so, the patient should be more composed, and the procedure can resume.

Third, whether or not the provider takes breaks in the procedure, he or she should periodically ask how the patient is doing. A 2007 observational study of "everyday" patients (ie, not restricted to anxious patients) included "checking in and noticing" among five comforting strategies.[41] (Other strategies were environmental distractions, pharmacologic comfort, structuring the interaction, and addressing patient anxiety.) The study found that dentists provided comfort in only 44.3% of visits and hygienists provided comfort in only 40.6%, but the frequency of comforting instances varied widely.

Checking in with patients shows concern, which is more difficult to do in the clinical phases of the appointment than in the initiating and interviewing or treatment presentation phases. Simply asking if the patient is comfortable or needs anything helps build on the strong relational foundation established during the first part of the appointment.[42] Checking in also allows the patient to verbalize distress, which could be important if the patient's nonverbal behavior does not express any anxiety, discomfort, or pain.

Question of ethics: Cleanings, examinations, and dental procedures can require long periods of time in which patients are unable to speak. Providers can address all six functions of communication and still find they have long periods of silence while they work. Many providers use this time to discuss social topics or self-disclose a bit about themselves. Such talk can relieve stress for both provider and patient, but—depending on what is shared—it can also make the patient uncomfortable. Mentioning your upcoming plans to go fishing is ethical. Mentioning your marital dissatisfaction is not. Draft a short policy describing your boundaries for which topics and opinions are acceptable to share with a patient and which are not.

Narrating

Communication during dental procedures and examinations can also function to provide an up-to-the-moment description of what the provider is doing. For a number of reasons, patients rarely see what is involved in clinical dentistry. Narrating the procedure helps to demystify it. First, the provider should describe what he or she is doing while doing it. This strategy can either complement or replace the strategy of providing benchmarks. The provider need not maintain a constant running commentary, nor is it necessary to describe mundane tasks repeatedly, but the patient should be kept abreast of the progress: "Now I'm working to smooth the edges of this amalgam filling so it will feel smooth instead of rough." This information not only helps the patient to keep track of the appointment's progress but may also let the patient know the value of the treatment received. For instance, a 2008 study found that few African Americans (who are at elevated risk for oral cancer) realized they were receiving an oral cancer screening every time they visited the dentist.[43] They were not informed that the examination of the tongue is a part of the oral cancer screening.

Second, the provider should describe what he or she is observing. The dental professional is privy to a view of the patient's mouth that is inaccessible to the patient. A brief, objective description of what the provider sees is a value-added service for the patient and lays a foundation for the presentation of a treatment plan: "I am seeing that the gum is receding a little bit, which likely is the cause of the sensitivity you reported."

One qualification, however, must be kept in mind. The provider should consider the language used to report conditions or findings in order to avoid alarming or insulting a patient: "That tooth is in such bad shape that I'm surprised you kept it as long as you did." Likewise, opinions and speculations should be shared only if they are supportive and positive. An example of an acceptable opinion to share might be, "We decided in the last visit to keep an eye on that back filling, and it looks to me like it is still going strong." An unacceptable opinion to share would be, "These nicotine stains tell me you failed to quit smoking. Again."

Third, the provider should offer praise and compliments when appropriate. The effectiveness of praise has been noted in the research on pediatric dentistry, but it can also facilitate relationships with adult patients.[44–47] Praise can focus on the patient's in-chair behavior: "This procedure has taken some time, and I appreciate your patience as we make that tooth as good as new." Praise can also focus on the patient's oral health and habits[48]: "Your plaque levels are really low. I wish all my patients took such good care of their teeth."

In addition to promoting preventive care and forging a closer relationship, praise may foster loyalty in some patients.[49,50] One study found that dental providers were significantly more likely to praise college-educated patients than patients with less education, so providers should make a deliberate effort to find something to praise about every patient regardless of his or her level of education.[51] Even if a patient's oral health is deplorable, the patient can be praised for showing an interest in improving it.

Educating

Patient-provider communication during a procedure or examination can also serve the function of educating the patient. Better informed patients may make better decisions regarding treatment. Patients—particularly anxious ones—are unlikely to be interested in hearing a lecture on periodontal disease, but they may find that dental information provided at a level they can understand is both interesting and useful. It can also save some time by reducing the amount of information provided and questions raised following the procedure.

Again, the provider should only discuss topics that will not agitate a patient. If, however, the patient seems interested and capable of understanding, information can be provided during the procedure. First, the provider should describe the etiology and risk factors of an observed problem: "Dental erosion happens when some sort of acid breaks down the tooth's surface. Often, diet is the cause: eating a lot of citrus or drinking lots of soft drinks or sport drinks. Vomiting, gastric problems, and low saliva flow can also put a person at risk."

Second, the provider should explain the consequences of permitting the condition to go untreated. This strategy should not be interpreted as a license to scare the patient into accepting a treatment plan. A gruesome description of the course of disease is likely to be counterproductive, as the patient will stop attending to the message. (Consider the low impact of antismoking campaigns that depend on photographs of cancerous oral cavities.) Instead, the provider should acknowledge that "do nothing" is often the default treatment option for patients—and it has been this way for most of human history. A description of what happens if no treatment is undertaken provides a baseline against which the patient can evaluate treatment options: "Dental erosion cannot be reversed. If nothing is done, the tooth will continue to wear away and we will not be able to restore it."

Third, the provider should mention preventive and/or restorative treatment options. The provider likely will be unable to give detailed descriptions of various treatment options while still working on a patient's mouth. Even so, the provider can mention that treatments are available. If there is time, the provider can briefly summarize what those options are. Of course, the provider will formally present treatment options later.

An earlier mention relieves the patient's anxiety that the condition may be untreatable and allows the patient more time to consider what may be the most appropriate treatment. The patient can be overwhelmed when presented with two or more treatment options at the end of an appointment. Within mere minutes, the patient is presented with a wealth of information in various forms (spoken, written, and with presentation aids) and feels pressured to weigh commitments of time, money, and discomfort and to make a quick decision. Telling the patient about the treatment options earlier in the appointment reduces the sense of pressure: "We can minimize or avoid further erosion by removing the causes: adjusting your diet or addressing vomiting or gastric issues, for instance. We also can restore what was lost to erosion by building up the teeth with restorative materials. I'll go over the treatment options when I'm done here."

Diagnosis and Prognosis

Providers find it tempting, in the name of efficiency, to skip straight from completing the examination or procedure to treatment planning. Unless patients have a full understanding of their condition, however, they cannot make an informed choice about appropriate treatment. Patient-centered care requires providers to communicate the results of examinations, procedures, and tests in a manner that patients can understand. To accomplish this task, providers must disclose what was confirmed or discovered during the examination or procedure (ie, the findings and the diagnosis) and what the future holds for the patient's oral health (ie, the prognosis). Relative to other forms of dental communication (eg, health history and treatment planning), little research has been conducted on diagnostic and prognostic communication in a dental context. The recommendations we make in this regard are primarily based on our own observations and experience.

In his communication research, Street[52] found that the amount of diagnostic information providers give patients is related to patients' anxiety, education level, and question-asking behavior. We have emphasized throughout this text that dental providers influence the first of these variables: patient anxiety levels. Although providers do not determine the education level of a patient, they do influence the amount of oral health knowledge and instruction patients receive. Regarding the third variable, Street[52] found evidence that providers influence question-asking behavior, saying,

"Patients' assertiveness and expressiveness were strongly influenced by physicians' use of 'partnership-building' utterances that solicited the patient's questions, concerns, and opinions." Other researchers have confirmed the influence of dental providers' communication behavior on patients' communication behavior.[53] Therefore, providers should understand the diagnostic portion of a consultation not as a one-way presentation of findings but rather as a two-way discussion of those findings. With this approach in mind, we recommend three steps in discussing results: *(1)* describe satisfactory and unsatisfactory conditions, *(2)* determine oral health and hygiene practices and risks, and *(3)* explain the consequences if no treatment is undertaken (Box 8-2).

Box 8-2	Steps in discussing examination findings

Step 1: Describe satisfactory and unsatisfactory conditions
- Start by praising or complimenting the patient.
- State (or restate) the diagnosis or areas of concern.
- Note any changes in oral health status over time.

Step 2: Assess the patient's risk for caries and other oral diseases
- Determine the patient's current oral hygiene practices.
- If appropriate, ask the patient to demonstrate his or her oral hygiene practices.
- Discuss behaviors that may place the patient at higher risk for oral health problems.

Step 3: Explain the consequences if no treatment or behavior change is undertaken
- Describe the likelihood of positive versus negative outcomes, using outcomes meaningful to the patient (cost, time, effort, and discomfort).
- Describe the short- and long-term consequences of negative outcomes.
- Mention that treatment options are available.

Step 1: Describe satisfactory and unsatisfactory conditions

The first step is required in all dental appointments. Immediately following the examination or procedure, the provider should describe what was observed or discovered. If the primary purpose of the appointment was a procedure rather than an examination, the results should focus on the conditions of the area on which the procedure was completed. For the reasons stated previously, the provider should begin the presentation of results by praising or complimenting the patient. Praise might address the following: low plaque scores, healthy gingiva, patience or helpfulness during the examination, previous dental work, or success in quitting tobacco. Examinations and procedures can be difficult or even traumatic, so transitioning to the diagnostic phase with a positive message may prepare the patient to hear what follows.

Activity 8-2

With some patients, finding an oral health condition or habit to praise is easy. For others, it can be a challenge. Make a list of 10 habits or conditions you could praise to a patient who takes good care of oral health. Then, make a list of 5 compliments you could pay to someone who clearly has a lot of work to do. Share your lists with colleagues and use the items on these lists to reinforce good oral hygiene habits in your patients.

The provider should then state any diagnosis or conditions of concern. A study of Australian dentists found that those who provide cost and treatment information to patients had patients with significantly lower diagnostic rates.[54] One potential implication is that such providers attract patients who prefer information and who may have fewer oral health problems to diagnose. Regardless, the patient paying for an examination or procedure is also paying for information. Professionalism includes an obligation to divulge diagnostic information in a way the patient can understand. If a provider is unable to provide a diagnosis based on the general examination, explaining what was observed and why a firm diagnosis cannot be offered should make a patient more agreeable to additional tests (eg, radiographs) or referral to a specialist.

In presenting both satisfactory and unsatisfactory conditions, the provider may have to repeat information previously provided during the actual examination or procedure. As in most cases in which a provider is giving information, repetition is desirable because it emphasizes what has been said and helps the patient to remember it. A written summary of findings would be even better, but most providers would not take the time to do this.

We offer one caveat on the subject of repetition: It is best for the provider to acknowledge that he or she is repeating information or questions. Otherwise, the patient begins to suspect that the provider cannot recall previous conversations. So the provider should begin with the following phrase: "As I said before…."

The provider should next note any changes in oral health over time. Specifically, the provider should mention whether general or specific conditions have changed since previous visits. Doing so helps to place the information into context and helps the patient know whether current behaviors are benefitting or harming his or her oral health.

If the purpose of the appointment was to complete a dental procedure, the provider should state plainly what was attempted and what was accomplished. In most cases, the procedure will have fixed whatever problem the patient wanted addressed. If the procedure did not entirely solve the problem, the provider should tell the patient so and provide a truthful reason for why the effort was unsuccessful.

Step 2: Assess the patient's risk for caries and other oral diseases

The second step in discussing results and findings with patients is to engage in a dialogue about any habits or behaviors that directly affect their risk for oral disease. This effort will help the provider determine the causes of existing conditions and will help the patient connect habits and risks to symptoms of oral disease. First, the provider should ask what the patient does to maintain oral health and how frequently he or she does it. Tooth brushing and flossing are obvious places to start, but the provider could also ask about mouthwash use, gum chewing, denture cleaning, and so on: "Receding gums sometimes come with aging, but I want us to do what we can to slow it down. Can you tell me what you do to take care of your teeth?"

Second, particularly if the patient's habits do not reveal causes of concern, the provider might ask the patient to demonstrate oral health practices. For instance, the patient may brush three or four times daily, but the technique used may cause damage to teeth, gingiva, or tongue. Asking for a description or a demonstration of how the patient brushes (or flosses or cleans dentures) may yield clues to the problems a patient is experiencing: "It sounds to me like you are brushing often enough, so that isn't the problem. Could you show me how you brush?"

Third, the provider should discuss the risks of engaging in behaviors that may lead to oral health problems. The provider may have elicited adequate risk information from the health history or may need to probe further. Ice chewing, for instance, may not emerge on a health history, but if the provider finds that a patient's teeth are prone to fracture, the provider can ask whether the patient crunches ice regularly. With most patients, the provider can avoid actual statistics and odds ratios but can speak in general terms about predispositions and risk factors: "The number of fillings you have already increases the risk of breaking teeth, and chewing ice only makes you more prone to breaking a tooth."

Step 3: Explain the consequences if no treatment or behavior change is undertaken

The third step in discussing results should be undertaken with all patients. The provider should present his or her best estimate of what will happen if no treatment is undertaken. If the patient is in good oral health and engages in practices supportive of continued health, the provider should offer an optimistic prediction: "If you continue your good home care practices and have regular checkups, you should be able to keep your teeth in good condition for many years." If, however, the examination or procedure revealed unsatisfactory results, the provider should translate those conditions or habits into outcomes meaningful to the patient. *Receding gingiva* and *eroded enamel* may mean little to a patient, but *bleeding* and *pain* are easy to understand.

This step actually overlaps with treatment planning but is included in the presentation of results because it helps the patient understand what a diagnosis means. First, in general terms, the provider should describe the likelihood of positive and negative outcomes: "Puffy and red gums that bleed easily are a sign of gum disease. I can make some recommendations to keep it from progressing." The next section of this chapter describes in greater detail strategies for translating diagnoses and prognoses into outcomes meaningful to the patient.

Second, the provider should describe short- and long-term consequences of negative outcomes. In doing this, the provider should take the patient's perspective and appreciate that the patient must weigh the consequences of no treatment against the investment of money, effort, time, and discomfort a given treatment may demand. The patient is likely to perform a quick calculation to compare the odds of a negative outcome against the severity of that outcome. Further, as with purchases from cars to boots, the patient may calculate whether it is possible to get by with the status quo for another season or year, until he or she has more resources to make the financial investment.

Although the provider can address financial commitments during the treatment planning phase of the appointment, during the diagnostic phase the provider should accurately summarize short-term and long-term consequences in both clinical and lay terms: "If you don't do anything, more redness and bleeding of the gums will be accompanied by destruction of the bone support of the teeth, resulting in bad breath and eventual tooth loss. In the long term, advanced gum disease is associated with heart disease and stroke."

Finally, the provider should conclude the diagnostic phase and prepare the patient for treatment planning by noting that treatment options are available.

Question of ethics: Because knowledge is power, dental providers hold some power over patients in knowing how bad a condition is and what the likely consequences are. Providers therefore can emphasize or even exaggerate negative conditions to persuade patients to undergo treatment. Is it ethical to do this if the recommendation is for costly restorative treatment? Is it ethical to do this if the recommendation is for inexpensive preventive treatment? As a child, did anyone try to scare you into brushing or flossing by predicting dire consequences if you neglected these practices? If so, do you think that person made an ethical lapse?

Understanding Patient Motivations

A key to effective and appropriate dental treatment is to identify the preventive or restorative treatments acceptable to individual patients. To determine what patients find acceptable, the dental provider must understand their motivations for oral health care.[55] Arriving at this understanding can require both communication skills and time, because patients seek care for a variety of reasons that they may not fully understand themselves and that may change over time.[56] Determining patient motivations therefore is much easier when providers have developed long-term relationships with their patients. Providers who have a fuller appreciation of patient motivations are better able to interpret diagnoses, prognoses, and treatment options in terms that are most relevant to patients.

In the following paragraphs, we discuss four of the most common motivations for seeking oral health care (Box 8-3): pain and pain relief, esthetics, function, and cost. This list is not exhaustive, and patients can have two or more reasons for seeking care. Some patients arrive at a dental practice out of habit. Some arrive because they have been motivated by others. Physicians and speech therapists refer patients. Romantic partners nag their significant others to take care of themselves. Parents insist that their children receive examinations.

Providers should keep in mind these common motivations as they communicate with patients. They should ask patients what they want from their dental health care. Arnett and Worley[57] even developed the Treatment Motivation Survey, which can be administered following a health history and examination. Providers should pay attention to what their patients say about their teeth and note any evaluation regarding their oral health status. Finally, providers should track patient motivations using notations in patients' files. Discussing and monitoring motivations is a characteristic of patient-centered care and shows patients that the provider takes seriously their reasons for seeking care through the provider's practice.

| Box 8-3 | Common motivations for seeking oral health care |

Pain and pain relief
- Toothache or jaw pain
- Tightness or pinching
- Rough edges

Esthetics
- Discoloration or stains
- Crooked or overlapping teeth
- Gingival problems
- Bad breath

Function
- Problematic occlusion
- Loose-fitting prostheses
- Problems chewing, eating, or speaking
- Difficulty cleaning teeth or dentures

Cost
- Expenditures on over-the-counter remedies
- Costs of various treatments
- Potential costs if treatment is delayed
- Opportunity costs

Pain and pain relief

Across ethnic and age groups, dental pain is associated with dental care utilization.[58] Simply put, patients often access dental care after they feel some sort of discomfort or pain. The disadvantage of this motivation is that patients (especially children) can come to associate dental visits with oral pain. Dental professionals can work this motivation to their advantage, however, by objectively diagnosing the cause of the pain and offering relief in the form of treatment. Patients who seek help for pain will be most responsive to information that addresses pain rather than esthetics or function.

Patients often live with pain for weeks or months before seeking help. One study of rural patients found that only half contacted a dental clinic within several days of the onset of their pain.[59] Most of them first attempted to manage the pain using lay techniques. A separate 2009 study found that the lay techniques patients use include over-the-counter medicines, home remedies, and prayer.[60] Perhaps patients believe these lay techniques will be effective or the pain will abate on its own. Or perhaps they cannot afford care. Even symptoms of oral cancer are minimized by patients who postpone seeking help.[61] Therefore, in their diagnosis and prognosis, providers should emphasize what is causing the pain, how the condition will progress, and how treatment will relieve the pain.

Esthetics

For decades, cosmetic dentistry was available primarily to the wealthy and those whose income depended on their appearance (eg, actors and models). In the past 30 years, cosmetic dentistry has become much less painful and less expensive. Now general practitioners can perform many routine cosmetic procedures such as tooth whitening and bonding. A 2006 survey of general dentists found that 77.8% perceived an increased demand for tooth whitening following the broadcast of makeover shows such as *Extreme Makeover* and 54.8% perceived an increased demand for veneers.[62] Respondents reported that women's magazines had the highest impact on patient perceptions of cosmetic dentistry.

The result of the general awareness and availability of services is that many patients, particularly younger ones, arrive with idealized expectations for their dental appearance. Relatively few of them may be willing to go through life with functional but crowded teeth. Even patients whose primary motivation is pain relief or function may be concerned with esthetics. For instance, today's patients may prefer a tooth-colored restoration (eg, composite resin or ceramic) rather than amalgam. Or they may prefer gold, as esthetic standards vary by culture and individual preference. In general, however, many patients want teeth that are whiter, straighter, and perfectly shaped. Providers should note such variations objectively and suggest treatments if patients indicate after being asked: "Are you happy with your smile? Many patients feel as though whitening their teeth is a 'smile-booster,' and if you are interested, I can explain how that is done."

Studies repeatedly find that esthetics is the reason most commonly cited by both patients and parents for seeking orthodontic treatment.[63,64] In younger adolescents, the esthetic motivation is associated with teasing by peers.[64,65] This reason suggests the profound influence dental appearance has on social adjustment. A study of adult orthodontic patients found appearance a key motivation, with participants mentioning a desire for straighter teeth and an improved smile.[66] Esthetic dental treatment is associated with significant increases in self-esteem.[67] Although adolescent patients are often motivated, studies find that parents of orthodontic patients are more motivated than the patients.[63,68] One reason given by parents for their high motivation is concern that their children may eventually resent not having the opportunity to have orthodontic treatment.

Providers should remain aware of the possibility that patients may have an unhealthy esthetic motivation for cosmetic dentistry.[65] One study found that patients preoccupied with a physical defect were nine times more likely to consider tooth whitening and six times more likely to consider orthodontic treatment.[69] An esthetic motivation is harmless in itself, but these patients were also five times more likely to be dissatisfied with their most recent treatment, illustrating the downside of the preoccupation with defects and the reason it is a feature of body dysmorphic disorder. This negative aspect of esthetic motivation demonstrates that providers must discern patient expectations and must clarify what dental treatment can and cannot accomplish.[70,71]

In addition to appearance, another esthetic consideration is odor. Patients may be ashamed of halitosis, believing it suggests poor hygiene and being unaware it is a symptom of various dental or systemic conditions. (Providers' diagnostic communication should address this misperception.)

Finally, patients may be too embarrassed to acknowledge either their esthetic shortcomings or their preoccupation with them. They may also forget to ask about the appearance of various treatments, although the esthetic outcome may determine their ultimate satisfaction. Therefore, providers should routinely mention esthetic aspects of diagnosis and treatment, providing more detail for those patients who communicate a desire for it.

Function

Patients may be motivated to seek help to address a functional problem, usually with eating or speaking. A 1980 study examined patient expectations prior to orthognathic surgery. It found that their expectations were restricted to improved function (39%), esthetics (17%), or both (44%).[13] Although not a key motivation, function (eg, "improve the bite") was mentioned as a secondary motive by adult orthodontic patients.[66]

As with other motivations, dental providers may not be aware of functional problems unless patients disclose them. Any major problems may be discovered during the health history. Providers may also uncover functional problems by observing the way patients speak or move their jaws. During an examination, if a problem is suspected, providers should ask directly about function while probing oral health habits during the diagnosis and prognosis stage of the appointment.

Cost

Access to health care is a prerequisite to care, and in the United States access to dental care is limited primarily by the cost of treatment. A 2007 study of low-income patients with dental pain showed that these patients clearly preferred to visit a dentist, but they postponed the expenditure until their financial concerns were overcome by the severity of their pain.[72] That study was conducted before the 2008 recession, which may have exacerbated the tendency to postpone treatment.

The costs of self-care may motivate patients to seek help if continued expenditures on over-the-counter and lay treatments cost more than the cost estimate for professional treatment. Similarly, the symptoms of dental problems may result in missed work days and lost wages—an **opportunity cost** that may exceed the cost of treatment. A study of participants reporting toothaches within the previous 12 months found that 44.3% had experienced more than five toothaches in the previous 10 years and 38.7% said it limited "a lot" their ability to work at their job.[60]

Perhaps more commonly, patients will delay treatment to maximize the value received when they eventually seek help. One study found that patients with oral cancer symptoms sometimes delayed addressing the problem until they had another reason for visiting a clinic.[73] Presumably, they were seeking to address multiple symptoms for the cost of one visit.

Providers should remain aware that few patients are unconcerned with the cost of dental care. Nevertheless, patients may refrain from directly addressing the costs of a diagnosis or various treatment options, even though it is a primary concern and may determine their treatment choice. Rarely is cost not a variable in treatment planning, so the topic will be taken up in more detail in the next chapter. During the discussion of diagnosis and prognosis, however, providers should habitually forecast any cost of declining treatment: "If it isn't causing you too much discomfort, you could simply leave it alone. Ignoring it, however, runs a substantial risk that you will face a very costly procedure in 3 or 4 years."

Activity 8-3

Imagine you have conducted an examination and discovered evidence of periodontal disease. Ask a colleague to assume the patient role and select which of the four motivations is primary (pain and pain relief, esthetics, function, or cost). Deliver the diagnosis and prognosis in a way that addresses both the primary motivation and one of the remaining three. Then assume the patient role and have the colleague deliver a diagnosis and prognosis of dental erosion.

Instruction Strategies for Routine Care

In the course of an examination or during the subsequent assessment of patients' oral hygiene practices and risks, providers may become aware of deficiencies in patients' routine care. Sometimes the way patients brush, floss, or clean their braces or dentures does not accomplish the goal. In some cases, the way patients implement these skills actually undermines their oral health. If patients are performing routine care inadequately or incorrectly, providers should instruct them in proper oral hygiene during the diagnosis and prognosis discussion. We view instruction in routine care (eg, how to brush properly) separately from preventive treatment planning (eg, how to stop smoking). The latter entails a more significant change in patient behavior. The strategies presented in this section can be used for both instruction and treatment planning, although preventive treatment planning usually entails additional strategies such as those recommended for motivational interviewing.

All of providers' verbal and nonverbal skills should be brought to bear when instructing patients on routine care. Of particular use are presentation aids, described in detail in chapter 6. When teaching patients how to effectively incorporate oral health skills into their daily routine, providers may require more complex strategies. In this section, we present four instructional strategies for teaching patients proper routine care: tell-show-do, teach-back, hand-over-hand, and chaining (Box 8-4). Simple spoken instruction may suffice for adults with adequate cognitive processing and literacy skills. For patients who have cognitive or literacy limitations that compromise their ability to process spoken instructions (eg, children and those with dementia), these strategies can reinforce spoken instructions.

Box 8-4 | **Instruction strategies for routine oral health care**

Tell-show-do
- Instruct the patient how to implement the practice.
- Illustrate the practice on yourself, the patient, or a model.
- Have the patient perform the practice satisfactorily.

Teach-back
- Describe and demonstrate the practice.
- Ask the patient to teach you how to do it.

Hand-over-hand
- Tell the patient what you are about to do.
- Place your hands on the patient's hands and perform the practice.
- Narrate the process.

Chaining
- Tell the patient what you are about to do.
- Teach the first task in a complex practice.
- After the first task is mastered, teach the second.
- Continue until the patient can perform the practice independently.

Unfortunately, dental providers use too few of the simple and complex strategies available to them.[74] Patients' proficiency at taking care of their routine oral health needs likely suffers.

Tell-show-do

The **tell-show-do technique** is a simple way to reinforce and illustrate verbal instructions in routine care, but it is also often used to teach a child how to cooperate during a dental examination or procedure. First the provider tells the patient what to do. Then the provider demonstrates how the skill is implemented. The demonstration can be carried out on the provider, on the patient, or on a model. The nature of the instruction and the preference of the provider should determine which is most appropriate. Finally, the provider asks the patient to demonstrate what has been explained to confirm that the patient both understands the skill and is capable of doing it.

Tell-show-do is a behavioral management technique with a long record of effectiveness when used with children and patients with special needs.[75] It remains a technique favored by pediatric dentists.[76,77] Further, parents often rate it more highly than any other behavioral management technique used by providers.[78–80] Its effectiveness can perhaps be enhanced if providers provide positive reinforcement when patients correctly demonstrate their newly acquired skills.[81] A member survey of the American Academy of Pediatric Dentistry indicates that 99% use tell-show-do and positive reinforcement.[82]

Teach-back

A similar way to teach proper routine care to a patient is the **teach-back method**. First, the provider instructs and/or demonstrates an oral health skill. When the provider believes the patient understands—or should understand—the instruction, the provider asks the patient to teach the skill back to the provider. For instance, after giving a brief lesson, the provider may say: "Now let me make sure that I explained denture care thoroughly. Can you explain to me how you are going to clean them every day?"

This technique is used by fewer than a quarter of dentists, but is easy to implement and can be useful when attempting to determine whether a patient truly understands what has been said.[74] For this reason, it is particularly useful for patients with low health literacy or little proficiency in English.[83] Even if patients have no cognitive or language limitations affecting understanding, teach-back is an effective way to help patients remember what they are supposed to do. For instance, the scheduling and dosage of some medications can be difficult for patients to remember, but teach-back can help patients recall how often and how much medication they should take: "Please tell me when you are going to take this medication and how much you will take." The communication strategy increases patient recall by 37.3% and is also associated with increases in patient satisfaction.[84]

Question of ethics: Some people seem better suited to treat patients with disabilities or communication limitations. Perhaps they have better communication skills or more patience. If you feel ill-equipped to treat challenging patients, is it ethical to refer them to a colleague? Is this fair to the patient? Is this fair to the colleague? Do providers have an ethical obligation to develop an adequate level of skill in treating patients who present challenges?

Hand-over-hand

The **hand-over-hand strategy** is as simple as it sounds. The provider teaches proper technique by placing his or her hands over the patient's hands and performing the task. The instruction is repeated until the patient can perform the task independently. The provider should narrate the instruction and offer positive feedback while carrying out the hand-over-hand technique: "This is the way you should brush your teeth, using small circles. Yes…I think you are doing it right. Great job! Now I'm going to turn your hand loose, and I want to see you do it by yourself."

Because this strategy is so directive and involves touching (in a low-contact culture), it is usually reserved for patients with significant cognitive limitations, such as those with intellectual disabilities or dementia.[85–87] In fact, it is often used by and recommended for geriatric nurses and nursing assistants in long-term care facilities to help residents learn or relearn repetitive self-care tasks such as brushing their teeth.[88] It has also been used successfully to teach oral hygiene skills to visually impaired elementary school children.[89] The patient populations who would most benefit from the hand-over-hand instructional technique generally have higher unmet oral health care needs, so—even if they rarely use it—providers should make the effort to incorporate this strategy into their repertoire.

Chaining

A fourth instructional strategy is **chaining**, in which the skill to be taught is first broken down into component tasks. For instance, one of the instruction strategies websites listed at the end of this chapter separates toothbrushing into 18 sequential tasks. The provider should explain what he or she is about to do and then teach the first of the tasks to the patient. Only after the patient has mastered the first task should the provider move to the next task. After all the component tasks have been mastered, the provider should ask the patient to perform the entire behavior independently. A variation of this technique is backward chaining, in which the patient is taught the last step first. As with other techniques, positive reinforcement can facilitate the instruction.

As with hand-over-hand, chaining can be very useful when providers are treating patients with dementia or Alzheimer disease.[86,90] It can also be useful for teaching autistic patients and patients with intellectual disabilities.[91,92] Providers should employ a trial-and-error approach and should combine instructional techniques to adapt the communication approach to the needs of particular patients. When providers exhibit enthusiasm, tenacity, and patience, their efforts will be rewarded by understanding.

Activity 8-4

The first step in using the chaining technique is to break a behavior into its component tasks. Doing this can help you think deliberately about the way patients might best receive complex information. Imagine you are going to use the chaining technique to instruct someone on how to floss properly. List the independent steps involved in the flossing behavior. Compare your list to those of your colleagues, noting that there is no correct number of steps. Different patients may require different levels of instruction.

Although treating patients with special needs can be challenging, doing so can also hone providers' communication skills by making them consider carefully how they present information—something they may be less aware of when treating fully functioning adults. Good dental providers with thriving practices will form long-term relationships with a variety of patients. Through accident or age, even the healthiest of patients may develop cognitive and physical limitations. To sustain patient relationships following such changes, providers must develop proficiency in alternative ways of presenting information.

Chapter Checklist ☑

Communication during procedures
☐ Remain aware that patient communication occurs even when the provider is not speaking or listening.
☐ Make sure that the patient sees you wash your hands and don your gloves.
☐ Notify the patient before you recline the chair or adjust the head or arm rests.
☐ Coordinating: Practice smooth patient handoffs from one practitioner to another.
☐ Coordinating: Disclose oral health status clearly, discreetly, nonjudgmentally, and in the presence of the patient.
☐ Coordinating: Treat the patient as a member of the dental team.
☐ Coordinating: Avoid overuse of the first person plural (ie, we).
☐ Coordinating: Say nothing in a patient's presence that would alarm or offend.
☐ Coordinating: Acknowledge the patient's presence and use eye contact to indicate when you are speaking to the patient.
☐ Coordinating: Minimize interruptions.
☐ Instructing: Determine the patient's control preferences and politely direct a patient who has lower control preferences.
☐ Instructing: Tell the patient what is expected of him or her, clarifying specific expectations.
☐ Instructing: Politely instruct the patient on how to facilitate the procedure, avoiding single-word commands.
☐ Instructing: Soften vocal tone, say please, and apologize when a mistake is made.
☐ Calming: Project calmness and confidence during the procedure.
☐ Calming: Minimize nervous behaviors and avoid internalizing a patient's anxiety.
☐ Calming: Empathize with the patient's anxiety, but model confidence.
☐ Calming: Avoid negative comments and criticism during the procedure.
☐ Calming: Provide encouragement and benchmarks on the procedure's progress.
☐ Monitoring: Observe the patient's nonverbal behavior for signs of distress.
☐ Monitoring: Offer breaks when needed.
☐ Monitoring: Designate a hand signal for the patient to request a break.
☐ Monitoring: Periodically ask how the patient is doing and if the patient would like a break.
☐ Narrating: Describe what you are doing as you do it.
☐ Narrating: Describe what you are observing, unless it will cause distress.
☐ Narrating: Offer praise and compliments on every patient's in-chair behavior or oral health and habits.
☐ Educating: Avoid dental topics that will agitate the patient.

❑ Educating: Describe the etiology and risk factors of the observed problem.
❑ Educating: Explain the consequences if no treatment is undertaken.
❑ Educating: Mention that preventive and/or restorative treatment options are available and summarize them.

Diagnosis and prognosis
❑ Describe conditions: Start by praising or complimenting the patient.
❑ Describe conditions: Describe what was observed and state or restate any diagnosis or areas of concern.
❑ Describe conditions: If a firm diagnosis cannot be offered, explain why.
❑ Describe conditions: Repeat information and acknowledge the repetition.
❑ Describe conditions: Note any changes in oral health status over time, stating plainly what was attempted and accomplished.
❑ Assess caries and disease risk: Determine the patient's current oral hygiene practices.
❑ Assess caries and disease risk: If appropriate, ask the patient to demonstrate his or her oral hygiene practices.
❑ Assess caries and disease risk: Discuss behaviors that may place the patient at higher risk for other oral health problems.
❑ Explain the consequences if no treatment or behavior change is undertaken: Describe the likelihood of positive versus negative outcomes, using outcomes meaningful to the patient (cost, time, effort, and discomfort).
❑ Explain the consequences if no treatment or behavior change is undertaken: Describe short- and long-term consequences of negative outcomes.
❑ Explain the consequences if no treatment or behavior change is undertaken: Mention that treatment options are available.

Understanding patient motivations
❑ Ask the patient what he or she wants from dental health care, keeping in mind common motivations.
❑ Note the patient's evaluations regarding health care and record motivations in the patient's records.
❑ Pain and pain relief: Remain aware that the patient may have lived with pain for weeks or months before seeking help.
❑ Pain and pain relief: Emphasize what causes the pain, how the condition will progress, and how treatment would alleviate the pain.
❑ Esthetics: Objectively note variations in tooth color, alignment, or integrity and mention available treatments.
❑ Esthetics: Remain aware of unhealthy esthetic motivations, discern the patient's expectations, and clarify what dental treatment can and cannot accomplish.
❑ Esthetics: Routinely mention esthetic aspects of diagnosis and treatment.
❑ Function: Address functional problems disclosed during the health history or observed in the way the patient speaks or moves the jaws.
❑ Function: Ask directly about function while probing oral health habits.
❑ Cost: Remain aware that few patients are unconcerned with the cost of dental care.
❑ Cost: Remain aware that the patient may refrain from directly addressing cost.
❑ Cost: Forecast any cost of deciding against treatment.

> **Instructions for routine care**
> ❑ Instruct the patient in proper oral hygiene during the discussion of diagnosis and prognosis.
> ❑ Provide spoken instruction to an adult with adequate cognition and literacy skills.
> ❑ Use positive reinforcement, which enhances all instruction strategies.
> ❑ When determining which strategy to use, employ a trial-and-error approach and combine instructional techniques.
> ❑ Tell-show-do: Tell the patient what to do, demonstrate the skill, and then ask the patient to demonstrate.
> ❑ Teach-back: Teach and/or demonstrate a skill and then ask the patient to teach the lesson.
> ❑ Hand-over-hand: Place your hands over the patient's hands, perform the task, and narrate the instructions with positive feedback.
> ❑ Chaining: Break the skill into component tasks.
> ❑ Chaining: Tell the patient what you are about to do and then teach each component.
> ❑ Chaining: Move to the next component when the previous one is learned.
> ❑ Chaining: Ask the patient to perform the entire skill independently.

For More Information

Communicating during examinations and procedures
- http://www.juniordentist.com/use-dental-hand-signs-in-clinics-for-communication-during-procedures.html
- http://www.dentaleconomics.com/articles/print/volume-100/issue-2/columns/comprehensive-case-acceptance/communicating-so-patients-understand.html
- http://www.dentalheroes.com/communicate-dental-patients

Communicating diagnosis and prognosis
- http://www.dentistrytoday.com/management-tips/4790-ten-steps-for-an-efficient-stress-free-recall-exam
- http://www.ncbi.nlm.nih.gov/pmc/articles/PMC3107733
- http://ukpmc.ac.uk/articles/PMC1955302

Patient motivations for dental care
- http://dental-work-needed.aidpage.com
- http://www.quintpub.com/PDFs/book_preview/B9015.pdf
- http://www.nycdentist.com/dental-information/38/Listen-to-the-Chief-Complaint-in-Dentistry
- http://www.ncbi.nlm.nih.gov/pmc/articles/PMC2690262
- http://www.sanedentist.com/why-people-ignore-dental-health.html

Instruction strategies
- http://www.dentalfearcentral.org/help/psychology/tell-show-do
- http://www.kevinmd.com/blog/2011/11/teaching-clinicians-teachback-patient-education.html
- http://engagingthepatient.com/2011/10/10/teach-back-the-benefits-and-challenges
- http://www.bbbautism.com/aba_shaping_and_chaining.htm
- http://abaappliedbehavioranalysis.weebly.com/chaining.html
- http://ocw.tufts.edu/Content/56/learningunits/675434

References

1. Friedman S. Diagnosis and treatment planning. Dent Clin North Am 1977;21:237–247.
2. Sandell R, Camner LG, Sarhed G. The dentist's attitudes and their interaction with patient involvement in oral hygiene compliance. Br J Clin Psychol 1994;33:549–558.
3. Eitel K. The hygiene handoff: A fail-proof way to increase productivity and decrease stress. Dent Today 2008;27(10):178–180.
4. Ceib P. Patient-centered outcomes in surgical and orthodontic treatment. Semin Orthod 1999;5:223–230.
5. Clark MS, Campbell SA, Clark AM. Technique for the administration of nitrous oxide/oxygen sedation to ensure psychotropic analgesic nitrous oxide (PAN) effects. Int J Neurosci 2006;116:871–877.
6. Wang RR, Olmsted LW. A direct method for fabricating tongue-shielding stent. J Prosthet Dent 1995;74:171–173.
7. Kinsman H, Roter D, Berkenblit G, et al. "We'll do this together": The role of the first person plural in fostering partnership in patient-physician relationships. J Gen Intern Med 2010;25:186–193.
8. Rouse RA. A paradigm of intervention: Emotional communication in dentistry. Health Commun 1989;1:239–252.
9. Irwin JY, Torres-Urquidy MH, Schleyer T, Monaco V. A preliminary model of work during initial examination and treatment planning appointments. Br Dent J 2009;206:E1.
10. Law A, Logan H, Baron RS. Desire for control, felt control, and stress inoculation training during dental treatment. J Pers Soc Psychol 1994;67:926–936.
11. Baron RS, Logan H. Desired control, felt control, and dental pain: Recent findings and remaining issues. Motiv Emotion 1993;17:181–204.
12. Levin R. Measuring patient satisfaction. J Am Dent Assoc 2005;136:362–363.
13. Olson RE, Laskin DM. Expectations of patients from orthognathic surgery. J Oral Surg 1980;38:283–285.
14. Milgrom P, Spiekerman C, Grembowski D. Dissatisfaction with dental care among mothers of Medicaid-enrolled children. Community Dent Oral Epidemiol 2008;36:451–458.
15. Sinha PK, Nanda RS, McNeil DW. Perceived orthodontist behaviors that predict patient satisfaction, orthodontist-patient relationship, and patient adherence in orthodontic treatment. Am J Orthod Dentofacial Orthop 1996;110:370–377.
16. Lester GW, Smith SG. Listening and talking to patients. A remedy for malpractice suits? West J Med 1993;158:268–272.
17. Coy K, Stratton R. Avoiding your greatest fear--malpractice. J Okla Dent Assoc 2002;93(2):18–27.
18. Jangland E, Gunningberg L, Carlsson M. Patients' and relatives' complaints about encounters and communication in health care: Evidence for quality improvement. Patient Educ Couns 2009;75:199–204.
19. Schwartz B. Errors in dentistry: A call for apology. J Am Coll Dent 2005;72(2):26–32.

20. Wei M. Doctors, apologies, and the law: An analysis and critique of apology laws. J Health Law 2007;40:107–159.

21. Poorsattar SP. Recognizing and managing dental fears: Anxiolysis from the perspective of a dental student. J Dent Educ 2010;74:397–401.

22. Schoenewolf G. Emotional contagion: Behavioral induction in individuals and groups. Mod Psychoanal 1990;15:49–61.

23. Lara A, Crego A, Romero-Maroto M. Emotional contagion of dental fear to children: The fathers' mediating role in parental transfer of fear. Int J Paediatr Dent 2012;22:324 330.

24. Bush JP, Melamed BG, Sheras PL, Greenbaum PE. Mother-child patterns of coping with anticipatory medical stress. Health Psychol 1986;5:137–157.

25. Hatfield E, Rapson RL, Le YCL. Emotional contagion and empathy. In: Decety J, Ickes W (eds). The Social Neuroscience of Empathy. Cambridge, MA: MIT Press, 2009:19–30.

26. Curtin S, Hammond S. Placing dental clinicians within the normative base regarding vicarious response. Eur J Dent Educ 2012;16:6–11.

27. Stouthard MEA, Hoogstraten J. Ratings of fears associated with twelve dental situations. J Dent Res 1987;66:1175–1178.

28. Rouse RA, Hamilton MA. Dentists' technical competence, communication, and personality as predictors of dental patient anxiety. J Behav Med 1990;13:307–319.

29. Okawa K, Ichinohe T, Kaneko Y. Anxiety may enhance pain during dental treatment. Bull Tokyo Dent Coll 2005;46(3):51–58.

30. Zhou Y, Cameron E, Forbes G, Humphris G. Systematic review of the effect of dental staff behaviour on child dental patient anxiety and behaviour. Patient Educ Couns 2011;85:4–13.

31. Moore R, Brødsgaard I, Rosenberg N. The contribution of embarrassment to phobic dental anxiety: A qualitative research study. BMC Psychiatry 2004;4(1):1–11.

32. Öhrn K, Hakeberg M, Abrahamsson KH. Dental beliefs, patients' specific attitudes towards dentists and dental hygienists: A comparative study. Int J Dent Hyg 2008;6:205–213.

33. Melamed BG. Assessment and management strategies for the difficult pediatric dental patient. Anesth Prog 1986;33:197–200.

34. Wilson TG. Compliance and its role in periodontal therapy. Periodontol 2000 1996;12:16–23.

35. Corah NL, O'Shea RM, Skeels DK. Dentists' perceptions of problem behaviors in patients. J Am Dent Assoc 1982;104:829–833.

36. Maytan LM, Terenzi GM. Fear and anxiety management for the special needs patient. In: Weiner AA (ed). The Fearful Dental Patient: A Guide to Understanding and Managing. Ames, IA: Wiley-Blackwell, 2011:241–264.

37. Tandon S, Garg R, Agrawal P. Dentists: Your back requires back-up now!!! WebmedCentral Dentistry 2010;1(9):WMC00573. http://www.webmedcentral.com/wmcpdf/Article_WMC00573.pdf. Accessed 8 February 2015.

38. Harp H, Hook E, Solberg E, Anderson D. A patient's perspective on how hygienists can decrease patient anxiety. J Dent Hyg 2000;74:322.

39. Coleman H, Burton J. Aspects of control in the dentist-patient relationship. Int J Sociol Language 1985;1985(51):75–104.

40. Dougall A, Fiske J. Access to special care dentistry. 2. Communication. Br Dent J 2008;205:11–21.

41. Abbe M, Sudano JJ Jr, Demko CA, et al. Revisiting comfort: Strategies observed in the direct observation study. Gen Dent 2007;55:420–425.

42. Levin RP. Creating true customer service. J Am Dent Assoc 2010;141:337–338.

43. Choi Y, Dodd V, Watson J, Tomar SL, Logan HL, Edwards H. Perspectives of African Americans and dentists concerning dentist-patient communication on oral cancer screening. Patient Educ Couns 2008;71:41–51.

44. Levin RP. The interpersonal factor. J Am Dent Assoc 2008;139:986–987.

45. Nash DA. Engaging children's cooperation in the dental environment through effective communication. Pediatr Dent 2006;28:455–459.

46. Patil MS, Patil SB. Geriatric patient—Psychological and emotional considerations during dental treatment. Gerodontology 2009;26:72–77.

47. Barenie J, Ripa L. The use of behavior modification techniques to successfully manage the child dental patient. J Am Dent Assoc 1977;94:329–334.

48. Azrin NH, Nunn RG, Frantz-Renshaw SE. Habit reversal vs negative practice treatment of self-destructive oral habits (biting, chewing or licking of the lips, cheeks, tongue or palate). J Behav Ther Exp Psychiatry 1982;13:49–54.

49. Fleming S, Demko CA, Lalumandier JA. Patient retention: What keeps them coming back? Presented at the IADR/AADR/CADR 87th General Session and Exhibition, Miami, April 4, 2009.

50. Corah NL. The dental-practitioner and preventive health behavior. Health Educ Behav 1974;2:226–235.

51. Milgrom P, Weinstein P, Melnick S, Beach B, Spadafora A. Oral hygiene instruction and health risk assessment in dental practice. J Public Health Dent 1989;49:24–31.

52. Street RL. Information-giving in medical consultations: The influence of patients' communicative styles and personal characteristics. Soc Sci Med 1991;32:541–548.

53. Klages U, Sergl HG, Burucker I. Relations between verbal behavior of the orthodontist and communicative cooperation of the patient in regular orthodontic visits. Am J Orthod Dentofacial Orthop 1992;102:265–269.

54. Brennan DS, Spencer AJ. The role of dentist, practice and patient factors in the provision of dental services. Community Dent Oral Epidemiol 2005;33:181–195.

55. Fox C. Evidence summary: What do we know from qualitative research about people's care-seeking about oral health? Br Dent J 2010;209:225–231.

56. Giddon DB, Anderson NK. Psychosocial factors in motivation, treatment, compliance, and satisfaction with orthodontic care. In: Krishnan V, Davidovitch Z (eds). Integrated Clinical Orthodontics. Chichester, England: Blackwell, 2012:69–82.

57. Arnett GW, Worley CM. The Treatment Motivation Survey: Defining patient motivation for treatment. Am J Orthod Dentofacial Orthop 1999;115:233–238.

58. Davidson PL, Andersen RM. Determinants of dental care utilization for diverse ethnic and age groups. Adv Dent Res 1997;11:254–262.

59. Stoller EP, Gilbert GH, Pyle MA, Duncan RP. Coping with tooth pain: A qualitative study of lay management strategies and professional consultation. Spec Care Dentist 2001;21:208–215.

60. Cohen LA, Bonito AJ, Akin DR, et al. Toothache pain: Behavioral impact and self-care strategies. Spec Care Dentist 2009;29:85–95.

61. Scott SE, Grunfeld EA, Main J, McGurk M. Patient delay in oral cancer: A qualitative study of patients' experiences. Psychooncology 2006;15:474–485.

62. Theobald AH, Wong BK, Quick AN, Thomson WM. The impact of the popular media on cosmetic dentistry. N Z Dent J 2006;102(3):58–63.

63. Wędrychowska-Szulc B, Syryńska M. Patient and parent motivation for orthodontic treatment—A questionnaire study. Eur J Orthod 2010;32:447–452.

64. Fleming PS, Proczek K, DiBiase AT. I want braces: Factors motivating patients and their parents to seek orthodontic treatment. Community Dent Health 2008;25:166–169.

65. Klages U, Zentner A. Dentofacial aesthetics and quality of life. Semin Orthod 2007;13:104–115.

66. Pabari S, Moles DR, Cunningham SJ. Assessment of motivation and psychological characteristics of adult orthodontic patients. Am J Orthod Dentofacial Orthop 2011;140:e263–e272.

67. Davis LG, Ashworth PD, Spriggs LS. Psychological effects of aesthetic dental treatment. J Dent 1998;26:547–554.

68. Daniels AS, Seacat JD, Inglehart MR. Orthodontic treatment motivation and cooperation: A cross-sectional analysis of adolescent patients' and parents' responses. Am J Orthod Dentofacial Orthop 2009;136:780–787.

69. De Jongh A, Oosterink FMD, van Rood YR, Aartman IHA. Preoccupation with one's appearance: A motivating factor for cosmetic dental treatment? Br Dent J 2008;204:691–695.

70. Marzola R, Derbabian K, Donovan TE, Arcidiacono A. The science of communicating the art of esthetic dentistry. 1. Patient-dentist-patient communication. J Esthet Dent 2000;12:131–138.

71. Derbabian K, Marzola R, Arcidiacono A. The science of communicating the art of dentistry. J Calif Dent Assoc 1998;26:101–116.

72. Cohen LA, Harris SL, Bonito AJ, et al. Coping with toothache pain: A qualitative study of low-income persons and minorities. J Public Health Dent 2007;67:28–35.

73. Scott SE, Grunfeld EA, Auyeung V, McGurk M. Barriers and triggers to seeking help for potentially malignant oral symptoms: Implications for interventions. J Public Health Dent 2009;69:34–40.

74. Rozier RG, Horowitz AM, Podschun G. Dentist-patient communication techniques used in the United States. J Am Dent Assoc 2011;142:518–530.

75. Lyons RA. Understanding basic behavioral support techniques as an alternative to sedation and anesthesia. Spec Care Dentist 2009;29:39–50.

76. Allen KD, Stanley RI, McPherson K. Evaluation of behavior management technology dissemination in pediatric dentistry. Pediatr Dent 1990;12:79–82.

77. Crossley ML, Joshi G. An investigation of paediatric dentists' attitudes towards parental accompaniment and behavioural management techniques in the UK. Br Dent J 2002;192:517–521.

78. Murphy MG, Fields HW Jr, Machen JB. Parental acceptance of pediatric dentistry behavior management techniques. Pediatr Dent 1984;6:193–198.

79. Alammouri M. The attitude of parents toward behavior management techniques in pediatric dentistry. J Clin Pediatr Dent 2006;30:310–313.

80. Eaton JJ, McTigue DJ, Fields HW, Beck FM. Attitudes of contemporary parents toward behavior management techniques used in pediatric dentistry. Pediatr Dent 2005;27:107–113.

81. Marshall J, Sheller B, Mancl L, Williams BJ. Parental attitudes regarding behavior guidance of dental patients with autism. Pediatr Dent 2008;30:400–407.

82. Adair SM, Waller JL, Schafer TE, Rockman RA. A survey of members of the American Academy of Pediatric Dentistry on their use of behavior management techniques. Pediatr Dent 2004;26:159–166.

83. Horowitz AM, Kleinman DV. Oral health literacy: The new imperative to better oral health. Dent Clin North Am 2008;52:333–344.

84. Bertakis KD. The communication of information from physician to patient: A method for increasing patient retention and satisfaction. J Fam Pract 1977;5:217–222.

85. Chalmers JM. Conducting geriatric dental research with cognitively impaired adults. Gerodontology 2000;17:17–24.

86. Chalmers JM. Behavior management and communication strategies for dental professionals when caring for patients with dementia. Spec Care Dentist 2000;20:147–154.

87. Cumella S, Ransford N, Lyons J, Burnham H. Needs for oral care among people with intellectual disability not in contact with community dental services. J Intellect Disabil Res 2000;44(pt 1):45–52.

88. Jablonski RA. Examining oral health in nursing home residents and overcoming mouth care-resistive behaviours. Ann Long-Term Care Clin Care Aging 2010;18(1):21–26.

89. Chang CH, Shih YH. Teaching oral hygiene skills to elementary students with visual impairments. J Vis Impair Blind 2005;99:26–39.

90. Prajer R, Kacerik M. Treating patients with Alzheimer's disease. Dimens Dent Hygiene 2006;4(9):24–26.

91. DeQuinzio JA, Townsend DB, Poulson CL. The effects of forward chaining and contingent social interaction on the acquisition of complex sharing responses by children with autism. Res Autism Spectr Disord 2008;2:264–275.

92. Jerome J, Frantino EP, Sturmey P. The effects of errorless learning and backward chaining on the acquisition of Internet skills in adults with developmental disabilities. J Appl Behav Anal 2007;40:185–189.

Presenting Treatment Plans

Why Treatment Planning Matters

Treatment planning is the phase of treatment that most clearly distinguishes patient-centered care from other approaches to health care delivery. The traditional model tends to be disease centered: Providers present the treatment plan most effective in removing the cause or relieving the symptoms of the diagnosed problem.

A common alternative to patient-centered care is the business-centered approach: Providers enhance the profitability of their practice by encouraging patients to pursue restorative and cosmetic treatments, particularly if those treatments are paid through insurance. Many practice consultants and resources are available to enhance the "productivity" of a dental practice. Some of their recommended strategies are transparent attempts to persuade or frighten patients into accepting treatment they do not need or cannot afford, with the result that patients are increasingly suspicious of the motives of dental providers who recommend any treatment. The problem of unnecessary treatment recommendations is widespread enough to prompt a movement (minimum intervention dentistry) and, in Great Britain, an investigation by the Committee of Enquiry into Unnecessary Dental Treatment.[1]

Practices must, of course, remain financially healthy if they are to continue providing care. Given this obligation, providers must rely on their own professionalism and ethical commitments to present options and plan treatments that meet their financial obligations, the patient's clinical needs, and the terms of the patient-provider relationship. Patient-centered care first acknowledges that not all appointments require treatment planning. Patients exhibiting good oral health and good health habits have no need of treatment beyond regular examinations. Esthetic treatment options can be presented, but any attempt to pressure patients unreceptive to esthetic procedures threatens to undermine the relationship: Patients do not like being told by professionals that their appearance is inferior. With patients who require no treatment or who require additional diagnostic tests or consultations with a specialist, providers should implement communication strategies for ending an appointment, provided in the last section of this chapter.

Many patients, however, do require treatment. Both preventive and restorative treatments require planning and patient adherence to provider recommendations. Although providers believe that patient adherence is vital to successful treatment, they rate most patients as moderate in treatment plan adherence.[2] One study found that patient adherence is significantly affected by personality factors, negative motives (eg, avoiding pain), and positive motives (eg, improving health).[3]

Such patient-focused studies, however, neglect the influence of providers in shaping awareness, motives, and expectations in their patients. The primary reasons for nonadherence cited by providers are patients' lack of awareness of problems, patients' lack of motivation, and patients' personal problems.[2] A 2009 meta-analysis of 127 studies found that the rate of nonadherence was 19% higher among patients of physicians with poor communication skills than among patients of physicians with good communication skills.[4] The same study found that communication training of providers increased patient adherence 1.62 times. Thus, patient-provider communication plays a key role in treatment planning. This chapter presents patient-provider communication strategies for effective treatment planning and implementation.

Strategies for Categorizing Treatment

Prescribed and discretionary treatment

In 1995, Bader and Shugars[5] reviewed the available research on treatment planning and found little agreement among dental professionals on what oral conditions required treatment and what that treatment should be: "Even when differences in patients are controlled, variation in dentists' clinical decisions is ubiquitous."

Two years later, *Reader's Digest* ran an article titled "How Honest are Dentists?" written by a Pulitzer Prize–winning journalist.[6] The author visited 50 dentists in 28 states, showed each a set of radiographs, and asked them for an examination and treatment recommendation. Despite having only one immediate problem (a crown needed on the mandibular first molar), he received varied diagnoses, and the cost of recommended treatments ranged from $500 to $30,000. The author concluded that his employer's direct reimbursement policy appealed to many of the dentists because insurance companies would not question their work or their charges. This conclusion suggests the central role insurance (or its absence) plays in treatment decisions that should more appropriately be determined by patients and dental teams. The article reinforced the suspicion that dentists are greedy. The article did not appear in a peer-reviewed dental journal, but—for better or worse—patients are more likely influenced by infomation about dentistry that appears in popular media outlets like *Reader's Digest* or the *Dr Oz Show*.

A 1996 study found that the recommended treatment option offered to 37 patients averaged three times the cost of the least expensive option offered.[7] The authors, however, found little evidence that a few greedy dentists were the cause of the cost discrepancies. Instead, they concluded that cost differentials were a result of inconsistencies in both the determination of which teeth required treatment and the selection of appropriate treatment. Providers routinely differ in the decision to treat and in the treatment recommended, but such variation could be interpreted by patients as evidence that some dentists are motivated more by money than by clinical considerations.

Christensen[8] noted the rapid expansion of treatment options available and observed, "It is very difficult for patients to know whether suggested treatment is mandatory or elective." The term *mandatory* is problematic and contradictory to patient-centered care. In reply to Christensen's article, Jensen[9] noted that nearly all treatment is elective: "The reality is, people can and do live with these pathological conditions constantly."

Dental care providers who have spent years studying ways to treat oral health problems—and more years implementing those treatments—find it challenging to realize that patients may have reasons for opting out of treatment. The reasons may not seem legitimate to providers, but because they belong to the decision-makers (ie, the patients), they must be respected. Therefore, the first treatment option presented should be "do nothing," followed by an accurate prognosis. Only after patients understand their prognosis can they make an informed decision regarding their options.

In an effort to promote patient-centered thinking in treatment planning, providers should reconsider using the words *mandatory* and *elective*. It is true that patients always retain the option of rejecting treatment, but treatments that are urgently needed or have irrefutable evidence of effectiveness are not necessarily *elective*, a word that connotes a take-it-or-leave-it attitude. To help patients better understand the importance of treatment, we suggest using the words *prescribed* or *discretionary*. Treatments in both categories can be recommended by providers, but the former bears the weight of evidence-based practice, whereas the latter term suggests that patient preferences play more of a role than clinical urgency.

> Q **Question of ethics:** In the *Reader's Digest* article[6] that was mentioned, the reporter noted that some dentists praised his former dental work, while others criticized the unknown dentists who performed it. In the course of your career, you will witness treatment recommendations or procedures you would not have offered. Do you have a professional obligation to mention to a patient the unnecessary or sub-optimal care delivered by another professional? Or do you have an obligation to support the professional judgment of a peer?

Restorative and preventive treatment

In addition to telling patients whether recommended options are prescribed or discretionary, providers should clarify whether treatment options are restorative or preventive. From the perspective of patients, **restorative treatment** generally refers to intensive clinical or behavioral interventions and their attendant follow-up care. **Preventive treatment** seeks to avert more intensive or invasive procedures by changing or improving patient's oral health–related behaviors.

As indicated in Table 9-1, every treatment option should be described by the presence of a problem (restorative or preventive) and the strength of the provider recommendation (prescribed or discretionary). Providers require the detail and background presented in treatment planning textbooks.[10–12] Few patients, however, need that level of detail. What all patients require is an honest discussion providing them an understanding of whether they have a problem yet and how important treatment is.

Table 9-1 Categories of treatment plans

Restorative	Preventive
Prescribed	
Primary goal: to relieve pain or restore lost function Examples: root canal treatment, tooth extraction, and prosthetics	Primary goal: to reduce the risk for severe oral health problems Examples: tobacco cessation and other beneficial behavioral changes
Discretionary	
Primary goal: to enhance cosmetic appeal Examples: tooth whitening, veneers, and bonding	Primary goal: to enhance or increase oral health–protective factors Examples: pit and fissure sealants and supplemental fluoride therapy

The need for discussion regarding restorative treatment is particularly important, given the variability in dentists' recommendations. A 1993 microlevel study found moderate interdentist reliability ($r = .62$) in recommending individual teeth for restorative treatment.[13] Reliability was lowest ($r = .43$) regarding previously restored teeth. A 1997 study found that variation in the use of crowns was significantly related to both age and geography.[14] Older patients were more likely to receive crowns, increasing the per-tooth treatment cost for this group by up to 33%. Regional variation increased per-tooth cost by up to 31%. Given this variation, providers should not only give some detail when communicating a diagnosis but also present a rationale for their restorative treatment options and recommendations.

Torabinejad and Goodacre[15] suggested that providers deciding between endodontic and dental implant therapy consider patient-related factors (eg, health, comfort, and perceptions of treatment), tooth- and periodontium-related factors, and treatment-related factors (eg, probability of complications and need for follow-up). We agree that this is good advice but would recommend that providers present the decision factors to patients at a level they can comprehend. When treatment options are discussed, involvement of the entire dental team (including specialists) can even lead to greater patient satisfaction.[16] Patients visit other dentists, receive second opinions, and compare their experiences with others in person and online. By providing context for their diagnosis and treatment recommendations, providers enhance their credibility with patients while simultaneously increasing patient ownership of the final treatment decision.

Activity 9-1	Imagine you have a patient with a tooth that requires either extraction or root canal therapy. In deciding between these options, you can find out only three things about the patient, either by asking questions or checking the chart. What three things would you want to know? Compare your answers to those of your colleagues.

Preventive treatment planning is, in many ways, similar to restorative treatment. It is an evidence-based response to an oral health problem or potential problem. Preventive treatments, however, are more likely to entail behavioral change on the part of the patient. Research increasingly reveals connections between systemic and oral health while also discovering connections between human behavior and health outcomes.[17] The ability to motivate and sustain behavioral change in patients entails principles of behavioral science that can seem foreign to clinicians trained in the natural sciences.[18] Unsurprisingly, research suggests that the amount of information provided to patients regarding preventive treatment depends more on provider-related variables than on patient-related variables.[19]

How comfortable are you discussing sensitive behavioral issues with patients? Consider various behavior-related risks to oral health: chewing tobacco, playing contact sports, remaining in a relationship with a violent partner, smoking, using methamphetamine, suffering an eating disorder, or drinking alcohol. Rank these from the easiest to the hardest to discuss with a patient. Does the difficulty lie in broaching the subject, in knowing what to say, or in having accurate information that can help the patient? If you learned to broach the subject, do you think you could grow comfortable with referring patients to specialists?

Activity 9-2

Fortunately, the field of dentistry now acknowledges the role dental professionals can play in promoting behavioral change as a way to minimize or avoid oral health problems.[20–22] Individual professionals, however, often feel uncomfortable or unskilled when communicating with a patient for whom a behavioral intervention is the treatment that would most effectively address a potential problem. As with restorative treatment, preventive treatment entails, at the very least, the professional obligation to discuss patients' risk status and to refer them to an appropriate specialist (eg, someone trained in smoking cessation or the treatment of alcoholism or bulimia). Communication technology is advanced enough that patients, dental providers, and specialists—whether medical or behavioral—can now plan treatments via teleconference.[23,24]

Ideally, providers should develop proficiency in the realm of behavioral dentistry. Doing so will help them handle a variety of challenges, including misbehaving children, anxious adults, and those needing assistance to overcome problems threatening their oral health. A variety of communication approaches can be effective in promoting patient acceptance of both restorative and preventive treatment recommendations while preserving providers' commitment to patient-centered care. In a systematic review of models of health promotion, Yevlahova and Satur[25] concluded that motivational interviewing is the most effective model for behavioral change in a clinical setting. Following a presentation of the steps in discussing a treatment plan, the basic elements of motivational interviewing will be reviewed.

Discussing a Treatment Plan

As mentioned, dental professionals and patients may differ in the perceived need for dental treatment. A 2005 survey study of dentists and parents of pediatric patients found that both groups recognized grossly carious maxillary primary incisors as unhealthy and unattractive and both groups found anterior steel crowns unacceptable for esthetic reasons.[26] There was less agreement that grossly carious teeth warranted extraction, with 92% of dentists agreeing but only 73% of parents. Even less agreement was found regarding treatment for carious teeth with sinus tracts. Dentists favored extraction, but parents favored fluoride application—illustrating the wide gap of knowledge between providers and patients/parents, given that fluoride treatment would never be effective for a carious tooth with a sinus tract. This study highlights something all dental providers quickly discover: Even when providers and patients agree on the need for treatment, they can disagree on the appropriate treatment.

As it relates to patient-provider communication, treatment planning is typically described as *presenting a treatment plan*. We are ambivalent about this terminology because it runs contrary to the tenets of patient-centered health care. It implies that providers are serving up a treatment plan that they have decided is the best for the patient—before the patient has a chance to consider various options or introduce important considerations into the treatment decision. A 1988 study indicated that only one-third of dentists considered patient factors or concerns when determining a treatment plan.[27] Therefore, we include treatment plan presentation as only the first part of a the process, preferring the terminology **discussing a treatment plan** because it better indicates the interchange between patient and provider that should take place when the best course of treatment for a specific patient is determined. Whether the potential treatment is restorative or preventive, or prescribed or discretionary, the provider should guide the treatment planning discussion through five steps (Box 9-1).

Box 9-1 | Steps in discussion of the treatment plan

Step 1: Present treatment options and recommendation
- Focus on the chief complaint or diagnosis.
- Mention treatment options or alternatives.
- Indicate which treatment is recommended.

Step 2: Outline details of treatment options
- Describe clinical details and time and cost commitments.
- Describe your responsibilities as provider as well as the responsibilities of the patient in each of the treatment options.
- Predict expected outcomes.

Step 3: Elicit input and questions
- Ask whether the patient needs clarification on any options.
- Ask whether the patient has concerns that have not been addressed.
- Listen to the patient.

Step 4: Respond to questions or concerns
- Provide truthful and comprehensive responses.
- Contextualize the patient's concerns.
- If you do not know the answers, seek further information.

Step 5: Secure commitment to treatment or schedule follow-up
- Ask the patient to commit to a treatment plan.
- Commit to your treatment obligation.
- If the patient wants to wait or think about it, schedule a time to follow up on the decision.

Step 1: Present treatment options and recommendation

The first step in the treatment plan discussion is for the provider to present options that address the diagnosis or chief complaint that prompted the appointment. The provider should open the discussion by simply mentioning the treatment options, describing them in comparative detail later: "If you decide to fix the broken tooth, two options would be a porcelain crown or a gold crown. Let me explain the advantages and disadvantages of each option and why I would recommend the porcelain crown."

Rarely can only a single treatment option address a patient's problem, so the provider should always try to present at least two treatment options. Doing so offers at least three benefits. First, presenting two options suggests to the patient that the provider has considered (and rejected) alternatives and did not simply select the most expensive. Second, having two options gives the patient some ownership in the decision. If only the recommended treatment is presented, the patient is not really provided with an option. In such cases, the only treatment option is "take it or leave it." With two treatment options to consider, the patient likely feels more invested in the decision and more committed to its implementation. Third, research by Kay and Nuttall[28] suggested that monitoring the patient's responses to various treatment options gives the provider an opportunity to gauge what is important to the patient (eg, pain and pain relief, function, esthetics, and cost).

> **Q** **Question of ethics:** Dental providers vary widely in the number of treatment options they offer patients. Further, they often consider a patient's background, culture, and circumstances when deciding which treatment options to recommend. A provider might recommend a crown for a regular patient or one who has insurance. If the same tooth was in the mouth of a patient without insurance or who has limited access to care, the provider might recommend extraction and might not mention a crown as an option. Is it more ethical to treat everyone the same or more ethical to consider each patient's particular situation? Could the second option lead to any conflicts of interest? Draft a short policy brief, summarizing how you decide how many treatment options to present and which one to recommend.

Step 2: Outline details of treatment options

Patients vary both in the number of options and the level of detail they prefer, so monitoring the responses of the individual patient is crucial. At minimum, the patient should know whether the options are prescribed or discretionary: "Fixing a broken tooth isn't just a cosmetic procedure. If patients postpone fixing the tooth, eventually the nerve and the gums are involved. What would have been a simple treatment may then require multiple procedures to fix your tooth."

The clinical details of the treatment options should be described in adequate detail for the patient to understand what is proposed. Presentation aids, particularly radiographs and models, can facilitate the presentation of options. Computer software, smartphone applications, even three-dimensional virtual treatment planning will increasingly shape patient expectations for treatment plan discussions.[29,30]

In addition to clinical details, the provider should compare and contrast the options in terms important to that particular patient: pain and pain relief, function, esthetics, and cost: "Although gold has a slight advantage in durability, the durability of porcelain has really caught up in recent years. I recommend porcelain because it looks better and it tends to be smoother." Providing a range is acceptable: "We can install the crown in two visits or three at most."

For most patients, cost and time are concerns, so these should be addressed in most treatment discussions. The patient has a right to an estimate of the amount of money and time various treatment options will require. If contingencies will determine the final cost of a procedure, the patient should be notified as well. When addressing issues of time, the provider should estimate how long a treatment or procedure will take and how long the results usually last.

The provider should also mention responsibilities of both patient and provider. With restorative treatment, such responsibilities are generally understood: The patient pays, and the provider performs the work. With preventive treatments, responsibilities should be explicitly detailed: "With this smoking cessation plan, you would be responsible for progressing through the American Lung Association's Freedom from Smoking web modules. I would follow up on your progress. If we decide that you need medication to help you quit for good, I'll make sure you get a prescription."

The provider should also predict expected outcomes, paying particular attention to those important to the patient. Again, it helps to offer ranges and speak in provisional language: "Your crown will feel just like a regular tooth when we are done. Although there are exceptions, with good home care habits crowns may last 10 years or more."

Step 3: Elicit input and questions

In patient-centered care, presentation of options and recommendations only initiates the treatment planning process. The next step is for the patient to contribute comments or concerns that influence the final decision. Patient involvement in the treatment planning process is significantly associated with patient satisfaction and one of the four most important factors determining whether a patient returns.[31]

The provider should first ensure that the patient understood everything that has been described: "Do you understand what your options are and why I made the recommendation I made?" After verifying or clarifying the patient's understanding of the discussion, the provider should elicit any concerns: "Do you have any concerns or want any more information about your treatment options?"

Patients vary in the degree of preferred participation in treatment planning. A patient who grew up with the previous models of health care delivery may be entirely satisfied if the dentist simply makes the treatment decision. A patient who has developed a trusting relationship with a provider may also prefer that the dentist make the decision. Even in such cases, presenting options and explaining why a given treatment is selected can enhance the provider's reputation and motivate the patient to adhere to the treatment plan.

Scarbecz[32] described how providers could use the **DISC (dominant, influencing, steady, cautious) system** to categorize patients according to the treatment discussion approach that would be most effective in motivating adherence. The DISC system was developed in 1928 by psychologist William Moulton Marston (also known for being co-creator of *Wonder Woman*).[33] According to Scarbecz,[32] **dominant patients** respond best to well-organized treatment plan presentations addressing what is needed, why, and what happens if treatment is not undertaken. **Influencing patients** may be more responsive to testimonials and anecdotal evidence than to statistics. **Steady patients** may respond best to assurances of safety and efficacy, and they may prefer traditional procedures to cutting-edge technology. Finally, **cautious patients** may prefer comprehensive details of each treatment option, and they may ask for time to consider their decision.

Even if the provider does not apply the DISC system, he or she should develop the habit of considering what type and level of treatment information a given patient will best accept. When eliciting patient feedback regarding the treatment options and recommendation presented, the provider should use active listening (see chapter 4).

Consider the DISC system described in the text. Additional DISC resources are available online. Categorize yourself as a dental patient according to this framework. Are you dominant, influencing, steady, or cautious? Next, categorize each member of your family. Consider different contexts of information seeking: Do you seek the same level and type of information from a dentist as you do from a produce vendor or mobile telephone salesperson? Are categorization frameworks useful, or do they fail to capture the complexity of human beings?

Step 4: Respond to questions or concerns

The provider should always take seriously the concerns voiced by the patient. While presenting treatment options, the provider should also monitor nonverbal cues emanating from the patient to determine whether the patient seems puzzled or concerned. For a variety of reasons, the patient may be reluctant to voice questions or concerns, and a provider who is an astute observer can identify and address such hesitation. The patient may be embarrassed to ask about pain or cost out of fear that such concerns will reflect badly on him or her.

In a dentistry setting, facing a provider in medical attire, a patient may develop anxiety when contemplating the prospect of dental treatment in much the same way many patients register elevated blood pressure due to environmental cues.[34] The anxiety may render the patient silent. The dental provider should therefore remain aware of "white coat syndrome" and gently press the patient to voice questions and concerns.

When a patient asks questions or expresses concerns, the provider should give accurate and comprehensive information. The provider's job is not to persuade the patient to accept unwanted treatment; the patient of today is likely to be fairly sensitive to marketing strategies. At all costs, the patient should never be misled. For instance, telling a patient that a painful procedure is painless—or that an expensive treatment is affordable—can quickly destroy the credibility of the provider.

All patient concerns are legitimate. The provider should acknowledge the concern, give an accurate assessment, and contextualize the issue. By **contextualize**, we mean enumerating the positive aspects of treatment to balance the (negative) focus or concerns of the patient: "A root canal can involve some discomfort, but the reputation of the procedure is far worse than the reality. We use ample anesthesia, so you feel numbness more than pain, and the drilling is over in a matter of minutes. I doubt it hurts as much as the tooth pain you are dealing with already, and that pain should go away forever when we are done." Cost concerns can be contextualized by comparing the cost of treatment to the cost of home remedies or the greater expense of more expensive and extensive dental work if the problem is not addressed.

The provider should seek more information when he or she does not know the answer to a patient's question. Answers can often be found while the patient is still in the dental office. If the issue cannot be resolved while the patient is in the office, the provider should indicate when he or she can get the information and follow up with the patient at that time.

Whether during the appointment or afterward, communication technology should be used to include the patient in pertinent discussions. Conference calling, Skype, texting, email, and various other media allow better information exchange among patients, dental providers, laboratories, primary physicians, pharmacists, and others.[35-37] Such media can also facilitate referral to a specialist, including specialists in the treatment of behavioral problems such as addiction or eating disorders.

In summary, the importance of establishing accurate patient understanding of treatment options, obligations, and outcomes cannot be overstated. From a legal standpoint, the patient must understand what he or she is agreeing to in order to provide informed consent. Beyond legal obligations, however, the provider can influence patient motivation and satisfaction through the discussion of treatment options. A 2010 study found that the more orthognathic surgery patients focused on functional and esthetic outcomes, the more satisfied they were with the surgery.[38] The same study found that such patients were also more satisfied following surgery if they were more energized prior to surgery. The provider's information and demeanor during treatment planning can therefore presumably influence both expectations for, and engagement with, treatment.

Step 5: Secure commitment to treatment or schedule follow-up

The fifth step in the treatment planning discussion is to come to some decision or agreement about the next phase of care. The provider should ask the patient to commit to a specific treatment: "Are we agreed, then, that we are moving forward with the porcelain crown?" In the spirit of reciprocity that distinguishes patient-centered care, the provider should likewise commit to the treatment obligations: "Great. I think we can schedule your first appointment within the next month. At that visit I'll take some x-rays, make an impression of the tooth, and seat a temporary crown. Then a couple of weeks after that, I'll swap the temporary crown for the permanent one." The provider should sustain and communicate enthusiasm for dentistry throughout an appointment, but particularly when the patient agrees to treatment. A provider who remains positive and focuses on the beneficial outcome can, through the process of emotional contagion, motivate the patient to follow through.

Frequently, the patient will want time to consider treatment options. The patient should be encouraged to think carefully about dental care. The provider must never pressure the patient to make an immediate decision he or she is reluctant to make. High-pressure strategies routinely backfire. If the patient does not absolutely own the treatment decision, the patient may be less satisfied with the outcome and more likely to blame the provider for any problems.

When the patient asks for time to think about the treatment options, the provider should schedule a time to follow up on the patient's decision: "Please take this literature with you and think about what you would like to do. Someone from the office will contact you next week to see if you have made a decision and answer any more questions you may have." It is important for the provider to follow up because it shows that the provider is both reliable and interested in the patient's oral health. The patient may opt for no treatment or to postpone treatment for reasons not shared with a provider. By involving the patient in treatment planning without pressuring for acceptance of treatment, the provider can help the patient become more accepting of treatment, whether that treatment takes place immediately or years later.

Motivational Interviewing

The traditional disease-centered model of health care delivery took for granted that patients shared the goals of providers: to achieve or improve health. Therefore, patients would agree, or at least defer, to the treatment plan determined by providers. One reason for the shift away from traditional health care delivery models is that delivery of treatment plans often faltered in the implementation phase. The process of the treatment planning discussion seeks to integrate the patient's concept of health and to address the patient's goals that may contribute to or compete with health: maintaining financial solvency, minimizing pain, enhancing esthetics, and improving function. Yet even when patients and providers achieve mutual understanding about goals and how best to achieve them, treatment plans can still falter in their implementation.

Although changes in patient circumstances may prompt a change in the implementation of treatment plans, patients more commonly falter in their motivation after they leave the dental chair. Patients may respond positively to dental providers who are enthusiastic about oral care and who engage the patient in a robust discussion of treatment options. But human beings are inconsistent and prone to distraction. After patients leave the office, enthusiasm can wane as the goals that compete with health begin to assert themselves.

This is true for patients who fail to follow up with restorative dental care requiring one or two subsequent visits. It is even more relevant for patients who agree to preventive care requiring ongoing behavioral change, because these changes require constant vigilance. It is difficult to quit smoking, stop drinking, overcome compulsive purging, or change diet. The field of dentistry, however, has long realized the negative impact such behaviors have on oral and systemic health. Dental professionals are now professionally obligated to help patients by developing and implementing preventive treatment entailing behavioral change. Fortunately, communication strategies have been developed in the past 30 years to facilitate such change.

Motivational interviewing (MI) was developed by Bill Miller[39] to help problem drinkers reduce their alcohol consumption. Following the work of psychologist Carl Rogers, Miller observed that dictating a treatment to patients (eg, "Stop drinking!") tended to elicit defensiveness or denial. MI, by contrast, is a process that helps patients to determine what their goals are and to recognize conflicts between those goals and their current behavior.

The effectiveness of MI in reducing patients' alcohol consumption led to rapid adoption of MI principles to treat a wide range of behavioral problems, including smoking, dietary issues, and eating disorders.[40–42] Recent reviews have supported the effectiveness of MI in both health care and oral health care.[43,44] MI has proven effective in achieving lower plaque scores, greater oral health knowledge, higher self-regulation, and fewer parental behaviors that contribute to early childhood caries.[45–47]

MI is a therapeutic approach to counseling that requires formal training and study.[48] Some of the effective elements of MI, however, can be incorporated into the treatment planning discussion or even the health history. Therefore, brief MI is now a routine component of training for many health care professionals.[49–52] We will present the four principles of MI (Box 9-2) and a brief discussion of four strategies for implementing MI. These principles and strategies can be most effectively used during the stages of treatment planning in which the provider is eliciting patient input and responding to questions and concerns.

Box 9-2	Principles of motivational interviewing

Express empathy
- "Simply acknowledging your eating disorder takes courage."
- "I understand why you are ambivalent about seeking help."

Support self-efficacy
- "Slips are expected. You were tobacco free for more than a week, which shows you can do this."
- "You made it through treatment once before, so you know you can do it again."

Roll with resistance
- "You aren't willing to stop drinking soft drinks, but can you try cutting down by one can a day?"
- "If you are too stressed to quit right now, can we discuss a quit-smoking date at your 6-month checkup?"

Develop discrepancy
- "From what you've observed, how will methamphetamine use affect your oral health?"
- "What concerns you most about the bulimia?"

Express empathy

MI attracted attention and adherents during the same period in which patient-centered care emerged as the dominant model of health care delivery. Both advocate a team approach to dealing with health-related problems, so provider empathy is central to the effectiveness of each. Yet even as the dental field increasingly acknowledges the centrality of empathy, dental schools seem to reduce the empathy students feel for their patients.[53–55] Perhaps the empathy gap widens as students develop the clinical detachment necessary to carry out their work. Perhaps it widens as students face the challenges of a professional life and career (eg, paying student loans and training staff) that differ from those of many patients (eg, drug addiction and smoking). Whatever the causes, dental professionals must work to navigate an appropriate boundary between clinical detachment and patient empathy. Such work comes in the form of communication.

As detailed in previous chapters, empathy is communicated both nonverbally and verbally. In the context of MI, the provider can quickly and easily demonstrate empathy nonverbally by sitting at the patient's level, making eye contact, nodding, and occasionally smiling a sympathetic smile.[56] The provider can communicate empathy verbally by using routine expressions that indicate an appreciation of the patient's perspective: "I understand that you…" or "I imagine you…" or "Tell me more about your…." Together, these deliberate verbal and nonverbal messages constitute active listening, and they become more important the more culturally dissimilar the patient and provider are.[56] To deploy active listening effectively, the provider must overcome the temptation to direct or advise the patient—a temptation that is particularly acute during treatment planning.

> **Q** **Question of ethics:** MI is promoted as a way to let patients, in consultation with their health care providers, decide which problems require treatment and what that treatment should be. Yet patients struggling with addiction or compulsive behaviors frequently make choices that seem unwise from a health care perspective, setting themselves up to fail. Alcoholics, for instance, may opt for an unpromising treatment of drinking only two drinks a day. If patients have a diminished capacity for choice, is MI still the best approach for treatment planning discussions?

Support self-efficacy

A second principle of MI, supporting self-efficacy, is implemented primarily through verbal communication. **Self-efficacy** reflects patients' beliefs that they can implement an agreed-upon treatment. Self-efficacy is associated with a wide range of behavioral health outcomes.[57] In oral health, self-efficacy predicts both tooth brushing and flossing behaviors.[58] Self-efficacy is significantly and negatively associated with dental neglect, suggesting that patients' belief in their ability to improve oral health is a prerequisite to oral health.[59] Further, interventions to enhance patient self-efficacy have been shown to improve oral care.[60]

From an MI perspective, providing treatment options is one way to enhance self-efficacy. The patient has experience on which to base a belief in his or her own ability to implement various treatments. Providing options allows the patient to choose the treatment he or she believes has the best chance of success and fosters a personal investment in the outcome. Because MI is nondirective, the provider should not simply tell the patient that he or she is capable of carrying out a difficult preventive treatment. Instead, the provider should help the patient explore any ambivalence by identifying concerns and examining experiences. A provider's optimism is necessary but not sufficient for successful treatment. The patient should emerge from the MI process with a firm belief in his or her capabilities, grounded in evidence and optimism.

Roll with resistance

Ambivalence is embraced in MI because it indicates that patients are realistic about the challenges they face. Patients who think it is easy to arrest an addiction or compulsion typically are those who have never tried it. When patient ambivalence tips into resistance to treatment, providers should accept resistance as a normal and rational response. What patients are responding to is usually either an undesired label or the challenge of changing the status quo.

When using MI principles during either the health history or treatment planning, the provider should not assign a label to a patient unless the patient first embraces the label. The patient can react negatively when labeled an addict, an alcoholic, or a bulimic by a health care worker. If those diagnoses are accurate, the provider might focus on treatment rather than labeling: "Would you be willing to talk to a specialist about how frequently you vomit?" In our experience, however, the patient with serious behavioral problems usually knows it and has struggled to address it. The patient will welcome acknowledgement of the problem far more often than a dental provider might expect, particularly if the provider can offer a solution.

The patient may be likely to resist changing the status quo, which is exactly what any kind of treatment is designed to do. The provider should interpret resistance to a treatment plan as a signal to change strategies. The provider who continues to advocate a single plan in a particular way elicits increasing defensiveness from the patient, who begins to feel threatened. This outcome makes behavioral change far less likely at the moment or in the future. To roll with resistance is to acknowledge that the patient has an intellectual or emotional reaction to what the proposed change represents. The provider might explore the resistance: "You are strongly opposed to telephone counseling. Can you tell me why?" Alternatively, the provider might propose other treatment options: "Would you be willing to try bupropion without the telephone support?"

Develop discrepancy

A fourth principle of MI is to develop discrepancy between patients' stated goals and their current behavior. MI was based in part on Leon Festinger's theory of cognitive dissonance.[61] **Cognitive dissonance** is the idea that people feel psychologic discomfort when they hold two conflicting beliefs. They can manage this discomfort by changing one of the beliefs or reducing its importance. So, for instance, patients will experience dissonance when they believe that *(1)* they practice good oral health habits and *(2)* their intake of sugared soft drinks is bad for their teeth. Such patients can reduce the importance placed on one of the beliefs: "So what if I drink sugared drinks?" Alternatively, such patients can change one of the beliefs: "Drinking sugared drinks doesn't matter if I brush regularly."

In MI, cognitive dissonance is a tool for motivating the patient to change behaviors. It relies on both the health history and patient education that precede the treatment plan discussion. During the health history, the provider should identify the patient's oral health goals and practices and note conflicts between the two. During the examination or procedure, the provider should clarify and emphasize the relevance of oral health practices to oral health outcomes. Ultimately, the provider is trying to increase cognitive dissonance by undermining the patient's tendency to believe untruths regarding oral health or by undermining the patient's tendency to minimize things he or she knows to be significant problems.

Developing discrepancy requires skill, as the provider should not impose his or her own beliefs but rather should allow the discrepant beliefs of the patient to surface: "You indicated that you want to avoid significant dental work. You also know that your drinking is likely causing your inflamed gums and precancerous lesions, which may eventually require surgery unless you reduce your intake."

OARS

Four communication strategies are particularly useful in implementing the MI principles described above. A useful mnemonic for remembering these strategies is **OARS**, which stands for **open-ended questions**, **affirmations**, **reflections**, and **summaries**. First, the provider should frequently ask open-ended questions, which are more likely to identify ambivalence and dissonance than are questions that elicit single-word answers (eg, *yes/ no* or numeric replies). Second, the provider should supply affirmations to the patient to minimize the threat of change and to increase self-efficacy. Third, the provider should reflect the patient's words and thoughts as an active listening strategy. Fourth, the provider should summarize what the patient says. By reflecting and summarizing what the patient is saying, the provider not only indicates that he or she is listening but also allows the patient to hear his or her own dissonant cognitions from a third person perspective.

Activity 9-4

Role-play with a colleague or friend a scenario in which you are a provider discussing treatment plans with a patient whose oral health is deteriorating because of methamphetamine abuse. First, have some fun by doing everything "wrong": hurl accusations, threaten, exaggerate, and bully the patient. Then, try it again using the treatment planning discussion steps and the MI principles and strategies. Finally, switch places in order to understand the experience of a patient in such a situation.

Ending the Appointment

Following the examination or procedure that was the primary purpose of the appointment, a treatment planning discussion may or may not be required. In either case, the appointment must end at some point. While concluding the appointment, providers must strive for effective and appropriate communication for two important reasons. First, effective, appropriate communication emphasizes the value of professional dentistry by reiterating what was accomplished and learned during the appointment.

Second, it reinforces the patient's commitment to complete the treatment plan or to sustain oral health practices. Poor communication at the end of the appointment not only fails to achieve these goals but also can undermine the relational and educational achievements that occurred during the appointment. The process of ending an appointment entails four steps: *(1)* review and preview, *(2)* ask and listen, *(3)* provide giveaways and takeaways, and *(4)* document and follow up.

Step 1: Review and preview

The provider should review the appointment and preview what will happen next. The provider should briefly review the completed clinical work and the agreed-upon treatment plan. A one-sentence summary should suffice for the review: "So, today I cleaned and examined your teeth and then we decided to place an amalgam filling in that molar."

To clarify the patient's obligations, the provider should preview the next actions required by the patient. Although the preview can be brief, it should also be specific, particularly when treatment is pending: "I'll see you again on Monday morning, May 14, at 9:30 am, and the restoration should be completed within an hour." If further tests are needed or if the provider is referring the patient to another specialist, that information should be repeated also. Even if no treatment is indicated, previewing the next step is appropriate: "On your way out, please have Alex schedule a routine cleaning in 6 months—and keep taking such good care of your teeth!"

Step 2: Ask and listen

The provider should give the patient a final opportunity to ask questions or provide feedback. That opportunity typically takes the form of a question. The question can relate to comprehension: "Is there anything we've done or said that you are unclear about?" The question can relate to comprehensiveness: "Is there anything else you'd like us to address today?" The question can relate to satisfaction: "Are you satisfied with what we've accomplished in today's appointment?"

Because the provider should have given the patient chances to pose questions and offer feedback throughout the appointment, the wording of the question is less important than the general attempt to elicit patient input. When the question is asked, the provider should pause a few seconds and listen closely to what the patient says. Doing so indicates that the provider values the patient's satisfaction and opinion.

Step 3: Provide giveaways and takeaways

In addition to giving oral instructions, the provider should ensure that the patient always leaves the office with something in his or her hands. Promotional items have a long history as marketing tools and elicit positive regard for the provider while cultivating a sense of reciprocal obligation.[62,63] In short, the patient will appreciate receiving complimentary samples and feel grateful to the person who distributes them.

Therefore, the dental provider should always give the patient a toothbrush and samples of toothpaste and floss. Because this is such a common practice, the patient may think poorly of a provider who does not follow suit.

In addition to these giveaways, the provider should repeat the takeaway message by providing two types of written information. First, the provider or scheduler should give the patient an appointment card noting the date and time of the next appointment. Second, the provider should give the patient brochures or other written information regarding the treatment options or treatment plan. After leaving the office, the patient may forget details he or she agreed to and understood while sitting in the chair. Written information helps the patient achieve clarity about the purpose and implementation of the treatment.

As the patient prepares to leave the operatory, the provider should end on a positive note by smiling, shaking hands, and saying "Goodbye."

Step 4: Document and follow up

The provider should use the patient's files to record brief pieces of information, in addition to clinical information, that will foster continuity when the patient returns. The provider should note a bit of personal information about the patient's life that can facilitate rapport: "Ask pt abt wife's surprise birthday party." If the patient is undertaking a rigorous preventive treatment plan, the provider should also note details of the treatment: "Ask if pt was able to eliminate sports drinks." A few impressive providers are able to remember such patient details without documentation, but most need reminders. The rewards of remembering even a few details about a patient far outweigh the minimal effort required to type them into a patient file.

Finally, to foster the patient-provider relationship and enhance patient understanding and motivation, providers increasingly use other forms of media to maintain patient contact between appointments.[23,36,64,65] The contact can be individualized (eg, a telephone call or postcard) or generalized (eg, newsletter or mass email).

Chapter Checklist ☑

Categorizing procedures
☐ Prescribed and discretionary: Acknowledge the patient's reasons for declining treatment.
☐ Prescribed and discretionary: First, present the do-nothing option, followed by the prognosis.
☐ Prescribed and discretionary: Use *prescribed* instead of *mandatory* and *discretionary* instead of *elective*.
☐ Restorative and preventive: Clarify whether treatment options are restorative or preventive.
☐ Restorative and preventive: Describe every treatment option in terms of the presence of a problem (restorative or preventive) and the strength of your recommendation (prescribed or discretionary).
☐ Restorative and preventive: Provide moderate detail in the diagnosis.
☐ Restorative and preventive: Provide a rationale for the restorative treatment options and recommendation.
☐ Restorative and preventive: Consider three factors in determining recommendation—patient-related factors, tooth-related factors, and treatment-related factors.
☐ Restorative and preventive: Present decision factors to the patient at a level he or she can comprehend.
☐ Restorative and preventive: Involve the entire dental team, including specialists, in the discussion.
☐ Restorative and preventive: Discuss risks of the patient's problematic behaviors and refer the patient to specialists.
☐ Restorative and preventive: Develop proficiency in the realm of behavioral dentistry.

Discussing a treatment plan
☐ Use the term *discussing* rather than *presenting* a treatment plan.
☐ Present options and recommendation: Focus on the chief complaint or diagnosis.
☐ Present options and recommendation: Mention at least two options.
☐ Present options and recommendation: Indicate which option you recommend.
☐ Outline option details: Tell the patient whether the options are prescribed or discretionary.
☐ Outline option details: Describe details of the treatment options in adequate detail.
☐ Outline option details: Compare and contrast the options in terms important to the patient (ie, pain and pain relief, function, esthetics, and cost).
☐ Outline option details: Estimate the amount of time and money each option requires.
☐ Outline option details: Estimate how long the treatment will take.
☐ Outline option details: Estimate how long the results will last.
☐ Outline option details: Mention your responsibilities as the provider and the responsibilities of the patient for each option.
☐ Outline option details: Summarize the expected outcomes, offering ranges and using provisional language.

❑ Elicit input and questions: Ask whether the patient needs clarification of any options.

❑ Elicit input and questions: Elicit any concerns that have not been addressed.

❑ Elicit input and questions: Consider what type and level of treatment information a given patient will best accept.

❑ Elicit input and questions: Listen to the patient's concerns, using active listening.

❑ Respond to questions and concerns: Monitor the patient's nonverbal cues for signs of white coat syndrome and gently press the patient to voice questions or concerns.

❑ Respond to questions and concerns: Take the patient's concerns seriously.

❑ Respond to questions and concerns: Provide truthful and comprehensive answers.

❑ Respond to questions and concerns: Contextualize the patient's concerns by listing positive aspects of treatment to balance the negative aspects or concerns.

❑ Respond to questions and concerns: If answers are not known, seek further information, including the patient in consultations with others.

❑ Secure commitment or schedule follow-up: Ask the patient to commit to a treatment plan.

❑ Secure commitment or schedule follow-up: Commit to your obligation.

❑ Secure commitment or schedule follow-up: Communicate enthusiasm when the patient agrees to treatment.

❑ Secure commitment or schedule follow-up: Avoid pressuring the patient.

❑ Secure commitment or schedule follow-up: If the patient delays the decision, suggest a time to follow up.

❑ Secure commitment or schedule follow-up: Follow up on schedule.

Motivational interviewing

❑ Express empathy: Find an appropriate balance between empathy for the patient and clinical detachment.

❑ Express empathy: Communicate empathy and active listening through both nonverbal and verbal channels.

❑ Express empathy: Avoid the temptation to direct or advise the patient.

❑ Support self-efficacy: Enhance self-efficacy by providing multiple treatment options.

❑ Support self-efficacy: Explore ambivalence rather than simply telling the patient that he or she is capable of carrying out behavioral change.

❑ Roll with resistance: Accept resistance from the patient as normal and rational.

❑ Roll with resistance: Avoid labeling the patient unless the patient embraces the label.

❑ Roll with resistance: When encountering resistance, change strategies.

❑ Roll with resistance: Acknowledge that the patient has intellectual or emotional reactions to the change.

❑ Roll with resistance: Explore resistance or propose other treatment options.

❑ Develop discrepancy: Identify the patient's oral health goals and note conflicts between goals and behaviors.

❑ Develop discrepancy: Clarify and emphasize the relationship between oral health practices and oral health outcomes.

❑ Develop discrepancy: Increase cognitive dissonance.

❑ Develop discrepancy: Avoid imposing your own beliefs on the patient.

❑ OARS: Ask open-ended questions, supply affirmations, reflect the patient's words and thoughts, and summarize what the patient says.

Ending the appointment
- ❏ Review and preview: Briefly review completed work and the treatment plan.
- ❏ Review and preview: Briefly and specifically, preview the next actions required by the patient.
- ❏ Ask and listen: Give the patient a final opportunity to ask questions or provide feedback.
- ❏ Ask and listen: Pause a few seconds and listen closely to what the patient says.
- ❏ Giveaways and takeaways: Ensure that the patient leaves with something tangible (eg, toothbrush, toothpaste, floss, etc).
- ❏ Giveaways and takeaways: Provide an appointment card with the date and time of the next appointment.
- ❏ Giveaways and takeaways: Provide brochures or other written information regarding treatment options or plans.
- ❏ Giveaways and takeaways: End on a positive note by smiling, shaking hands, and saying "Goodbye."
- ❏ Document and follow up: Foster continuity between appointments by noting a bit of personal information about the patient and details of preventive treatment.
- ❏ Document and follow up: Use other media to maintain patient contact between appointments (eg, telephone, email, newsletters, etc).

For More Information

Restorative and preventive treatment planning
- http://www.aapd.org/publications/brochures
- http://www.aae.org/treatmentoptions
- http://archive.ahrq.gov/research/findings/factsheets/costs/dentalcare/dentria.pdf

Presenting a treatment plan
- http://www.discusonline.com/udisc/default.htm
- http://www.dentalcare.com/en-US/dental-practice-management/patient-management/effective-treatment/effective-treatment.aspx
- http://www.dentalcare.com/en-US/dental-practice-management/dental-hygiene/treatment-plan/treatment-plan.aspx

Motivational interviewing
- http://www.motivationalinterviewing.org
- http://www.dentalcare.com/media/en-US/education/ce381/ce381.pdf
- http://www.tobacco-oralhealth.net/events/workshop2005/pdf/Undergraduate%20Education.pdf
- http://www.nova.edu/gsc/forms/mi_rationale_techniques.pdf

Ending an appointment
- http://www.mbsdental.com
- http://www.identity-links.com/professions/dental

- http://www.dentaleconomics.com/articles/print/volume-97/issue-8/features/patient-reminder-communciations-an-online-approach.html
- http://www.patientnews.com

References

1. Dawson AS, Makinson OF. Dental treatment and dental health. 1. A review of studies in support of a philosophy of minimum intervention dentistry. Aust Dent J 1992;37:126–132.
2. Bos A, Hoogstraten J, Prahl-Andersen B. Towards a comprehensive model for the study of compliance in orthodontics. Eur J Orthod 2005;27:296–301.
3. Egolf RJ, BeGole EA, Upshaw HS. Factors associated with orthodontic patient compliance with intraoral elastic and headgear wear. Am J Orthod Dentofacial Orthop 1990;97:336–348.
4. Zolnierek KB, Dimatteo MR. Physician communication and patient adherence to treatment: A meta-analysis. Med Care 2009;47:826–834.
5. Bader JD, Shugars DA. Variation in dentists' clinical decisions. J Public Health Dent 1995;55:181–188.
6. Ecenbarger W. How honest are dentists? Reader's Digest February 1997:50–56.
7. Shugars DA, Bader JD. Cost implications of differences in dentists' restorative treatment decisions. J Public Health Dent 1996;56:219–222.
8. Christensen GJ. Elective vs. mandatory dentistry. J Am Dent Assoc 2000;131:1496–1498.
9. Jensen JM. Mandatory or elective [letter]? J Am Dent Assoc 2001;132:145–146.
10. Bain CA. Treatment Planning in General Dental Practice: A Problem-based Approach. Philadelphia: Elsevier Health Sciences, 2003.
11. Dibart S, Dietrich T. Practical Periodontal Diagnosis and Treatment Planning. Ames, IA: Wiley-Blackwell, 2009.
12. Stefanac SJ, Nesbit SP. Treatment Planning in Dentistry. St Louis: Mosby, 2006.
13. Bader JD, Shugars DA. Agreement among dentists' recommendations for restorative treatment. J Dent Res 1993;72:891–896.
14. Shugars DA, Hayden WJ Jr, Crall JJ, Scurria MS. Variation in the use of crowns and their alternatives. J Dent Educ 1997;61:22–28.
15. Torabinejad M, Goodacre CJ. Endodontic or dental implant therapy: The factors affecting treatment planning. J Am Dent Assoc 2006;137:973–977.
16. Margolis MJ. Esthetic considerations in orthodontic treatment of adults. Dent Clin North Am 1997;41:29–48.
17. Kiyak HA. Age and culture: Influences on oral health behaviour. Int Dent J 1993;43:9–16.
18. Schou L. The relevance of behavioural sciences in dental practice. Int Dent J 2000;50(suppl 6 pt 1):324–332.
19. Hellman S. The dentist and preventive dental health information. Health Educ Monogr 1976;4:132–176.
20. Mostofsky DI, Forgione AG, Giddon DB (eds). Behavioral Dentistry. Ames, IA: Wiley-Blackwell, 2006.
21. Adair SM, Waller JL, Schafer TE, Rockman RA. A survey of members of the American Academy of Pediatric Dentistry on their use of behavior management techniques. Pediatr Dent 2004;26:159–166.
22. Milgrom P. The impact of behavioral technology on dental caries. J Dent Educ 2001;65:1102–1105.
23. Aziz SR, Ziccardi VB. Telemedicine using smartphones for oral and maxillofacial surgery consultation, communication, and treatment planning. J Oral Maxillofac Surg 2009;67:2505–2509.
24. Cook J, Austen G, Stephens C. Information technology: Videoconferencing: What are the benefits for dental practice? Br Dent J 2000;188:67–70.
25. Yevlahova D, Satur J. Models for individual oral health promotion and their effectiveness: A systematic review. Aust Dent J 2009;54:190–197.

26. Woo D, Sheller B, Williams B, Mancl L, Grembowski D. Dentists' and parents' perceptions of health, esthetics, and treatment of maxillary primary incisors. Pediatr Dent 2005;27:19–23.

27. Grembowski D, Milgrom P, Fiset L. Factors influencing dental decision making. J Public Health Dent 1988;48:159–167.

28. Kay E, Nuttall N. Clinical decision making—An art or a science? 5. Patient preferences and their influence on decision making. Br Dent J 1995;178:229–233.

29. Ackerman JL, Proffit WR. Communication in orthodontic treatment planning: Bioethical and informed consent issues. Angle Orthod 1995;65:253–261.

30. Swennen GRJ, Mollemans W, Schutyser F. Three-dimensional treatment planning of orthognathic surgery in the era of virtual imaging. J Oral Maxillofac Surg 2009;67:2080–2092.

31. Fleming S, Demko CA, Lalumandier JA. Patient retention: What keeps them coming back? Presented at the IADR/AADR/CADR 87th General Session and Exhibition, Miami, April 4, 2009.

32. Scarbecz M. Using the DISC system to motivate dental patients. J Am Dent Assoc 2007;138:381–385.

33. Marston WM. Emotions of Normal People. London: Routledge, 2005.

34. Celis H, Fagard RH. White-coat hypertension: A clinical review. Eur J Intern Med 2004;15:348–357.

35. Schleyer TKL, Spallek H, Bartling WC, Corby P. The technologically well-equipped dental office. J Am Dent Assoc 2003;134:30–41.

36. Levin RP. Creating true customer service. J Am Dent Assoc 2010;141:337–338.

37. Mendelson MR. Effective laboratory communication...It's a two-way street. Dent Today 2006;25(7):96–98.

38. Meade EA, Inglehart MR. Young patients' treatment motivation and satisfaction with orthognathic surgery outcomes: The role of "possible selves". Am J Orthod Dentofacial Orthop 2010;137:26–34.

39. Miller WR. Motivational interviewing with problem drinkers. Behav Psychother 1983;11:147–172.

40. Berg-Smith SM, Stevens VJ, Brown KM, et al. A brief motivational intervention to improve dietary adherence in adolescents. Health Educ Res 1999;14:399–410.

41. Koerber A, Crawford J, O'Connell K. The effects of teaching dental students brief motivational interviewing for smoking-cessation counseling: A pilot study. J Dent Educ 2003;67:439–447.

42. Treasure J, Schmidt U. Motivational Interviewing in the management of eating disorders. In: Arkowitz H, Westra HA, Miller WR, Rollnick S (eds). Motivational Interviewing in the Treatment of Psychological Problems. New York: Guilford Press, 2008:194–224.

43. Lundahl BW, Kunz C, Brownell C, Tollefson D, Burke BL. A meta-analysis of motivational interviewing: Twenty-five years of empirical studies. Res Soc Work Pract 2010;20:137–160.

44. Martins RK, McNeil DW. Review of motivational interviewing in promoting health behaviors. Clin Psychol Rev 2009;29:283–293.

45. Yeung CA. Motivational interviewing in an oral health promotion programme. Evid Based Dent 2010;11:14–15.

46. Williams K. Motivational interviewing: Application to oral health behaviors. J Dent Hyg 2010;84:6–10.

47. Freudenthal JJ, Bowen DM. Motivational interviewing to decrease parental risk-related behaviors for early childhood caries. J Dent Hyg 2010;84:29–34.

48. Rollnick S, Miller WR, Butler CC. Motivational Interviewing in Health Care: Helping Patients Change Behavior. New York: Guilford Press, 2007.

49. Croffoot C, Krust Bray K, Black MA, Koerber A. Evaluating the effects of coaching to improve motivational interviewing skills of dental hygiene students. J Dent Hyg 2010;84:57–64.

50. Lozano P, McPhillips HA, Hartzler B, et al. Randomized trial of teaching brief motivational interviewing to pediatric trainees to promote healthy behaviors in families. Arch Pediatr Adolesc Med 2010;164:561–566.

51. Martino S, Haeseler F, Belitsky R, Pantalon M, Fortin AH. Teaching brief motivational interviewing to year three medical students. Med Educ 2007;41:160–167.

52. White LL, Gazewood JD, Mounsey AL. Teaching students behavior change skills: Description and assessment of a new motivational interviewing curriculum. Med Teach 2007;29(4):e67–e71.

53. Sherman JJ, Cramer A. Measurement of changes in empathy during dental school. J Dent Educ 2005;69:338–345.
54. Yarascavitch C, Regehr G, Hodges B, Haas DA. Changes in dental student empathy during training. J Dent Educ 2009;73:509–517.
55. Nash DA. Ethics, empathy, and the education of dentists. J Dent Educ 2010;74:567–578.
56. Harrigan JA, Rosenthal R. Nonverbal aspects of empathy and rapport in physician-patient interaction. In: Blanck PD, Buck R, Rosenthal R (eds). Nonverbal Communication in the Clinical Context. University Park, PA: Pennsylvania State University Press, 1986:36–73.
57. Street RL, Makoul G, Arora NK, Epstein RM. How does communication heal? Pathways linking clinician-patient communication to health outcomes. Patient Educ Couns 2009;74:295–301.
58. Buglar ME, White KM, Robinson NG. The role of self-efficacy in dental patients' brushing and flossing: Testing an extended Health Belief Model. Patient Educ Couns 2010;78:269–272.
59. Lee JY, Divaris K, Baker AD, Rozier RG, Vann WF Jr. The relationship of oral health literacy and self-efficacy with oral health status and dental neglect. Am J Public Health 2012;102:923–929.
60. Kakudate N, Morita M, Fukuhara S, et al. Application of self-efficacy theory in dental clinical practice. Oral Dis 2010;16:747–752.
61. Festinger L. A Theory of Cognitive Dissonance. Stanford, CA: Stanford University Press, 1957.
62. Budden MC, Browning SR. The marketing of dental wellness. Health Mark Q 1990;7(3–4):23–32.
63. Rudzki REJ, Li S. The economic paradox of the "freebies" phenomena: How and why companies give stuff away for free. Direct Market Int J 2007;1:180–194.
64. Chestnutt IG, Reynolds K. Perceptions of how the internet has impacted on dentistry. Br Dent J 2006;200:161–165.
65. Downes P. Use of e-mail by dentists is increasing, mainly for inter-professional communications [abstract]. Br Dent J 1999;186:123.

Part IV

Communication Challenges

The background information and skill sets presented in the first three sections of this book are sufficient for any dental provider to communicate effectively with most patients. Most patients are like most dentists: adults with social, cognitive, and physical attributes adequate to the task of communicating what they wish to communicate. Communicating with such patients is fairly easy. Communication challenges emerge, however, when patients have attributes that may limit their ability or motivation to communicate. This section considers three types of communication challenges that dental providers will encounter: life span challenges (chapter 10), hearing and speaking challenges (chapter 11), and challenges related to stigma (chapter 12). This section does not exhaust the potential challenges that dental providers may face, but it presents several of the more common challenges so that providers are equipped to react appropriately when such challenges arise. This preparation also will help providers anticipate and address similar challenges that are not discussed here.

10

Managing Life Span Challenges

Why Planning for Life Span Challenges Matters

In theory, patient-provider communication would be much more effective if providers focused their practice on patients with whom they communicated well. To a limited extent, this happens. Some dentists specialize, and certain specializations (eg, pediatric dentistry or prosthodontics) target patients who have much in common. In practice, however, 85% of dentists do not specialize.[1] As a result, most patients are treated at family practices where the staff treats patients of all ages.

Treating patients of diverse ages is a sign of a healthy practice. It shows that patients who differ widely in age from the practice staff are nevertheless satisfied with the care they receive. It also indicates that patients are loyal to the practice as they age, and such loyalty is both a cause and consequence of effective patient-provider communication.

Patient-centered care is much easier to achieve if patients can see the same providers over time and develop relationships with them. This continuity of care benefits both patients and providers.[2] Patients benefit from the reduction in uncertainty. They learn to navigate a practice's physical and bureaucratic environment, and they learn to anticipate the way certain providers communicate. Providers benefit because they gain a better sense of patients' capabilities and motivations, and they are able to track conditions over time. In short, even if providers wanted to confine their practice to healthy adults with generous insurance policies, those providers who were most clinically and communicatively competent would find their patients growing older and having children—as healthy patients so often do.

In addition to the practical reasons for developing communication skills to accommodate life span challenges are professional and ethical reasons. For a variety of reasons related to access and cost, oral health disparities exist for both the young and the old.[3,4] Dental care is the most prevalent unmet health need among US children.[4] The most common childhood disease is dental caries, and dental-related illnesses cause children to miss more than 51 million school hours each year.[5] Oral health disparities are even more acute for low-income children. Among seniors, 30% of those 65 years or older are edentulous, and 23% have severe periodontal disease.[5] Oral health disparities are even more acute for low-income seniors and those in long-term care facilities.

Reducing these disparities will require concerted efforts on multiple fronts.[6] Communicating with children and seniors in a way that facilitates restorative treatment and promotes preventive care is crucial to minimizing such disparities. This chapter first addresses communication with those who often accompany children or seniors to their appointments. The next section describes communication challenges with young patients and the skills to deal with them. Particular attention is given to the common challenge of treating anxious or fearful children and the less common, but potentially more difficult, challenge of treating autistic children. Finally, the chapter ends by considering how providers can effectively communicate with seniors, particularly those suffering a decline in their cognitive or hearing abilities.

Communicating with Guardians and Caregivers

A shared feature of dental visits by children and senior adults is the common presence of a third party. Parents usually accompany young children and may accompany older children in special circumstances. Although many independent seniors make and attend their appointments alone, others may be accompanied as they grow older, by either relatives or professional caregivers. Discerning the relationships between patients and others who accompany them to the office or the operatory can prove challenging to dental providers. Finding a way to include such people in patient-provider communication can be even more challenging, as their presence in an operatory may compromise goals of privacy, consent, and patient-centered care. On the other hand, co-present others can provide sources of information and support that facilitate both patient-provider communication and clinical care. In the sections that follow, we present various considerations and strategies for providers who interact with those who accompany children or seniors.

Parents and guardians of children

Providers treating pediatric patients must first establish whether the person who brought the patient is the parent. If not, informed consent must be secured from custodial parents prior to treatment. Foster parents must show proof of guardianship when first bringing a child for treatment. Providers should also be aware that adult dependents between ages 18 and 26 years may remain on a parent's insurance but that the parent will no longer have access to any of the child's records without a signed release from the child. Dental providers should ensure familiarity and compliance with Health Insurance Portability and Accountability (HIPAA) regulations regarding parents and others who might accompany patients.

In communicating with the parent or guardian of a pediatric patient, the dental professional should rely extensively on observation and listening skills and should remain flexible in the approach taken. The presence of another person in the operatory can pose logistical challenges, as the provider must find a place for the adult to sit or stand and must direct attention and comments to both the patient and the parent. Beyond these logistical considerations, however, are the expectations and responses of the parent and child to the clinical experience, which may be similar or may be very different. The best pediatric appointments are those that involve a cooperative child and parent. By announcing the need for cooperation at the start of the appointment, the dental professional can shape the expectations of all involved and perhaps elicit more cooperation.

Quite often one or both parents will accompany a young child into the operatory, particularly when the child is seeing a dentist for the first time. Approximately 80% of pediatric dentists surveyed supported parental accompaniment, with more experienced dentists more supportive than newer dentists.[7] Although the parent is the legal guardian of the child and is responsible for treatment decisions, the provider should always remember that the child is the patient and the initial visits train the child how to engage in effective patient-provider communication. Therefore, the provider should address the child directly as "you" rather than address the parent and refer to the child in the third person.

As with standard appointments, the provider should seek rapport before collecting the health history. The parent can be particularly helpful with the health history, as he or she should know a great deal about the child's experiences and habits. Nevertheless, the provider should conduct the interview with the child as much as possible, eliciting answers and clarifications from the parent only when the child cannot answer.

In interactions with a pediatric patient, the provider should aim to teach the child to take responsibility for his or her own oral health—including participation in the clinical encounter. After a few visits, a healthy child should be able to complete a dental appointment without a parent in the operatory. This independence can yield benefits during the interviewing phase, as a child or adolescent may be more willing to disclose unhealthy behaviors such as smoking if the parent is not within earshot.

Of particular concern, about two-thirds of child abuse victims suffer injuries to the head, neck, face, and mouth—injuries that would be apparent to a dental professional.[8,9] Childhood sports and recreation injuries, however, are also apparent to the professional. The dental provider should always determine the cause of injuries and take appropriate steps to minimize their recurrence. The dental provider should ask the parent to wait in the reception area whenever the parent's presence in the operatory interferes with information gathering.

> **Q Question of ethics:** If you discover that a pediatric patient is engaging in an unhealthy behavior, do you have an ethical obligation to the patient to keep the information private or to the parent to disclose a condition or behavior that could affect the child's health? Does your answer change depending on the behavior (eg, chewing tobacco versus snorting methamphetamine)? Does your answer change depending on whether the patient disclosed it to you or you deduced the behavior based on a clinical examination?

In general, the parent is a source of comfort for children, particularly the anxious child and the child attending a first dental appointment. The parent can be encouraged to hold the child's hand or make other soothing gestures during the actual examination or procedure. A behavioral management technique growing in acceptance among providers is live modeling of appropriate dental behaviors by the parent.[10,11] Thus, beyond serving as a calming presence, the parent can actively participate during appointments: "Watch Dr Franklin place this other small mirror in Mommy's mouth!"

Not every parent, however, proves calming or helpful. Fear of dentistry on the part of a parent—particularly a mother—seems to cultivate dental fear in the child.[12,13] The presence of a fearful parent in the operatory during an examination or procedure may exacerbate anxiety in the pediatric patient and may interfere with the concentration of the dental team. A fearful parent should be asked to wait in the reception area.

Whether or not the parent remains in the operatory during examinations and procedures, he or she should probably be present during the treatment planning discussion, given that the parent is responsible legally, ethically, and financially for decisions regarding the child's health. However, because the pediatric patient ultimately undergoes any treatment—and lives with the outcome—the dental provider must accomplish the delicate communication task of simultaneously engaging both parent and child. According to Freeman,[14] problem-solving skills and negotiation skills are central to communicating within the patient-provider-parent triad.

Parental acceptance of restorative treatment plans depends primarily on trust, perceptions of dentist skill, and anticipated pain for the child.[15] Therefore, with both the parent and the patient, the provider should address trust, skill, and anticipated pain. In addition, the parent and the patient often have different expectations for restorative treatment, so the provider should clarify expected outcomes.[16]

Finally, parental neglect of preventive dental care is directly related to poor dental health in children. Numerous studies have shown motivational interviewing with parents to be effective in improving preventive care in children.[17–19]

Spouses, children, and caregivers of seniors

Older patients also are frequently escorted to dental appointments. In contrast to pediatric patients, who are usually accompanied by parents, the patient relationships and roles of those escorting seniors are more variable and therefore can be more difficult for the provider to discern. When anyone arrives with a patient, the provider should determine who the person is and how involved the patient wishes him or her to be. The provider can start this process by shaking hands and introducing himself or herself. After the identity and relationship of the escort are determined, the provider should briefly explain HIPAA regulations, determine the patient's wishes regarding the escort's participation in treatment and decision-making, and, if participation is desired, secure a signed consent form that should be entered into the electronic health record. If HIPAA regulations are met, the provider should let the patient decide whether he or she would like the escort present in the operatory. As the appointment proceeds, the provider should observe the patient's responses to gauge the level of escort participation that the patient is comfortable with. As long as the escort's presence does not interfere or distract, the patient's wishes should be accommodated.

<table>
<tr><td>

Activity 10-1

</td><td>

Interview a dentist or dental hygienist whose practice specializes in pediatric dentistry or gerodontics. Ask specifically about the provider's experience with people accompanying patients during examinations or procedures. Does the provider have horror stories about such experiences? Do parents or escorts help the patient? Does the practice or professional have a formal or informal policy regarding who may remain in the operatory? How does the provider ask a parent or escort to leave the operatory, when doing so is necessary? How often do issues of privacy and consent arise and how are they handled with respect to HIPAA compliance?

</td></tr>
</table>

In general, the level of escort participation in an appointment depends on the capabilities of the patient, the motivation of the escort, and the relationship between the two people. Often (but not always), privacy and consent are less problematic with older spouses. Spouses who have been together many years are generally comfortable disclosing health history information in each other's presence. A senior patient, for instance, sometimes needs an escort's assistance to recall prescription drug names and dosages. Like spouses, children of a senior patient often provide health history information a parent might have forgotten. Other escorts (eg, friends, professional caregivers, or volunteer drivers) may be less helpful in providing information. Regardless of an escort's presence, the provider should address health history questions to the patient and encourage the patient to answer but should thank an escort when he or she provides needed information.

In treatment planning discussions, senior patients often prefer their spouses to be present, listen to the treatment options, and contribute to the decision. When a married patient expresses this preference, the provider should address both patient and spouse. Some patients will even allow the spouse to make the decision, which is acceptable if the patient clearly consents to the decision. Children and caregivers of senior patients should also be encouraged to participate in the treatment planning discussion if the patient prefers. Particularly for a patient with memory, cognitive, or hearing deficits, the presence of another person can help the patient recall treatment details and make a more informed decision. A patient's child or caregiver, however, may have a vested (financial) interest in the treatment plan decision, so the provider should explicitly confirm that the patient understands the implications and consents to the treatment decision: "Mrs Richards, please confirm for me that you are choosing the extraction rather than having a root canal because of cost concerns. You understand that this may compromise your ability to chew some foods."

Finally, the spouse, child, or caregiver should be involved in preventive treatment planning discussions unless the patient objects. The escort may be integral to the effective implementation of a preventive treatment plan. He or she can help the patient remember details of the plan and often motivate or remind the patient to engage in preventive care. If the patient has a physical or cognitive limitation making self-care difficult, the provider should reach agreement regarding oral health tasks the spouse, child, or caregiver will perform on behalf of the patient (eg, ensuring dentures are washed or dry mouth is regularly addressed). With such a patient, subsequent patient visits should be scheduled with the person responsible for follow-up care.

Communicating with Children

The goals of treating adults are straightforward: delivery of excellent oral health care and development of a relationship supportive of patient-centered care. The goals of treating children are the same, with one additional goal: training children how to interact with dental providers so that they may get the best care during their visits. Dental providers, however, could do a better job with children on their first visit. In one survey, 72% of adults reported that their initial dentist visit was a negative experience.[20] Nevertheless, childhood dental visits among those same adults were associated with positive oral health attitudes and beliefs and with better oral health. The implication is that child patients are able to overcome the negativity associated with the first visit to forge a relationship with dentistry and dental professionals that fosters better oral health through their adulthood.

Activity 10-2

Write a brief account of your first trip to the dentist. Describe details of the reason for the visit, the reception area, the operatory, and the dentist and hygienist. Also include details about how you felt before, during, and after the visit. If you cannot remember your first visit, write a brief account about your relationships with your childhood dentist and hygienist and how your feelings regarding dentistry changed over the years.

Of course, negative experiences for the child may well prove to be negative experiences for the dental provider as well. Further, the child or parent, rather than the dental professional, may be the cause of the difficulty. Approximately one in four pediatric patients is difficult to manage.[21] The good news is that most children are easy to treat and professionals can simply adjust their communication style to suit the child's level of comprehension. The bad news is that professionals who are highly skilled at communicating with children may yet find some children challenging. In the following sections, we present communication strategies that should increase the likelihood that the first and subsequent dental visits will be positive experiences for the child. We first discuss children who are anxious about the dental visit, and then we consider children with an autism spectrum disorder. Providers who learn to address these challenges should be skilled enough to deal with nearly any child who needs treatment.

Anxious and fearful children

Dental fear in children is primarily a result of either a negative experience or an observation of fear modeled by someone else (eg, a mother).[22] The negative experience prompting fear is not necessarily pain related. Adults whose dental fear began in childhood report that the dentist's professional behavior was most accountable for their fear.[23] Explicitly mentioned were professionals who were heavy handed, critical, remote, and distant.

Because adults often feel entitled or obligated to correct bad behavior in children, even a provider who refrains from criticizing adults for lax oral health habits may be tempted to criticize children. With all patients, and especially children, the provider should resist the temptation to scold, because criticism raises communication barriers by making the patient less likely to disclose information. When commenting on insufficient oral health practices, the provider should describe what he or she observes but address the benefits of engaging in preventive behaviors. Because a child can be susceptible to emotional contagion, the provider should make an extra effort to smile and act enthusiastic about the child's visit. A provider who seems distracted or irritated may trigger or increase anxiety in a child.

When beginning clinical procedures during a child's first visit to a dental office, the provider should take some time to introduce the child to dentistry. The verbal introduction involves previewing the examination and explaining the rationale for what will happen. The nonverbal introduction involves showing the pediatric patient the various instruments and equipment. Allowing the child to handle some of the equipment—particularly the air and water—can make the environment seem less threatening. A child may find the mask intimidating, so playing with the mask or making a game out of putting it on may alleviate mask-related anxiety: "I don't want to sneeze on you so I'm going to put on my sneeze mask."

A 2011 systematic review on the effect of provider behavior on child anxiety and behavior provided evidence-based guidelines for avoiding or alleviating anxiety-related behavioral challenges in children.[24] Effective communication strategies included empathic communication with an appropriate level of touch. Empathy is communicated by acknowledging and addressing the patient's anxiety, experience, or concerns: "You seem a little anxious about this tooth cleaning, but your mother has done it, I've done it, and I am going to make sure you do it without any problems at all, OK?"

The authors also found that verbal explanations and reassurance were effective at eliciting cooperation: "This whirling thing I have is actually a toothbrush. I know it sounds loud and feels different from the toothbrush you use, but it polishes your teeth as it cleans them. Other kids I use this tooth polisher on actually laugh—they think it tickles!" The provider might even place the rubber cup from the handpiece on the child's thumb and let the brush rotate for a few seconds, saying, "See how that tickles?" These communication strategies (empathy, touch, explanations, and reassurance) seem most effective when used together.

Staff threats and punishment not only prompt anxiety but also reduce patient cooperation. When speaking to an inattentive child, the provider should use a firm and loud voice, which minimizes patient disruption without eliciting uncooperative behavior. Additional communication strategies for minimizing disruptions are presented in Box 10-1.

Box 10-1 | Strategies for communicating with anxious or fearful children

- **Make short appointments:** The younger the patient is, the shorter the appointments should be.
- **Encourage exploration:** "I am going to place this little straw in your mouth and let you feel how it is like a vacuum cleaner for your mouth."
- **Encourage cooperation:** "Today I want to make your teeth cleaner than they have ever been. Are you going to help me do that?"
- **Negotiate:** "If you can sit still for just a few more minutes, it will be time to pick out your prize from the prize basket."
- **Enlist parental help:** "If you can keep being a good helper, I will ask your mother to come over and sit next to you while we finish up."
- **Separate parent from child:** "Mrs Carter, having this many people in the operatory tends to distract me from my work. Would you mind waiting in the reception area? We'll call you back in about 15 minutes when we are ready to discuss the next stage of treatment."
- **Use technology:** "I want to show you a short cartoon on my tablet computer..." or "I'm going to let you pick the music we listen to during this appointment."

If the provider communicates effectively with a pediatric patient during an examination or procedure, the child should be calm enough to participate in the subsequent treatment planning discussion. Parents and adolescents differ in perceptions of adolescents' oral health and need for treatment.[25] Therefore, both the parent and child should be included in treatment planning so that everyone involved will have the same expectations. Furthermore, the child should never leave a dentist appointment without participating in a treatment planning discussion, as preventive care is crucial to oral health and the provider can motivate the patient in a way that the parent might not be able to.

The instruction strategies for routine oral health care (see Box 8-4) can be very useful with children: tell-show-do, teach-back, hand-over-hand, and chaining. With children, tell-show-do can be particularly effective.[26] Child-appropriate giveaways such as sugarless gum or fruit-flavored toothpaste may also promote good oral health habits. Providers, however, should not underestimate what children are capable of understanding or implementing. For instance, teenagers may be at higher risk for tongue piercings, "grills," or mouth jewelry, but the American Academy of Pediatric Dentistry recommends counseling patients regarding piercings when they are between 6 and 12 years.[27]

Question of ethics: Tongue and lip piercings, lip tattoos, "grills," and even split tongues can be very unhealthy, but in a sense they are as much a form of cultural expression as the lip plates favored by the Mursi tribe or the filed teeth of the Wapare. When patients want to make cosmetic changes to their mouth, what are the limits to professional advice? Should you set aside your own taste to address only the clinical risks, or should you also explore the social implications of such modifications? Does it make a difference if you are discussing modifications with an adult instead of a child?

Patients with autism

Autism rates have increased significantly in recent years, although the increase may reflect better screening and diagnosis procedures.[28,29] **Autism** and **autism spectrum disorders** refer to a cluster of developmental disorders that affect communication ability throughout life.[30] Autism symptoms appear in the first 3 years of life, but the identification of children as autistic occurs at a median age of 5.7 years.[31] Autism is not associated with income, education, or lifestyle factors, but boys are almost five times more likely to have the disorder than are girls.[32] The severity of autism and its symptoms vary widely, and many children (and adults) are highly functional. The Centers for Disease Control and Prevention estimates that the prevalence of autism spectrum disorders is 1 in 88.[32]

Autism may include any of a wide array of symptoms. For the dental professional, the most salient are those that compromise the patient's ability to remain still in the chair, to cooperate, and to communicate effectively. For instance, an autistic patient may be hypersensitive to stimuli, may communicate with gestures instead of words, and may avoid eye contact.[30] In their review of the research on treating autistic patients, Klein and Nowak[33] recommended that the provider learn as much as possible about a patient's behavior and communication patterns before undertaking treatment. A 2007 study identified five factors that can predict the level of cooperation the dental professional can expect from an autistic patient: *(1)* ability to read; *(2)* age; *(3)* toilet training; *(4)* expressive language; and *(5)* concurrent diagnoses.[34]

Activity 10-3

This activity is designed to help you understand how auditory and sensory stimulation interfere with communication for autistic people. Place earbuds from an MP3 player or radio in your ears and listen to a spoken podcast or news broadcast at a fairly high sound level. While you are listening, avert your eyes as a colleague gives you directions on how to drive to his or her old high school. When the colleague has finished, repeat the directions while the earbuds are still in and your eyes remain averted. Ask the colleague how accurately you replicated the directions.

Klein and Nowak[33] recommended that the provider employ the same communication strategies effective with nonautistic patients but emphasize that flexibility is essential. They explicitly mention frequent positive reinforcement, immediate verbal praise, and giveaways when the appointment ends. Also, the provider should issue short and clear commands and should ignore inappropriate behavior.

A 2008 study surveyed parents of autistic children to determine what dental communication techniques they perceived as both acceptable and effective.[35] A subset of responses came from parents who had observed the techniques in actual use, and those strategies are listed in Box 10-2.

Box 10-2	Effective strategies for communicating with autistic children*
Basic strategies • Positive verbal reinforcement • Tell-show-do • Rewards • Frequent breaks • Distraction • Mouth props	**Advanced strategies** • Stabilization device • Hand holding by staff • Hand holding by parent • Parental restraint • Staff restraint

*Information compiled and adapted from Marshall et al.[35]

Although parents of autistic children initially were less accepting of the use of a stabilization device such as an immobilizing Papoose board, 95% of those who allowed its use thought it was acceptable, and 96% found it efficacious.[35] The authors therefore emphasized that the provider should present the use of a stabilization device in a positive way and must secure consent. In addition to these specific strategies, the authors recommended more generally that the provider recognize that an autistic child is likely to require behavioral management techniques; involve the family in treatment; provide a supportive and structured environment; and maintain the continuity of the dental team in return visits.

Communicating with Seniors

Children's oral health and communication behaviors typically fall within a predictable and narrow range. As adult patients grow older, however, they may vary markedly from one another in their need for restorative treatment, their preventive oral health habits, and their ability and motivation to maintain their oral health. A common advantage is that older patients generally exhibit less dental fear than do younger ones.[36] A disadvantage is that older patients may be less able to feel or express pain than younger patients are.[37,38]

When treating new patients who are elderly, providers should acknowledge that the patients may have their own agenda items and should be careful not to condescend or treat them with paternalism.[39] The likelihood that this will happen drops if the provider has developed a relationship with the patient over many years, and such relationships help providers to understand individual patient perspectives and anticipate patient needs. When older patients are treated, empathy and perspective taking can be critical to effective treatment. Wetle[40] identified several ethical issues when dealing with the elderly: increased illness burden, sensory deficits, financial constraints, and ageism among both providers and patients.

Question of ethics: The primary obligation of health care providers is to care for their patients. For those requiring assistance from caregivers, however, the ability and willingness of the caregiver often determines whether a treatment is implemented effectively. For instance, working to preserve a patient's teeth may be better for the patient, but extractions may be easier for the caregiver who can better care for dentures than for teeth. To what degree should a caregiver's abilities or motivations inform the patient's treatment plan?

In reviewing oral health disparities in the elderly and those with cognitive impairments, Mouradian and Corbin[41] identified several themes, four of which should sensitize providers to the special needs of elderly patients. First, aging bodies often exhibit oral-systemic interactions that may require interprofessional collaboration. The elderly should not bear the entire burden of coordinating care across health professionals and health facilities. Dental providers should make the effort to include other health care providers in treatment planning discussions.

Second, the potential for diminished mental and physical abilities in the elderly may compromise self-care. In treatment planning, providers should remain aware of what patients are capable of doing.

Third, seniors may face multiple barriers to health care access. Providers should work within the constraints elderly patients may face: fixed incomes, lack of transportation, inadequate assistance from caregivers, and so on. A 2010 qualitative study of seniors' access to oral health care identified five major themes: need for information, service access, affordability, anxiety, and dentist relationships.[42]

Fourth, social and cultural factors may influence the care an elderly patient receives. For instance, providers should acknowledge and address the attitude of some older patients and their families that tooth loss is an acceptable indicator of aging. Behaviors and attitudes among gerodontology patients change slowly, and specific attitudes may be more difficult to change if they are culturally rooted.[43]

Providers who have developed relationships with aging patients over many years may be able to minimize barriers to care, but patient familiarity can also lead providers to assume that patients are unchanging in their habits and abilities. Providers should not become complacent in their observation skills as patients pass middle age. As long as traditional communication patterns are functional, they should be maintained—even to the end of a high-functioning patient's life. Yet providers should remain mindful that physical capabilities, cognitive processing, family structure, and financial resources can change rapidly for senior adults. Because the interval between visits can be several months, providers might notice changes more readily than close family members who interact with patients daily.

When an older patient's ability to communicate or participate in treatment is compromised, providers should adapt to the patient's abilities and anticipate the trajectory of oral health needs and abilities. In the following sections, we consider two conditions—one mental and one physical—that are common among older patients and that complicate communication.

Patients with dementia or Alzheimer disease

Among those aged 71 years and older in the United States, the prevalence of dementia is 13.9%, and the prevalence of Alzheimer disease (the most common cause of dementia) is 9.7%.[43] Risk increases with age, so more than a third of individuals older than 90 years have dementia. Furthermore, the early signs of Alzheimer disease relate directly to oral health and communication: Patients complain of memory loss, impairment of verbal expression, and dysphasia.[44] Alzheimer disease and dementia are progressive, and patients may eventually exhibit personality changes, mood disorders, and even psychosis.[45,46]

The result of advances in dentistry and access to oral health care is that more individuals—including those with Alzheimer disease and dementia—remain dentate into their old age and therefore require dental care. Oral health problems, however, are associated with these diagnoses. A 2008 study found that the mean number of root surfaces with caries in Alzheimer patients was 4.9, significantly higher than the number in patients with other forms of dementia (2.3) and those without dementia (1.7).[47] Many dental students do not feel well prepared for treating patients with special needs, but those with more confidence in their ability to do so have a greater intention of providing dental care to such patients.[48]

Question of ethics: Any patient may refuse dental care, but aging patients in cognitive and/or physical decline pose an ethical dilemma. If a healthy elderly patient refuses consent to treatment—for an abscessed tooth, for instance—would you proceed anyway? What if the refusing patient was clearly suffering from Alzheimer disease or dementia? What if he or she was in the early stages of dementia and lucid most of the time? Consider how you would determine whether a patient was capable of consent (or refusal) and what level of cognitive compromise would make consent irrelevant.

Suspected or diagnosed dementia does not indicate that a patient is incapable of participating in dental care. In 1997, a research team published the Dental Behavior Index, which proved useful in predicting an Alzheimer patient's level of participation in a dental examination (Box 10-3).[49] Interestingly, a number of patients were physically and cognitively more impaired than their score on the Dental Behavior Index would indicate, suggesting that the familiar routines of dentistry and oral health behavior may be retained even though the patient is incapable of more complex reasoning or behavior. In addition to previous dental memories and the stage of the disease, patient participation can also be influenced by personality and background.[50]

Box 10-3	The Dental Behavior Index*

Instructions: Observe the patient and assign a score for each item. The total score is the sum of the items, ranging from 0 to 20. Lower scores indicate greater impairment, with scores under 20 suggesting a reduced ability to cope with dental procedures and scores under 10 suggesting that the dementia affects treatment decisions and treatment planning.

Item 1: Familiarity
The patient recognizes the dental office or setting.

4 = Yes, immediately; 3 = after thinking; 2 = with prompting; 1 = probably; 0 = not at all.

Item 2: Behavior
Behavior during oral assessment with mirror and probe: The dentist introduces the action by stating that he or she is going to examine the patient's teeth and brings the instrument in front of the patient's mouth.

4 = Opens mouth spontaneously or on request; 3 = opens mouth after instruction; 2 = closes mouth involuntarily; 1 = refuses to open mouth, compresses lips; 0 = sucking behavior when lips are touched.

Item 3: Recognition
Recognition of a toothbrush: The dentist shows the patient a toothbrush and asks the patient if he or she recognizes what it is.

4 = Yes, immediately; 3 = after thinking; 2 = with prompting; 1 = probably; 0 = not at all.

Item 4: Brushing
The dentist dips the toothbrush in a glass of water and asks the patient to use it to brush his or her teeth. A kidney bowl is placed in front of the patient.

4 = Adequate function; 3 = impaired function; 2 = poor function; 1 = refuses; 0 = no reaction.

Item 5: Rinsing
Behavior in response to "I am going to rinse your mouth": The patient is asked to open his or her mouth, and water is squirted into the mouth. The patient is then asked to swish the water through the mouth and then to close his or her lips around the suction tip.

4 = Adequate function; 3 = after instruction; 2 = incorrect function; 1 = refuses; 0 = no reaction.

*Adapted from Nordenram et al[49] with permission.

Our late colleague Jane Chalmers focused her research on providing dental care to those with dementia, and that research yielded numerous practical suggestions.[51] First, many patients are more lucid in the morning and decline as the day goes on, so the provider should try to schedule the patient earlier in the day. Second, because dementia and Alzheimer disease are progressive, the provider should attempt to restore oral function quickly, before the patient's capabilities decline. Third, the patient with dementia often has to rely on others, so the provider should enlist the help of caregivers and family members who know best how to communicate with the patient. Such helpers bear a heavy burden, however, and transporting the patient can be an ordeal, in addition to being inconvenient. Therefore, fourth, the provider might schedule longer appointments to accomplish more during each visit. Fifth, instructional techniques such as tell-show-do, teach-back, hand-over-hand, and chaining can work well with a patient who is having difficulty understanding language. Sixth, a patient who lacks verbal skills may communicate pain through facial expression, so the provider should either monitor the patient's facial expressions during procedures or designate a dental team member to do so.[52]

A number of other explicit strategies that can facilitate care for patients with Alzheimer disease or dementia are listed in Box 10-4.

Box 10-4	**Strategies for communicating with patients with cognitive impairments***

Speech construction
- Begin by identifying yourself and using the patient's name or title.
- Use short words and simple sentences.
- Use nouns and not pronouns.
- Minimize questions for the patient.

Speech style
- Speak slowly and clearly and lower your tone.
- Use your normal voice (not baby talk).
- Ask one question at a time and wait for a response.
- Repeat questions exactly, when necessary.
- Never talk as though the patient were not there.
- Assume that the patient understands more than he or she can express.
- Minimize choices.
- Pace instructions and repeat them when necessary.

Nonverbal strategies
- Coordinate with verbal communication.
- Remain in the patient's line of sight.
- Maintain eye contact.
- Avoid sudden movements.
- Smile and use gentle touch.
- Allow rest periods.

Other strategies
- Use praise and positive response.
- Decrease the number of people in the room.
- Explain procedures before performing them.
- Enlist the patient's participation.

*Adapted from Chalmers[51] with permission.

Patients with hearing loss

In the United States, approximately one in five people older than 12 years of age has hearing loss in at least one ear significant enough to interfere with communication.[53] Further, the incidence is increasing, owing partly to the aging of the population.[54] The odds of hearing loss are 5.5 times greater for men than for women and 70% lower for blacks compared with whites.[55] Smoking is associated with earlier hearing loss. The prevalence of hearing loss rises dramatically with age. Among those aged 65 years or older, 27.8% had trouble hearing, and an additional 11.1% were deaf.[56] Therefore, dental providers who inspire loyalty can expect many long-term patients with good hearing to lose their hearing as they grow older.

Because hearing loss is significantly associated with a range of health disparities, health care providers are undertaking efforts to facilitate access to care for this population.[56–58] One such effort is to promote more effective communication with patients who struggle to hear.

Untreated hearing loss can make dental treatment difficult if patients are unable to hear or understand health history questions, requests and instructions during examinations or procedures, or treatment options and directions. Recognizing hearing loss in a patient can also pose challenges. Due to the association of hearing loss with old age in a youth-obsessed society, a social stigma persists for the hard of hearing. As a result, fewer than one in three senior adults (70 years or older) who would benefit from a hearing aid has ever worn one, a figure that drops to fewer than one in six for adults under 70 years old.[59] Patients who are losing their ability to hear may face an adjustment period during which they are unwilling to acknowledge a problem or may be in denial of their declining ability. Dentists should understand and accommodate these transitions.

Given the stigma some patients attach to hearing loss, the dental provider must be sensitive when attempting to determine a patient's ability to hear. We recommend three primary ways for identifying hearing loss in a patient. The easiest way to find out whether a patient has hearing loss is to ask. A question about hearing loss asked after a problem is suspected could cause the patient embarrassment, but the patient may volunteer the information if the question is phrased appropriately and asked as a routine part of the health history: "Have you ever been diagnosed with hearing loss?"

Second, even when the patient indicates that he or she has no hearing loss, the dental provider should note behaviors associated with hearing loss. Those behaviors include asking others to repeat comments, avoiding conversation, speaking too loudly, providing answers unrelated to questions asked, and not responding at all.

Third, as a health care provider, the dental professional can suggest screening. The National Institute on Deafness and Other Communication Disorders offers a brief online assessment for hearing loss that could be administered in the dental chair (http://www.asha.org/public/hearing/testing/assess.htm). The dental professional can also refer a patient to an audiologist or ear, nose, and throat specialist for evaluation.

This activity is designed to help you understand how hard-of-hearing patients experience life. While going about your daily activities, wear earplugs for a few hours. Wearing a stocking cap will add to the experience, because others will not realize that your hearing is compromised. Describe your interactions with others. Do you think you missed any information? Did you have to ask people to repeat what they said? Did you notice any frustration?

When treating a patient with acknowledged or unacknowledged hearing loss, the dental provider can employ several communication strategies to facilitate communication (Box 10-5). Most of these are fairly straightforward, while others may need some explanation. For instance, taking turns speaking is important because the patient with hearing loss may have difficulty locating the source of a sound. For this reason, the mask can prove problematic. The mask can also muffle voices and obscure moving lips, which cue the hard-of-hearing patient to listen.

The hard-of-hearing patient relies extensively on nonverbal cues, so important information should be given when the patient is sitting upright and when not wearing a dental dam, which can interfere with vision.

Because lower vocal ranges are easier to hear than higher ones, the dental provider—particularly anyone with a higher voice—should speak in a lower register.

Finally, using presentation aids is usually a good idea but may be even more important with a hard-of-hearing patient, who should be provided written treatment options or instructions so that the provider can ensure the patient understands the most crucial information.

Box 10-5	Strategies for communicating with hard-of-hearing patients

Ask what helps
- For an acknowledged hearing loss: "What can I do to help you hear and understand during the appointment?"
- For an unacknowledged hearing loss: "I realize that the clinic can be noisy. Can I do anything to help you to hear what I am saying to you?"

Reduce background noise
- Close operatory doors.
- Lower the volume of intercoms.
- Turn off background music.

Take turns speaking
- Avoid speaking simultaneously with the patient or other members of the dental team.
- Never interrupt a patient.

Remove the mask
- Exchange important messages before donning the mask.
- Pull down the mask when speaking is necessary.

Face the patient
- Remain at eye level when possible.
- Maintain eye contact.
- Remove the dental dam.

Modify speaking patterns
- Speak slowly.
- Lower your voice.
- Use short words and sentences.

Rephrase
- When repeating, use different words.
- Provide contextual information.

Use nonverbal communication
- Visual cues can be ineffective if the patient closes his or her eyes during treatment.
- Touch signals may be most effective.

Speak to the hearing ear
- Note in the patient's file which ear hears better.

Chapter Checklist ✓

Parents and guardians of children
❑ Rely on observation and listening skills.
❑ Remain flexible.
❑ Find a place for the parent or guardian to sit or stand in the operatory.
❑ Divide attention and comments between the patient and the parent or guardian.
❑ State the need for cooperation from everyone in the operatory.
❑ Remember that the child is the patient and address the child directly.
❑ Seek rapport before collecting the health history.
❑ Conduct the interview with the child as much as possible.
❑ Teach the child to take responsibility for his or her oral health.
❑ Determine the cause of any injuries and take steps to minimize recurrence.
❑ Ask the parent to wait in the reception area whenever his or her presence interferes with information gathering.
❑ Ask the fearful parent to wait in the reception area.
❑ Encourage the parent or guardian to participate in live modeling of appropriate dental behaviors.
❑ Address trust, skill, and anticipated pain.
❑ Clarify expected outcomes.
❑ Use motivational interviewing with the parent or guardian to encourage preventive care for the child.

Spouses, children, and caregivers of seniors
❑ Determine the relationship between the escort and the senior and determine how involved the patient wishes the escort to be.
❑ Shake hands with the escort and introduce yourself.
❑ Ask the patient whether he or she would like the escort present in the operatory.
❑ Observe the patient's responses to gauge the level of escort participation the patient is comfortable with.
❑ Understand that the level of escort participation depends on the patient's capabilities, the escort's motivations, and the relationship between patient and escort.
❑ Address health history questions to the patient and encourage the patient to answer.
❑ Thank the escort who provides needed information.
❑ If a patient prefers, address both the patient and the spouse.
❑ Explicitly confirm that the patient understands the treatment options and consents to the treatment decision, particularly when the escort has a financial interest in the decision.
❑ Involve the spouse, child, or caregiver in preventive treatment planning discussions unless the patient objects.
❑ Reach agreement regarding any oral health tasks the spouse, child, or caregiver will perform on the patient's behalf.
❑ Try to schedule subsequent appointments to include the person responsible for follow-up care.

Anxious children
❑ Set a goal of training the child patient in how to interact with the dental provider.
❑ Resist the temptation to scold.
❑ Describe observed problems, but emphasize the benefits of preventive behaviors.

☐ Smile and act enthusiastic about the child's visit.
☐ Preview the examination and explain the rationale for what will happen.
☐ Show the child various instruments and allow him or her to handle some of the equipment.
☐ Play with the mask to distract or reassure a frightened child.
☐ Practice empathic communication and appropriate touch.
☐ Acknowledge and address patient anxiety, experience, or concerns.
☐ Provide verbal explanations and reassurance.
☐ Use a firm, loud voice.
☐ Make short appointments.
☐ Encourage exploration.
☐ Encourage cooperation.
☐ Negotiate.
☐ Enlist parental help to alleviate anxiety or foster cooperation.
☐ Separate the parent from the child if doing so will alleviate a child's anxiety.
☐ Use technology by showing cartoons or playing music the child selects.
☐ Include both the parent and the child in treatment planning.
☐ Use instructional techniques: tell-show-do, teach-back, hand-over-hand, and chaining.
☐ Provide rewards and giveaways such as sugar-free gum and fruity toothpaste.
☐ Avoid underestimating a child's understanding or capabilities.
☐ Begin counseling the patient before he or she reaches the age of lip and tongue piercings.

Patients with autism
☐ Learn as much as possible about a patient's behavior and communication patterns.
☐ Remain flexible in your approach to communication and treatment.
☐ Practice positive reinforcement through immediate verbal praise and giveaways.
☐ Issue short and clear commands.
☐ Ignore inappropriate behavior as much as possible.
☐ Use tell-show-do to instruct the autistic patient.
☐ Take frequent breaks.
☐ Ask the parent or a dental team member to hold the patient's hand.
☐ Ask the parent to restrain the child.
☐ If necessary, suggest the use of a stabilization device in a positive way and secure consent.
☐ Recognize that the autistic patient is likely to require behavioral management techniques.
☐ Involve the family in treatment.
☐ Provide a supportive and structured environment.
☐ Maintain continuity of the dental team in return visits.

Senior patients
☐ Acknowledge that the senior patient may have items he or she wishes to discuss.
☐ Avoid treating the senior patient with condescension or paternalism.
☐ Cultivate empathy for the senior patient through perspective taking.
☐ Include other health care providers in treatment planning.
☐ Remain aware of the patient's capabilities.

❑ Work within the common constraints of the senior patient: fixed income, lack of transportation, inadequate caregiver assistance, and so on.

❑ Acknowledge and address the attitude that tooth loss is acceptable among seniors.

❑ Avoid becoming complacent in observing the longtime patient as he or she ages.

❑ Remember that physical capabilities, cognitive processing, family structure, and financial resources can change rapidly for the senior patient.

❑ Adapt to the patient's abilities and anticipate oral health needs and abilities.

Patients with dementia or Alzheimer disease

❑ Administer the Dental Behavior Index to gauge the patient's degree of dementia.

❑ Schedule the patient earlier in the day.

❑ Attempt to restore function quickly, before capabilities decline further.

❑ Enlist the help of the caregiver and family members.

❑ Schedule longer appointments.

❑ Use instructional techniques: tell-show-do, teach-back, hand-over-hand, and chaining.

❑ Monitor or designate a team member to monitor the patient's facial expressions during procedures.

❑ Speech construction: Begin by identifying yourself and using the patient's name and title.

❑ Speech construction: Use short words and simple sentences.

❑ Speech construction: Use nouns instead of pronouns.

❑ Speech construction: As much as possible, avoid questioning the patient.

❑ Speech style: Speak slowly, clearly, and in a lower tone.

❑ Speech style: Use your normal voice, avoiding baby talk.

❑ Speech style: Ask one question at a time and wait for a response.

❑ Speech style: Repeat questions exactly, when necessary.

❑ Speech style: Never talk as though the patient were absent.

❑ Speech style: Assume that the patient understands more than he or she can express.

❑ Speech style: Minimize choices.

❑ Speech style: Pace instructions and repeat them when necessary.

❑ Nonverbal: Coordinate nonverbal and verbal communication.

❑ Nonverbal: Remain in the patient's line of sight.

❑ Nonverbal: Maintain eye contact.

❑ Nonverbal: Avoid sudden movements.

❑ Nonverbal: Smile and use gentle touch.

❑ Nonverbal: Allow frequent breaks.

❑ Use praise and positive reinforcement.

❑ Decrease the number of people in the room.

❑ Explain procedures before performing them.

❑ Enlist the patient's participation.

Patients with hearing loss

❑ Diagnosis: Be sensitive to perceived stigma when gauging a patient's hearing ability.

❑ Diagnosis: Ask about hearing loss during the health history.

❑ Diagnosis: Note behaviors associated with hearing loss (eg, asking people to repeat comments, avoiding conversation, speaking too loudly, and so on).

❑ Diagnosis: Suggest a hearing screening.

❑ Give important information when the patient is upright and not wearing a dental dam.

❏ Speak in a lower register.
❏ Use presentation aids.
❏ Ask what helps.
❏ Reduce background noise by closing doors and lowering intercom or music volume.
❏ Take turns speaking and never interrupt the patient.
❏ Remove the mask, particularly when important information is given.
❏ Face the patient, maintaining eye contact at eye level.
❏ Modify speaking patterns by using short words and sentences.
❏ Rephrase when repeating information, using different words and providing context.
❏ Use nonverbal communication, particularly touch.
❏ If the patient hears better in one ear, speak to that ear.

For More Information

Parents and caregivers
- http://www.aapd.org/assets/1/7/FastFacts.pdf
- http://www.aapd.org/resources/frequently_asked_questions
- http://www.cdc.gov/fluoridation/safety/infant_formula.htm
- http://kidshealth.org/parent/general/teeth/healthy.html
- http://www.alsa.org/als-care/resources/publications-videos/factsheets/fyi-oral-care.html
- http://www.nidcr.nih.gov/OralHealth/Topics/DevelopmentalDisabilities/Dental-CareEveryDay.htm

Young patients
- http://www.chickmoorman.com/dentalTalk/agesAndStages.pdf
- http://www.aapd.org/media/Policies_Guidelines/G_Adoleshealth.pdf
- http://www.cdc.gov/oralhealth/publications/factsheets/childrens_oral_health/brushup.htm

Patients with autism
- http://www.autismspeaks.org/family-services/tool-kits/dental-tool-kit
- http://www.nidcr.nih.gov/OralHealth/Topics/DevelopmentalDisabilities/PracticalOralCarePeopleAutism.htm
- http://dentalresource.org/topic55autistic.html
- http://www.autismcenter.org/dental-care-indivduals-autism-level-1
- http://www.autismtoday.com/library-back/DentalDilemma.htm
- http://summerlinpediatricdentist.com/autism-dental-center

Senior patients
- http://www.aafp.org/fpm/2006/0900/p73.html
- http://www.cdc.gov/nchs/data/ahcd/agingtrends/03oral.pdf
- http://www.ouhsc.edu/geriatricmedicine/education/Oral_Health/Geriatric_Dentistry.htm
- http://www.toothwisdom.org/resources/entry/visiting-the-dentist-a-caregivers-guide

38. Kaasalainen S. Pain assessment in older adults with dementia: Using behavioral observation methods in clinical practice. J Gerontol Nurs 2007;33(6):6–10.
39. Greene MG, Adelman RD, Friedmann E, Charon R. Older patient satisfaction with communication during an initial medical encounter. Soc Sci Med 1994;38:1279–1288.
40. Wetle T. Ethical issues in geriatric dentistry. Gerodontology 1987;6:73–78.
41. Mouradian WE, Corbin SB. Addressing health disparities through dental-medical collaborations. 2. Cross-cutting themes in the care of special populations. J Dent Educ 2003;67:1320–1326.
42. Slack-Smith L, Lange A, Paley G, O'Grady M, French D, Short L. Oral health and access to dental care: A qualitative investigation among older people in the community. Gerodontology 2010;27:104–113.
43. Plassman BL, Langa KM, Fisher GG, et al. Prevalence of dementia in the United States: The aging, demographics, and memory study. Neuroepidemiology 2007;29:125–132.
44. Ghezzi EM, Ship JA. Dementia and oral health. Oral Surg Oral Med Oral Pathol Oral Radiol Endod 2000;89:2–5.
45. Chung JA, Cummings JL. Neurobehavioral and neuropsychiatric symptoms in Alzheimer's disease: Characteristics and treatment. Neurol Clin 2000;18:829–846.
46. Galasko D. New approaches to diagnose and treat Alzheimer's disease: A glimpse of the future. Clin Geriatr Med 2001;17:393–410.
47. Ellefsen B, Holm-Pedersen P, Morse DE, Schroll M, Andersen BB, Waldemar G. Caries prevalence in older persons with and without dementia. J Am Geriatr Soc 2008;56:59–67.
48. Vainio L, Krause M, Inglehart MR. Patients with special needs: Dental students' educational experiences, attitudes, and behavior. J Dent Educ 2011;75:13–22.
49. Nordenram G, Ryd-Kjellen E, Ericsson K, Winblad B. Dental management of Alzheimer patients. A predictive test of dental cooperation in individualized treatment planning. Acta Odontol Scand 1997;55:148–154.
50. Nordenram G, Ryd-Kjellen E, Ericsson K, Winblad B. Unexpected dental behavior in five Alzheimer patients. Differences between cognitive and functional capacity, graphic performance, and dental behavior. Acta Odontol Scand 1995;53:381–388.
51. Chalmers JM. Behavior management and communication strategies for dental professionals when caring for patients with dementia. Spec Care Dentist 2000;20:147–154.
52. Sheu E, Versloot J, Nader R, Kerr D, Craig KD. Pain in the elderly: Validity of facial expression components of observational measures. Clin J Pain 2011;27:593–601.
53. Lin FR, Niparko JK, Ferrucci L. Hearing loss prevalence in the United States. Arch Intern Med 2011;171:1851–1852.
54. Pleis JR, Lethbridge-Cejku M. Summary health statistics for U.S. adults: National Health Interview Survey, 2006. Vital Health Stat 10 2007(235):1–153.
55. Agrawal Y, Platz EA, Niparko JK. Prevalence of hearing loss and differences by demographic characteristics among US adults: Data from the National Health and Nutrition Examination Survey, 1999–2004. Arch Intern Med 2008;168:1522–1530.
56. Schoenborn CA, Heyman K. Health disparities among adults with hearing loss: United States 2000–2006. Atlanta, GA: National Center for Health Statistics, 2008. http://www.cdc.gov/nchs/data/hestat/hearing00-06/hearing00-06.htm. Updated February 26, 2010. Accessed 16 February 2015.
57. Barnett S, Franks P. Health care utilization and adults who are deaf: Relationship with age at onset of deafness. Health Serv Res 2002;37:103–118.
58. Barnett S. Communication with deaf and hard-of-hearing people: A guide for medical education. Acad Med 2002;77:694–700.
59. National Institute on Deafness and Other Communication Disorders. Quick statistics. Bethesda, MD: National Institutes of Health, 2014. http://www.nidcd.nih.gov/health/statistics/Pages/quick.aspx. Updated 3 October 2014. Accessed 16 February 2015.

11

Managing Hearing and Speaking Challenges

Why Planning for Hearing and Speaking Challenges Matters

Throughout this book we have emphasized that effective patient-provider communication is a prerequisite of patient-centered care.[1,2] Communicating with patients in a consultative context entails communication challenges that are absent in a social context. Common communication barriers include patients' pain and anxiety and providers' multitasking and clinical focus. For both the provider and the patient, training and experience can minimize these barriers and facilitate effective communication most of the time. Most of the training provided up to this point has presumed that patients and providers can both hear each other and

The **postlingual deaf** lose their hearing after they begin to speak, and they can be very comfortable communicating with hearing individuals, provided they are able to see the face of their conversation partner. Evidence suggests differences in health access and outcomes between the prelingual and postlingual deaf; the prelingual deaf visit the doctor less frequently, but the postlingual deaf may have greater health problems.[25,26]

Regardless of the age of onset, the deaf who use ASL share a language. For many deaf people, ASL is their first language. Native users of ASL resemble native speakers of other foreign languages in that they share a meaning system and therefore a common way of experiencing the world and of expressing their experiences. The result is a strong sense of community among the deaf—a culture, in fact.[27] Increasingly, health care workers are encouraged to perceive deafness as a **cultural characteristic** requiring cultural competence rather than a **hearing impairment**, a term many deaf people reject.[28] The rationale is that a perception of deaf patients as physically compromised may contribute to a perception that treating them is difficult. In fact, among a menu of patient "disabilities," health care providers report that those with communication limitations (such as deafness) are the most difficult to serve.[29]

The perception that deaf patients are difficult may contribute to the significant disparities in health and health care access for this population.[30] A survey of deaf participants regarding their health care experiences found that communication challenges were "ubiquitous" and marked by fear and mistrust.[31] The prevalence of fair or poor health increases with the degree of hearing loss.[20] The deaf are also more likely to smoke, drink alcohol, and suffer from obesity.[20,32]

Regarding oral health care access, 60% of hearing patients visited the dentist in the previous year, but fewer than half of the deaf had done so.[25] Deaf patients who use ASL report significantly lower rates of preventive treatment when they have a provider who does not use ASL.[33] To address these disparities, professionals both within and outside the field of dentistry have called for greater efforts and training to facilitate communication between providers and deaf patients.[34–38]

Activity 11-2

Deaf people must develop keen powers of perception to thrive in a hearing world. To better appreciate this fact, find a brief instructional video on YouTube (https://www.youtube.com) and watch it with the sound muted. Search "how to make a paper gun" or "how to shuck an oyster" or something similar. After watching the instructions once, do you believe you could complete the task effectively? Does this activity give you a fuller appreciation of the potential—and limits—of nonverbal communication when you are providing instruction or treatment options to deaf patients?

Communication strategies

The key to successful treatment of a deaf patient is preparation, and efforts to accommodate deafness begin with appointment setting. Automated telephone menu systems should be eliminated, or the touchtone options should be minimized. Simple alternatives to the telephone should be made available, including the option for the patient to schedule an appointment by email, text, or fax. **Telecommunications device for the deaf (TDD)** is the term for a number of assistance devices, including the telephone typewriter (TTY), which allows users to type to one another using telephone lines. The interaction is similar to instant messaging and texting, which are rapidly replacing TDDs. The practice can place free calls to a deaf patient using http://www.SprintRelay.com. This service, which relies on an assistant to relay messages between the hearing and deaf, is useful for both scheduling and confirming appointments; the service is available in Spanish as well as English.

After the appointment is made, the provider should follow up any telephone communication with written confirmation and instructions detailing what can be expected during the visit.

Before beginning the appointment, the provider should confer with the patient to determine what communication aids or services might be needed. The patient is the best source of information about his or her own needs, so the provider should first ask about the type and source of assistance the patient requires. A 2010 study found that patients who do and do not rely on speech in everyday life differ in their preferences for communication in a clinic setting, and the provider's degree of "deaf awareness" affected their preferences.[39] The provider should remain aware that treating a deaf patient might take more time than treating a hearing patient, so the schedule should be adjusted accordingly.

When the patient checks in, the receptionist or provider should speak slowly, loudly, and clearly, as some deaf patients have limited hearing ability. A patient's name should not be called across a waiting room. Instead, a staff member should approach and escort the patient to the operatory. The provider should avoid shouting and never share health information that can be overheard by others.

The provider should maintain eye contact with the patient, as many deaf patients rely on lip reading and nonverbal cues to facilitate understanding. Written instructions with clear illustrations should be provided to indicate what procedures and tests will be undertaken during the appointment. The reception area, as well as the operatory, should maintain good lighting so the patient can clearly see the faces of the staff.

In an article on health care interactions with the deaf, Meador and Zazove[40] noted two communication characteristics of deaf culture that the provider should keep in mind. First, in deaf culture, information is freely shared, so the provider should be forthcoming with information even when it does not directly relate to the deaf patient. To withhold information is considered rude. Thus, if someone knocks at the door, the provider should tell the patient someone is knocking. If dental team members are speaking to each other, the patient should be told what the conversation entails.

Second, contrary to the usual custom, the deaf often begin conversations abruptly then drag out the farewell, so the provider should get straight to the point but not leave before the patient is satisfied. For instance, during treatment planning, a deaf patient may ask the same question multiple times.

A variety of strategies are available to enhance chairside communication with a deaf patient, and the correct approach depends on the nature of the appointment and the needs of the patient. Deaf patients report that more positive health care experiences are characterized by the use of ASL interpreters, providers who know ASL, and providers who make an effort to improve communication with deaf patients.[31] For a provider who is not fluent in ASL, relying on a certified ASL interpreter is the standard of care and ensures accurate and private patient-provider communication. A 1995 study, however, found that writing is the method physicians use most often to communicate with deaf patients, even though many deaf patients have limited reading skills and although 63% of physicians acknowledge that signing should be the primary method used with deaf patients who sign.[41]

Other communication strategies may substitute for or complement certified ALS interpreters in some circumstances: during an emergency appointment, when the interpreter does not arrive on schedule, or if the patient is comfortable with lip reading, for instance. Box 11-1 reviews various commonly used communication strategies, indicating the benefits and drawbacks of each.

Box 11-1	Strategies for communicating with a deaf patient

Lip reading
- Few deaf people can read lips.
- Even a proficient lip reader can miss or misunderstand more than half of what is said.
- Unfamiliar dental terminology can make lip reading challenging.

Note writing and texting
- Note writing can be slow.
- Many deaf patients struggle with written English.
- Unfamiliar dental terminology can make note reading challenging.

Prepared materials
- Many deaf patients struggle with written English.
- Providing forms, instructions, and descriptions in advance can shorten appointment time and allow others to help the deaf patient prepare.

Prepared visual aids
- Visual aids can be understood even by a patient who does not read well.

Computer-aided support
- A large and growing number of resources are available online to illustrate the spectrum of dental problems and treatments.
- Many online videos and photographs are free and include closed-captioned or subtitle options.

Video remote interpreting
- Video remote interpreting is the second-best option when a medical interpreter is unavailable.
- An interpreter may be unfamiliar with dental terminology.
- Streaming technology compromises privacy.

Chairside certified interpreter
- A chairside certified interpreter is the standard of care for treating a deaf patient.

Although cochlear implants facilitate lip reading, only a small percentage of deaf people can lip read. Even the most proficient can miss more than half of what is spoken. Therefore, lip reading alone is rarely an adequate means of communicating about health care. Even skilled lip readers can misunderstand questions and comments. The situation is further complicated by unfamiliar dental terminology.

When treating a patient who prefers lip reading, the provider should face the patient and maintain eye contact. The provider should not speak while looking down at a file or washing at a sink. When speaking to a deaf patient, the provider should lower the mask[42] and remove anything in or near his or her mouth, such as gum or pencils. The provider should speak at regular volume and use regular lip movements. The provider's face should be illuminated and not in shadow; overhead light is best for this purpose. Finally, the provider should use simple terms and avoid dental jargon.

Deaf patients also vary in their abilities and preferences for written communication. For the patient who prefers to write notes during an appointment, the provider should allow extra time for the slower pace of writing. The provider should write short phrases and avoid dental jargon. Writing implements should be kept on hand; small whiteboards can serve this purpose. The patient may be quicker and more comfortable typing or texting a message. If so, the provider should have a keyboard accessible or prepare to exchange notes on a personal digital assistant or texts on a mobile phone.

Providing written forms, instructions, and descriptions in advance not only saves appointment time but also can enhance patient understanding. Written materials provided before the appointment allow even a patient who does not read well to seek input and explanations so that he or she arrives better prepared with information and appropriate questions regarding treatment. The scheduler should mail, email, or fax the health history form and descriptions of the anticipated schedule and procedures to the deaf patient. Too often, the health care provider does not share or explain findings to the deaf patient, so the patient may be unaware of significant aspects of his or her health status. Providing forms in advance allows the deaf patient time to locate records and information. Illustrated descriptions of the schedule and procedures to be accomplished during the appointment help a patient to arrive prepared. Many descriptions of conditions and procedures are available online from the American Dental Association.

The syntax of ASL differs so much from written and spoken English that many deaf people consider English their second language. As a result, deaf patients vary widely in their literacy skills. Dental providers should rely on visual aids to better communicate with all patients, but particularly so with deaf patients. Visual aids can include models, radiographs, pictures, and drawings (including wall posters and flipbooks). Even gestures can be used to illustrate messages. A mirror and pointing, for instance, can be used to indicate an area of concern.

Increasingly, visual aids are available online, so an available Internet connection and monitor in the operatory can enhance communication. Similarly, DVDs and digital video files can be played on a monitor. Closed-captioning is particularly useful in such instances. The American Dental Association has placed numerous videos and a few animations online. Although not all are closed-captioned, many include useful illustrations and text.

Video remote interpreting uses teleconferencing equipment and the Internet to allow a professional sign language interpreter to interpret messages via streaming video. The National Association of the Deaf, however, suggests this option only when a chairside certified interpreter is unavailable.[43] An interpreter is privy to sensitive health information. Disclosing that information via digital technology to a person the patient has never met clearly compromises the patient's rights to privacy. The ideal auxiliary service for a deaf patient is a chairside certified interpreter of ASL. We devote the next section to strategies for effectively working with such an interpreter.

Question of ethics: A variety of conditions can lead to hearing loss and deafness, and dental providers are not immune. In fact, researchers have long sought to determine whether environmental noise in a dental office increases the risk of hearing loss. If you were to lose your hearing, do you believe you could continue to provide adequate dental care to your patients? If so, do you believe they would have an ethical obligation to remain loyal to you, even if their appointments might take longer and require more effort to overcome the communication barrier? Regarding deafness-related communication challenges, do you think most dental professionals' willingness to accept deaf patients is equivalent to their expectation that hearing patients would accept a deaf provider?

Using an ASL interpreter

Dental providers might reasonably wonder why relatives or friends of a deaf person cannot supply the needed ASL interpretation services for free. After all, such people commonly accompany patients into the operatory, and their familiarity with each other should minimize miscommunications. Family and friends are inappropriate choices as interpreters for four good reasons. First, dental vocabulary is somewhat specialized, and amateur interpreters cannot be expected to know all the correct terminology or how to sign it. Second, the health history may reveal sensitive information deaf patients would prefer not to disclose to family or friends. Third, family and friends may have an emotional interest in the diagnosis or a conflict of interest regarding treatment planning, placing them in a difficult position. They may be tempted to withhold some information or encourage one treatment option over another. Fourth, unreliable interpreting compromises the ability of patients to consent to treatment. For these reasons, providers should decline any patient's recommendation to pay a friend or family member and should hire a professional interpreter.

Professional ASL interpreters can be located through the Registry of Interpreters for the Deaf (RID) website (http://www.rid.org). Alternatively, an Internet search using the terms *deaf services* and the city or state should yield a link to nearby interpreters. Professional interpreters may need several days' notice, so advance planning is important. Interpreters' fees can vary widely, but the more qualified generally charge more. At present, RID does not offer a specialization in medical interpreting, but providers should insist on general certification from RID. In most regions, providers can expect to pay between US$30 and US$70 per hour.

Box 11-2 presents several strategies for using an ASL interpreter after one has been hired. First, the provider should confer with the interpreter in advance of the patient appointment. If this meeting takes place immediately prior to the appointment, ample time should be allowed to discuss financial and contractual arrangements, to inform the interpreter what is expected to take place, and to agree on responsibilities. Often, the interpreter will be an excellent source of advice, should the provider have questions. Because the purpose of this meeting is for the interpreter and provider to become familiar with each other and to settle business details, the patient should not be present.

Second, when the patient is seated, the provider should position the ASL interpreter in front of the patient, and the provider should sit or stand beside the interpreter. The line of sight is very important for a deaf patient, and the patient should always retain a clear view of the interpreter's hands. (In this way, ASL interpreters differ from foreign language interpreters, who generally stand behind the patient.) In a small operatory, positioning can pose challenges: One or more providers must have adequate room to maneuver, and the interpreter must have adequate room to sign in the sight of the patient. Once the chair reclines, positioning can become even more challenging, so the provider should determine the best operatory and positioning before the patient arrives.

Third, after the patient is seated and the interpreter is positioned, the provider should introduce everyone in the room. If the practice is in a city with a cohesive deaf community, the patient and interpreter may know each other. As mentioned previously, deaf culture generally discourages the withholding of information, so the provider should introduce all staff members who walk into the operatory during the appointment—even those who will not be participating in care. As the appointment gets underway, the provider should be polite to the interpreter but should remember that rapport building is focused on the patient.

Fourth, the provider should face the patient while speaking and listening, maintaining eye contact and normal facial expression. The deaf patient will rely on a combination of lip reading, nonverbal communication, and ASL to understand what is being said and to assess the provider's comprehension of what the patient has expressed. The mask is an obvious barrier to communication via facial expression, so the provider should pull down the mask when speaking. In addition, the reclining position may complicate the patient's observation, and a dental dam may obscure the view of the provider's face. Therefore, important information should be communicated when the patient is upright and not wearing a dam. Facing the patient is also beneficial because it allows the provider to observe the patient's nonverbal expression, which may indicate dental anxiety or other important information.

Box 11-2 | Strategies for working with an ASL interpreter

Confer in advance
- Inform the interpreter of the appointment's purpose.
- Ask the interpreter for any advice to make the appointment proceed smoothly.

Position yourself and the interpreter
- The patient must be able to see the interpreter.
- You must have room to work.

Introduce everyone
- Familiarity facilitates communication.
- Engage in typical rapport-building communication with the patient.

Face the patient
- The patient relies on lip reading and facial expression.
- Lower your mask whenever speaking.
- Communicate important information when the patient is sitting up and not wearing a dental dam.

Communicate with the patient
- Resist the urge to talk to the interpreter.
- During the appointment, the interpreter should be regarded as a communication medium.

Preview and narrate
- The standard communication strategies of previewing and narrating are even more important for deaf patients.
- Do not mistake lack of eye contact for disinterest.

Ask for feedback
- Use open-ended questions and encourage suggestions for improved communication.
- Request that the patient summarize what has been said.

Fifth, the provider should communicate directly with the patient, treating the interpreter as a medium of communication. Treating a present person impersonally can seem awkward or even rude, but professionalism requires the interpreter to unobtrusively and objectively communicate everything that is being communicated between two or more people. The provider should focus on the deaf patient to the same degree as a hearing patient. Therefore, the provider should not turn to the interpreter and say, "Ask him when he last saw a physician." Instead, the provider should look at the patient and ask, "When did you last see a physician?" Then, the provider should watch the patient as the response is conveyed through the interpreter.

Sixth, the provider should preview what will happen during the appointment and should narrate the procedures as they occur. These communication strategies should be common practice with every patient, but they are especially important with a deaf patient. A provider who is unaccustomed to being around deaf people may find it awkward to talk and receive no vocal response. The provider should resist the temptation to stop talking and proceed in silence. The provider may also find it unusual to speak to a patient whose gaze is frequently (and necessarily) focused on the interpreter. The provider should resist the impulse to interpret the lack of eye contact as a lack of interest. Spoken information is very important, and when speaking, the provider should use simple words and short phrases whenever possible.

Finally, the provider should consistently ask for feedback, using open-ended questions and encouraging suggestions for improved communication. For instance, "How frequently do you floss?" Or, "Is there anything else we can do to help you see the interpreter while I'm working?"

Also, to ensure understanding, the provider should ask the deaf patient to summarize what has been said. Instructional methods such as tell-show-do and teach-back can be especially useful when treatment instructions are given to a deaf patient. Not only do these methods reinforce the message by delivering it verbally and visually, but they also confirm that the deaf patient understands everything that has been said.

Activity 11-3

How important is it to have a health care provider who understands your background and needs? Consider this question from a deaf person's perspective and find the nearest dentist who caters to the deaf community. How did you carry out this search? How far away is the dentist you found? Does the dentist advertise the practice as deaf friendly? What sorts of accommodations does the practice offer to make appointment experiences positive for deaf patients? Did this activity teach you anything about health care access barriers and health disparities for deaf patients?

Communicating with LEP Patients

Prevalence and health disparities

In addition to language accommodation mandated for recipients of federal funds by the Civil Rights Act of 1964, the US Department of Health and Human Services has issued 15 national standards on Culturally and Linguistically Appropriate Services (CLAS).[44] Four of the standards deal explicitly with the provision of language services by health care organizations:

- Standard 5: Offer language assistance to individuals who have LEP and/or other communication needs, at no cost to them, to facilitate timely access to all health care and services.
- Standard 6: Inform all individuals of the availability of language assistance services clearly and in their preferred language, verbally and in writing.
- Standard 7: Ensure the competence of individuals providing language assistance, recognizing that the use of untrained individuals and/or minors as interpreters should be avoided.
- Standard 8: Provide easy-to-understand print and multimedia materials and signage in the languages commonly used by the populations in the service area.

According to the US Census Bureau, 20% of the US population older than the age of 5 years speak a language other than English in their home.[45] Although most of these people speak English well, 13.5 million either do not speak well or do not speak English at all. Because the majority of those who speak a language other than English at home are Spanish speakers, this discussion will focus on Hispanic patients who have LEP. The remaining 36% speak a language other than English or Spanish. Given the numbers of this population—nearly 21 million people—providers should be prepared to address a variety of language needs.

Preparation is necessary because of the relationship between language and health care access and because of the challenges of language barriers. Language barriers often result in reduced access to care, quality of care, and satisfaction with care. Distinguishing the health disparities tracing to race or ethnicity from those tracing to language can be challenging.[46,47] Hispanics access care less often than white and black people do, and they are less satisfied with the health services they do access.[48] The reasons for these disparities are both cultural and linguistic. Derose and Baker[49] found that English proficiency among Hispanics was not related to seeing a physician in the previous 3 months but, among those who had seen a physician, LEP was associated with 22% fewer physician visits. The influence of LEP on the number of physician visits was similar to the influence of having no insurance or no regular source of care.

Evidence for an effect of LEP on general health care is mixed. A 2002 review of the research in the previous decade found that 55% of studies reported that LEP adversely affected access and 86% found that LEP adversely affected quality of care.[50] A large-scale 2007 study found that Hispanics who did not speak English at home were less likely to receive health care services for which they were eligible; the discrepancy was even greater among those who were uncomfortable speaking English.[51] Researchers have acknowledged that more work must be done to determine the impact of LEP on access and care.[52]

The research on language-related disparities in oral health care is similarly mixed, but results suggest that language likely contributes to some disparities. A 2008 study of health care access found that multiple disparities among children were associated with the language spoken at home.[53] Children in non–English-speaking households were more likely to have teeth in fair or poor condition (27% versus 7%), to lack dental insurance (39% versus 20%), and to have made no preventive dental visits in the previous year (14% versus 6%). These disparities persisted even after data were controlled for sociodemographic variables. In a 2009 study, on the other hand, researchers controlled for sociodemographic factors among Hispanic adults and found that language was not a significant predictor of a dental visit in the previous year.[54]

Access aside, a body of evidence indicates that language barriers interfere with health care processes and satisfaction. Compared with English-language patients, LEP patients are significantly more likely to report problems understanding medical situations, bad medication reactions, and trouble reading labels.[55] A survey of safety-net dental clinics in North Carolina found that 13% of dental providers reported differences in treatment recommendations for LEP patients and 19% reported differences in treatment provided.[56]

One survey found that Hispanic patients who responded to their health care providers in Spanish were significantly less satisfied with their providers' communication than were Hispanics or non-Hispanic white patients responding in English.[57] Specifically, 29% of those responding in Spanish rated providers' listening as fair to very poor (versus 17% of Hispanics responding in English and 13% of non-Hispanic whites responding in English). They also expressed significantly higher dissatisfaction with obtaining answers to questions (27% versus 19% and 14%, respectively), with explanations about prescriptions (22% versus 19% and 14%, respectively), with explanations about procedures or test results (36% versus 21% and 17%, respectively), and with reassurance and support (37% versus 23% and 18%, respectively). Next, we will discuss several communication strategies that should help reduce LEP patients' dissatisfaction with their dental care.

Volunteer at a community health or dental clinic and observe how the providers interact with patients who have LEP. Draft a brief report outlining your observations. What differences, if any, did you notice in the way providers communicated with LEP patients compared with patients who spoke English fluently? Did you notice any differences in the treatment provided to LEP versus English-fluent patients? Were any clinicians or staff members available to interpret? What other strategies did providers use to overcome language barriers, and were those strategies effective?

Communication strategies

Hearing- and speech-related communication barriers are similar in many respects, and similar solutions can overcome them. Yet the strategies presented in Box 11-3 differ in some respects from strategies presented for communicating with deaf patients, because the regulations for communicating with LEP patients are not as stringent as those for communicating with deaf patients and because the greater diversity of cultures among patients with LEP requires a greater diversity of responses.

When determining which strategy or combination of strategies will work best, the provider should bear in mind three situational variables. First, the language skills of patient and provider will influence the choice of strategy. A patient who is semifluent in English may be able to understand everything if the provider is careful. A provider who is fluent in the patient's native language may also have no trouble delivering care. Second, treatment urgency plays a role in the strategy chosen. Scheduled care allows for more preparation than emergency care. Third, treatment complexity is also a factor. Routine care that entails little new information may be easier to carry out with simple strategies, whereas complicated procedures likely require more elaborate efforts.

Box 11-3	Strategies for communicating with a patient who has LEP

- **Nonprofessional interpreters:** The patient may be comfortable with a family member, friend, or even a bilingual stranger.
- **Brochures, websites, and videos:** Printed materials in Spanish are widely available. In addition, many presentation aids include drawings, photographs, and diagrams that are not language specific. Some videos offer closed-captioning in other languages.
- **Translation websites and software:** Computer programs can now translate English-language instructions.
- **Aided augmentative communication (AAC) boards:** These boards allow the provider and patient to point to words such as *yes, no, rinse,* and *pain.* Tablet computers now allow the provider to generate and adapt a virtual AAC board.
- **Bilingual staff members or trained volunteers:** Staff members and volunteers are likely to know the terminology.
- **Off-site interpreters:** Interpretation is available via telephone and Internet.
- **Certified medical interpreters:** Professional interpreters now can be certified to indicate their specialization in medical vocabulary.

First, family members and friends of the patient can perform interpretation services. In an emergency situation, so can a bilingual stranger. A survey of dental students in California found that they perceived that LEP patients were more difficult to treat but that amateur interpreters worked adequately.[58] Australian dentists reported amateur interpreters as their preferred method for overcoming language barriers with LEP patients.[59] In that same survey, however, 29% of respondents said that language barriers compromised consent.

The consent problem was one of several noted in the previous discussion regarding amateur ASL interpreters. Other problems relate to privacy, misunderstandings due to interpreting skill deficits, and potential conflicts of interest. Nevertheless, a patient from a culture that values family intimacy over individual privacy may prefer to allow an amateur family member to interpret rather than a professional stranger.

Second, brochures, websites, and videos in the patient's language should be available for the patient with LEP. Many free resources in various languages are now available online. In fact, the American Dental Association provides Spanish translations for many of its resources depicting dental conditions and procedures. They can be viewed online, printed, or ordered in hard copy. Websites and videos in other languages are also available, and some videos (online or on DVD) have a closed-caption feature for common languages such as Spanish and French. Not all patients are highly literate, so presentation aids with many photographs can be helpful.

Third, translation websites and software now allow the provider to instantly translate English-language phrases and materials into a wide array of foreign languages. Not only can these programs facilitate the translation of materials, but they can be accessed from a handheld device such as a smartphone so that the chairside provider can find foreign language phrasing for simple instructions or requests. Internet sites such as Google Translate (https://translate.google.com) and Babelfish (http://www.babelfish.com) offer translation of phrases and entire websites into a variety of languages. Their frequent inaccuracy in translating dental terminology suggests that these should only be used as supplements to other communication aids.

Activity 11-5

> Verify the accuracy of an online translation program such as Google Translate (https://translate.google.com). Type a simple phrase in English (eg, "I am going to polish your teeth.") and translate it into one foreign language. Cut and paste the result so that you can translate the phrase into another language; cut and paste again to translate the phrase back to English. How closely does the final phrase resemble the original? Try it with other languages and more complex dental vocabulary and instructions.

Fourth, the aided augmentative communication (AAC) board is a useful tool for any number of challenging communication situations, and children particularly like it. It is a portable board that includes written words and matching illustrations so that the patient and provider can point to symbols indicating ideas such as *pain* or instructions such as *rinse*. It is a useful low-technology solution, and although AAC boards are available for purchase, they are easy to make. We have found that Velcro backing works well to allow quick modification of the AAC board with concepts and instructions specific to a given patient. The proliferation of tablet computers now permits a high-technology adaptation of the concept, which can even be supplemented by simple spoken words in English and a foreign language, when a patient or provider touches the screen.

Fifth, staff members and volunteers who are fluent in a patient's first language can be an enormous help. Their familiarity with dental terminology makes them more reliable interpreters than friends and family members. Any staff members or volunteers must be trained in Health Insurance Portability and Accountability Act (HIPAA) regulations regarding patient privacy, and the patient must consent to their assistance. Even if consent is granted, however, the patient may be uncomfortable with a stranger's presence in the operatory. This is another reason that the patient should always be consulted about his or her preferences prior to arrival.

Sixth, technology now allows off-site interpreters to provide services via telephone or over the Internet. Some insurers, including Delta Dental, and some commercial services, including LanguageLine (http://www.languageline.com), provide interpreters both via telephone and in person. Telephone interpreting services have long been perceived as inferior to in-person interpreting, due to a lack of personalization and visual nonverbal cues. With the online proliferation of inexpensive voice-and-video services such as Skype (http://www.skype.com/en), video remote interpreting is increasingly seen as a better option than telephone interpreting. Both options require special equipment, so again preparations must be made in advance.

Finally, as with ASL interpreting, professional interpreters are the standard—and with good reason. A study found that when routine interpreting services were introduced to a health maintenance organization, use of clinical services significantly increased.[60] Findings from another study indicated that patients receiving interpretation services did not significantly differ from those speaking the same language as their provider in their ratings on most measures of communication.[61] Further, those who rated the interpretation services highly also rated their care highly.

Satisfactory interpreting services are perhaps more widely available now that certification is available for language interpreters through the National Board of Certification for Medical Interpreters. The Board's website (http://www.certifiedmedical interpreters.org) now has a registry that is searchable by language and state. Box 11-4 outlines six strategies to facilitate work with a medical interpreter.

Box 11-4	Strategies for working with a language interpreter

Allow time
- Patient visits requiring an interpreter may require much more time because verbal communication must be repeated and understanding should be verified.
- Simultaneous interpreting takes less time than consecutive interpreting, but you might find that it interferes with concentration.

Clarify the interpreter's role
- Introduce yourself, the patient, and the interpreter.
- Clarify the scope of the interpreter's responsibilities.
- Encourage feedback if dental terminology or cultural concerns interfere with understanding.

Position the interpreter behind the patient
- Have the interpreter stand behind the patient.
- Look at and speak to the patient, not to the interpreter.

Use short phrases and simple language
- The patient might understand some English.
- Simpler words are easier for the translator to render in a different language than are technical terms.

Listen to the patient
- Although you do not share a language, listen to the patient and provide nonverbal feedback cues such as eye contact.
- Watch the patient's nonverbal cues, which may indicate understanding, anxiety, or pain.

Ask the patient to summarize
- At the end of the appointment, ask the patient to briefly summarize his or her understanding of what he or she is expected to do.

Chapter Checklist ☑

Legal obligations
❏ Become familiar with state regulations regarding the provision of services to deaf and LEP patients.
❏ ADA: Providers must provide services to any (potential) patient with a hearing-related disability.
❏ ADA: Providers' communication with deaf patients must be as effective as communication with hearing patients.
❏ ADA: Consult with deaf patients on a case-by-case basis to determine the most effective auxiliary aid or service.
❏ ADA: The dental practice must absorb any cost for auxiliary aids and services.
❏ Civil Rights Act: Providers receiving federal funds may not discriminate against patients with LEP.
❏ Civil Rights Act: Meaningful access for LEP patients is based on the number of individuals with LEP likely to be encountered, the frequency of their contact with the practice, the importance of the practice to the individuals, and the resources available to the provider.
❏ Civil Rights Act: Providers may work out with LEP patients the best approach to communication.
❏ Civil Rights Act: Providers receiving federal funds are required to pay for communication assistance.

Preparing to treat deaf patients
❏ Frame deafness as a cultural characteristic and avoid the term *hearing impairment*.
❏ Eliminate automated telephone menu systems.
❏ Schedule appointments via email, text, or fax.
❏ Use TDDs, including TTYs, or opt for instant messaging or texting.
❏ Place calls to a deaf patient using http://www.SprintRelay.com.
❏ Follow up telephone communication with written confirmation and instructions.
❏ Confer with the patient in advance to determine needed aids and services.
❏ Understand that treating a deaf patient may take more time than treating a hearing patient.
❏ Speak slowly, loudly, and clearly.
❏ Avoid calling for the patient across a reception area but instead approach the deaf patient and escort him or her to the operatory.
❏ Avoid shouting or sharing health information in a voice that can be overheard.
❏ Maintain eye contact.
❏ Provide written instructions with clear illustrations indicating what procedures and tests will be undertaken in the appointment.
❏ Maintain good lighting in the reception area and operatory.
❏ Be forthcoming with information, even when it does not directly relate to the deaf patient.
❏ Address points quickly, but be prepared for lingering goodbyes.

Communication strategies with deaf patients
❏ A certified ASL interpreter at chairside is the standard of care, but other strategies may supplement interpreting or substitute for interpreting if the patient consents.
❏ Lip reading: Face the patient and maintain eye contact.

❑ Lip reading: Avoid speaking while looking down.

❑ Lip reading: Lower the mask when speaking.

❑ Lip reading: Remove anything in or near the mouth when speaking.

❑ Lip reading: Speak at regular volume using regular lip movements.

❑ Lip reading: Ensure that your face is illuminated and not in shadow.

❑ Lip reading: Use simple terms and avoid dental jargon.

❑ Note writing: Allow extra time in the schedule for writing.

❑ Note writing: Write short phrases and avoid dental jargon.

❑ Note writing: Keep writing implements on hand (eg, whiteboards, notepads, keyboards, or mobile telephones).

❑ Prepared materials: Provide the health history forms and illustrated descriptions of the anticipated schedule and procedures.

❑ Prepared materials: Mail, email, or fax the forms and information in advance, if possible, to prepare the patient.

❑ Visual aids: Use models, radiographs, pictures, and drawings, including wall posters and flipbooks.

❑ Visual aids: Use gestures and the mirror to indicate areas of concern.

❑ Computer-aided support: Locate and prepare online visual aids, DVDs, and digital video files.

❑ Computer-aided support: Use closed-captioned visual aids, if possible.

❑ Video remote interpreting: Use video remote interpreting only if a chairside interpreter is unavailable.

Working with an ASL interpreter

❑ Decline any patient's recommendation to pay a friend or family member to interpret.

❑ Locate certified interpreters through the Registry of Interpreters for the Deaf or via an Internet search for interpreters in your area.

❑ Plan for communication needs several days in advance.

❑ Prior to the appointment, discuss with the interpreter the financial and contractual arrangements, the expectations for the appointment, and the interpreter's and your responsibilities.

❑ Position the interpreter in front of the patient and beside yourself.

❑ Before the appointment, determine the best operatory and positioning for everyone.

❑ Introduce everyone in the room and any staff members who enter the operatory.

❑ Focus rapport-building efforts on the patient and not on the interpreter.

❑ Face the patient when speaking and listening.

❑ Maintain eye contact and normal facial expression.

❑ Pull down the mask when speaking.

❑ Communicate important information when the patient is upright and not wearing the dental dam.

❑ Observe the patient's nonverbal expressions.

❑ Communicate directly with the patient, treating the interpreter as a medium of communication.

❑ Focus on the deaf patient to the degree you would focus on a hearing patient.

❑ Preview what will happen and narrate procedures as they happen.

❑ Resist the temptation to lapse into silence.

❑ Do not interpret lack of eye contact as a lack of interest.

❑ Use simple words and short phrases whenever possible.

- ❑ Ask for feedback using open-ended questions and encourage suggestions to improve communication.
- ❑ Ask the patient to summarize what you said.
- ❑ Use instructional methods such as tell-show-do and teach-back.

Patients with LEP

- ❑ Prepare to address a variety of language needs.
- ❑ Consider three situational variables when determining (with the patient) appropriate communication strategies: the language skills of the patient and your own language skills, treatment urgency, and treatment complexity.
- ❑ Nonprofessional interpreters: Discourage the use of friends and family members as interpreters.
- ❑ Brochures, websites, and videos: Keep materials in the patient's language on hand.
- ❑ Brochures, websites, and videos: Find materials with photographs and illustrations because not all patients are highly literate, even in their native language.
- ❑ Brochures, websites, and videos: Search for videos with closed-captioning in the patient's language.
- ❑ Translation websites and software: Locate websites and software that offer quick, accurate translation of typed messages or other relevant websites.
- ❑ Aided augmentative communication board: Construct a low-technology AAC board in advance using cardboard and Velcro.
- ❑ Aided augmentative communication board: Adapt the AAC concept to a tablet computer or smartphone.
- ❑ Bilingual staff members or trained volunteers: Consult the patient beforehand to address any privacy concerns regarding strangers interpreting sensitive health information.
- ❑ Off-site interpreters: Opt for video remote interpreting over telephone interpreting to provide nonverbal visual cues.
- ❑ Certified medical interpreters: Certified medical interpreters are the standard of care.

Working with a language interpreter

- ❑ Allow time: Understand that appointments with an interpreter require much more time than regular appointments.
- ❑ Allow time: Realize that simultaneous interpreting takes less time than consecutive interpreting.
- ❑ Clarify the interpreter's role: Introduce everyone, clarify the scope of the interpreter's responsibilities, and encourage feedback.
- ❑ Position the interpreter behind the patient: Look at and speak to the patient and not the interpreter.
- ❑ Use short phrases and simple language.
- ❑ Listen to the patient: Provide nonverbal feedback such as eye contact.
- ❑ Listen to the patient: Monitor the patient's nonverbal cues for signs of understanding, anxiety, or pain.
- ❑ Ask the patient to summarize: At the appointment's end, confirm the patient's understanding of what he or she is expected to do.

For More Information

ADA and Civil Rights Act
- http://www.ada.gov
- http://www.csda.com/docs/default-source/regulations/americans-with-disabilities-act.pdf
- http://www.ada.gov/moddentpro.htm
- http://paul-burtner.dental.ufl.edu/disability-links
- http://www.hhs.gov/ocr/civilrights/resources/laws/revisedlep.html
- http://www.archives.gov/eeo/laws/title-vi.html
- http://www.hhs.gov/ocr/civilrights/resources/specialtopics/lep/factsheetguidanceforlep.html
- http://www.lawhelp.org/documents/383231nhelp.lep.state.law.chart.final.pdf

Deaf patients
- http://www.nidcd.nih.gov
- http://www.mass.gov/eohhs/docs/dph/com-health/oral-communicate-dental-health-deaf.pdf
- http://depts.washington.edu/pfes/PDFs/DeafCultureClue.pdf
- http://www.dss.cahwnet.gov/forms/english/pub391.pdf
- http://www.sprintrelay.com
- http://www.nad.org/issues/technology/vri
- http://courses.washington.edu/intro2ds/Readings/Deafness_as_culture.pdf

Using an interpreter
- http://www.ncihc.org
- http://www.imiaweb.org
- http://www.rid.org
- http://www.languageline.com
- http://www.certifiedmedicalinterpreters.org/registry

Patients with LEP
- http://www.lep.gov
- http://www.nnoha.org
- https://www.youtube.com/user/AmericanDentalAssoc/playlists
- https://oralhealth.thinkculturalhealth.hhs.gov
- http://babelfish.com
- https://translate.google.com
- http://www.hablamosjuntos.org
- http://www.patientprovidercommunication.org/index.cfm/bibliography.htm

References

1. Wanzer MB, Booth-Butterfield M, Gruber K. Perceptions of health care providers' communication: Relationships between patient-centered communication and satisfaction. Health Commun 2004;16:363–384.
2. Dutta-Bergman MJ. The relation between health-orientation, provider-patient communication, and satisfaction: An individual-difference approach. Health Commun 2005;18:291–303.
3. Americans with Disabilities Act of 1990. United States of America. Pub L No. 101-336, 104 Stat 328 (1990).
4. Civil Rights Act of 1964, Pub L No. 88-352, 78 Stat 241 (1964).
5. White D. Deaf patient sues doctor under ADA. Tex Dent J 1994;111:31.
6. Schwartz MA. Limits on injunctive relief under the ADA: Rethinking the standing rule for deaf patients in the medical setting. J Health Care Law Policy 2008;11:163–214.
7. American Dental Association. American Dental Association Principles of Ethics and Code of Professional Conduct. Chicago: American Dental Association, 2012. http://www.ada.org/~/media/ADA/About%20the%20ADA/Files/code_of_ethics_2012.ashx. Accessed 26 February 2015.
8. American Dental Hygienists' Association. Bylaws: Code of Ethics. Chicago: American Dental Hygienists' Association, 2014. http://www.adha.org/resources-docs/7611_Bylaws_and_Code_of_Ethics.pdf. Accessed 26 February 2015.
9. Sfikas PM. Treating hearing-impaired people: A look at the use of sign interpreters in dentistry. J Am Dent Assoc 2000;131:108–110.
10. Sfikas PM. Serving the hearing-impaired: An update on the use of sign-language interpreters for dental patients and their families. J Am Dent Assoc 2001;132:681–683.
11. US Department of Health and Human Services, Office of Civil Rights. Guidance for federal financial assistance recipients regarding Title VI prohibition against national origin discrimination affecting limited English proficient persons. Washington, DC: US Department of Health and Human Services, 2003. http://www.hhs.gov/ocr/civilrights/resources/laws/revisedlep.html. Accessed 16 February 2015.
12. Sfikas PM. Serving those with little or no knowledge of English: An examination of language-assistance requirements issued by the U.S. Department of Health and Human Services. J Am Dent Assoc 2004;135:1616–1618.
13. Hughes RJ, Damiano PC, Kanellis MJ, Kuthy R, Slayton R. Dentists' participation and children's use of services in the Indiana dental Medicaid program and SCHIP: Assessing the impact of increased fees and administrative changes. J Am Dent Assoc 2005;136:517–523.
14. McBroome K, Damiano PC, Willard JC. Impact of the Iowa S-SCHIP program on access to dental care for adolescents. Pediatr Dent 2005;27:47–53.
15. Bisgaier J, Cutts DB, Edelstein BL, Rhodes KV. Disparities in child access to emergency care for acute oral injury. Pediatrics 2011;127:e1428–e1435.
16. Graham EA, Jacobs TA, Kwan-Gett TS, Cover J. Health services utilization by low-income limited English proficient adults. J Immigr Minor Health 2008;10:207–217.
17. Lessard G, Ku L. Gaps in coverage for children in immigrant families. Future Child 2003;13(1):101–115.
18. Perkins J, Youdelman M. Summary of State Law Requirements Addressing Language Needs in Health Care. Washington, DC: National Health Law Program, 2008.
19. Ku L, Flores G. Pay now or pay later: Providing interpreter services in health care. Health Aff 2005;24:435–444.
20. Schoenborn CA, Heyman K. Health disparities among adults with hearing loss: United States 2000–2006. Atlanta, GA: National Center for Health Statistics, 2008. http://www.cdc.gov/nchs/data/hestat/hearing00-06/hearing00-06.htm. Updated 26 February 2010. Accessed 16 February 2015.
21. Mitchell RE. How many deaf people are there in the United States? Estimates from the Survey of Income and Program Participation. J Deaf Stud Deaf Educ 2006;11:112–119.
22. Mitchell RE. Can you tell me how many deaf people there are in the United States? Washington, DC: Gallaudet University, February 15, 2005. https://research.gallaudet.edu/Demographics/deaf-US.php. Accessed 16 February 2015.

23. Freel BL, Clark MD, Anderson ML, Gilbert GL, Musyoka MM, Hauser PC. Deaf individuals' bilingual abilities: American Sign Language proficiency, reading skills, and family characteristics. Psychology 2011;2:18–23.
24. Musselman C. How do children who can't hear learn to read an alphabetic script? A review of the literature on reading and deafness. J Deaf Stud Deaf Educ 2000;5:9–31.
25. Barnett S, Franks P. Health care utilization and adults who are deaf: Relationship with age at onset of deafness. Health Serv Res 2002;37:103–118.
26. Barnett S, Franks P. Deafness and mortality: Analyses of linked data from the National Health Interview Survey and National Death Index. Public Health Rep 1999;114:330–336.
27. Padden C, Humphries TL. Inside Deaf Culture. Cambridge, MA: Harvard University Press, 2005.
28. Hoang L, LaHousse S, Nakaji M, Sadler G. Assessing deaf cultural competency of physicians and medical students. J Cancer Educ 2011;26:175–182.
29. Bachman SS, Vedrani M, Drainoni ML, Tobias C, Maisels L. Provider perceptions of their capacity to offer accessible health care for people with disabilities. J Disabil Policy Stud 2006;17:130–136.
30. Harmer L. Health care delivery and deaf people: Practice, problems, and recommendations for change. J Deaf Stud Deaf Educ 1999;4:73–110.
31. Steinberg AG, Barnett S, Meador HE, Wiggins EA, Zazove P. Health care system accessibility: Experiences and perceptions of deaf people. J Gen Intern Med 2006;21:260–266.
32. Guthmann D, Sandberg K. Assessing substance abuse problems in deaf and hard of hearing individuals. Am Ann Deaf 1998;143:14–21.
33. McKee MM, Barnett SL, Block RC, Pearson TA. Impact of communication on preventive services among deaf American Sign Language users. Am J Prev Med 2011;41:75–79.
34. National Council on Disability. The Current State of Health Care for People with Disabilities. Washington, DC: National Council on Disability, 2009.
35. Alsmark SS, Garcia J, Martinez MR, Lopez NE. How to improve communication with deaf children in the dental clinic. Med Oral Patol Oral Cir Bucal 2007;12:E576–E581.
36. Crabb JJ. Communication with deaf people in the surgery setting [comment]. Br Dent J 1990;168:93.
37. Crabb JJ. Deafness and dentistry [comment]. Br Dent J 1993;175:280.
38. Holt RD. Deafness and dentistry. Br Dent J 1993;175:120–121.
39. Middleton A, Turner GH, Bitner-Glindzicz M, et al. Preferences for communication in clinic from deaf people: A cross-sectional study. J Eval Clin Pract 2010;16:811–817.
40. Meador HE, Zazove P. Health care interactions with deaf culture. J Am Board Fam Med 2005;18:218–222.
41. Ebert DA, Heckerling PS. Communication with deaf patients. Knowledge, beliefs, and practices of physicians. JAMA 1995;273:227–229.
42. Davis L. Facemasks [letter]. Br Dent J 2008;204:112.
43. Civil Rights Subcommittee of the Public Policy Committee. Advocacy statement: Use of VRI in the medical setting. National Association of the Deaf, April 2008. http://nad.org/issues/technology/vri/advocacy-statement-medical-setting. Accessed 26 February 2015.
44. Office of Minority Health, US Department of Health and Human Services. National Standards for Culturally and Linguistically Appropriate Services (CLAS) in Health and Health Care. Rockville, MD: US Department of Health and Human Services, 2013. https://www.thinkculturalhealth.hhs.gov/pdfs/EnhancedNationalCLASStandards.pdf. Accessed 16 May 2015.
45. Shin HB, Kominski RA. Language Use in the United States: 2007. American Community Survey Reports, ACS-12. Washington, DC: US Census Bureau, 2010.
46. Cooper LA, Powe NR. Disparities in Patient Experiences, Health Care Processes, and Outcomes: The Role of Patient-Provider Racial, Ethnic, and Language Concordance. New York: The Commonwealth Fund, 2004.
47. Pérez-Stable EJ. Language access and Latino health care disparities. Med Care 2007;45:1009–1011.
48. Saha S, Arbelaez JJ, Cooper LA. Patient-physician relationships and racial disparities in the quality of health care. Am J Public Health 2003;93:1713–1719.

49. Derose KP, Baker DW. Limited English proficiency and Latinos' use of physician services. Med Care Res Rev 2000;57:76–91.

50. Timmins CL. The impact of language barriers on the health care of Latinos in the United States: A review of the literature and guidelines for practice. J Midwifery Womens Health 2002;47:80–96.

51. Cheng E, Chen A, Cunningham W. Primary language and receipt of recommended health care among Hispanics in the United States. J Gen Intern Med 2007;22:283–288.

52. Jacobs E, Chen AH, Karliner LS, Agger-Gupta N, Mutha S. The need for more research on language barriers in health care: A proposed research agenda. Milbank Q 2006;84:111–133.

53. Flores G, Tomany-Korman SC. The language spoken at home and disparities in medical and dental health, access to care, and use of services in US children. Pediatrics 2008;121:e1703–e1714.

54. Jaramillo F, Eke P, Thornton-Evans G, Griffin S. Acculturation and dental visits among Hispanic adults. Prev Chronic Dis 2009;6(2)A50.

55. Wilson E, Chen AH, Grumbach K, Wang F, Fernandez A. Effects of limited English proficiency and physician language on health care comprehension. J Gen Intern Med 2005;20:800–806.

56. Hammersmith KJ, Lee JY. A survey of North Carolina safety-net dental clinics' methods for communicating with patients of limited English proficiency (LEP). J Public Health Dent 2009; 69:90–94.

57. Morales LS, Cunningham WE, Brown JA, Liu H, Hays RD. Are Latinos less satisfied with communication by health care providers? J Gen Intern Med 1999;14:409–417.

58. Itaya LE, Glassman P, Gregorczyk S, Bailit HL. Dental school patients with limited English proficiency: The California experience. J Dent Educ 2009;73:1055–1064.

59. Goldsmith C, Slack-Smith L, Davies G. Dentist-patient communication in the multilingual dental setting. Aust Dent J 2005;50:235–241.

60. Jacobs EA, Lauderdale DS, Meltzer D, Shorey JM, Levinson W, Thisted RA. Impact of interpreter services on delivery of health care to limited–English-proficient patients. J Gen Intern Med 2001;16:468–474.

61. Green AR, Ngo-Metzger Q, Legedza ATR, Massagli MP, Phillips RS, Iezzoni LI. Interpreter services, language concordance, and health care quality. J Gen Intern Med 2005;20:1050–1056.

Managing Stigma Challenges

Why Planning for Stigma Challenges Matters

Chapter 3 addressed the topic of culturally competent communication, and one section explored stigma as a culturally embedded phenomenon. In other words, the physical or behavioral characteristics that are stigmatized vary from one culture to another or even from one social context to another within a culture. In the past century, health care has made great strides toward becoming a stigma-free context for patients. Although not eliminated, discrimination by health care workers against homosexual, obese, or mentally ill patients is not as common as it once was. Yet perceptions of stigma persist even within the health care field. For instance, a 2002 study found that only 22% of medical students with depression sought help, and 30% cited the stigma associated with help-seeking as a barrier.[1]

The tenets of patient-centered care require that all patients be treated with respect, both because human dignity demands it and because effective treatment is compromised when stigmatized patients are unwilling to trust their providers.[2–4] The research literature provides ample evidence that many stigmatized patients would rather suffer from mental illness, incontinence, HIV, and multiple other problems rather than disclose them to a health care worker.[5–7] A cultural shift toward more openness about physical and mental illness is facilitating care in advanced nations. Yet stigmatizing attitudes are widespread in some developing nations and even among a minority of dental providers in the United States. For instance, when dental and dental hygiene students were asked about obese patients, 17% said that it was difficult to feel empathy for them and 14% were uncomfortable examining them.[8] Larger proportions of these students had negative attitudes about obese patients (eg, perceiving them as lazy and lacking willpower) and felt uncomfortable discussing dietary habits and appetite-suppressant use.

For several reasons, providers of dental care should work to make every patient relationship free of stigma. First, all health care providers have a professional obligation to treat all patients with dignity and respect, and this professionalism requires that the provider minimize or eliminate negative personal attitudes toward patient characteristics or behaviors.[9–11] Second, many stigmatized characteristics or behaviors (such as HIV or eating disorders) are a cause or consequence of poor oral health. Therefore, oral health workers must be prepared to address them. Third, even stigmatized conditions that have no obvious connection to oral health may affect oral health. For instance, major depressive disorder is often associated with rampant dental caries, and medication used to treat it can magnify associated xerostomia.[12] Finally, the type of communication advocated in this manual fosters patient disclosure of sensitive personal information, so providers should be prepared to respond to disclosures of stigmatized conditions. Research indicates that both patient-centered communication and the length of time spent with a patient are associated with increases in patient trust.[13] Furthermore, patients who perceive providers as simultaneously trustworthy, competent, and objective may seek help from providers rather than family and friends, who may be too judgmental or emotionally invested.

Ultimately, stigmatized conditions affect oral health, and oral health problems often cannot be treated effectively until more pressing non–oral health problems are dealt with. Chapter 3 offered brief suggestions for communicating with patients stigmatized with eating disorders and HIV/AIDS. This chapter first offers suggestions for preparing to treat patients with stigmatized conditions. Then it explores treating smokers, because smoking now carries a stigma and communication with smoking patients can serve as a template for communicating about a variety of stigmatized conditions. The subsequent section explores the stigma of substance use disorder. The chapter concludes with a discussion about treating patients who may be victims of intimate partner violence.

Communication Strategies for Addressing Stigma

Overcoming barriers to treatment

Researchers have published many studies on stigmatized patients' perceptions of health care and the reasons they do not access services.[14,15] A number of studies also examined health care providers' perceptions of specific stigmatized conditions and their reluctance to treat patients with specific conditions.[16–18] Little research, however, explores the reluctance of providers to address or treat stigmatized conditions as a general phenomenon. The research that comes closest to discussing general barriers to addressing and treating stigmatized conditions is the literature on the inverse care law.[19,20] As originally articulated by Hart[19] in 1971, the **inverse care law** holds that "The availability of good medical care tends to vary inversely with the need for it in the population served." Although the law initially explained the economic barriers that denied health care to those more likely to need it (eg, the poor), the fact that financial vulnerability is itself a stigma in developed nations indicates that the law can be applied to other forms of stigma. In short, those with health-related stigmatized conditions (eg, smoking, addiction, or intimate partner violence) may simultaneously have greater need of treatment and be less likely to receive it.

In 2005, Fiscella and Shin[21] elaborated the inverse care law to include its effects on specific stigmatized populations: the homeless, those with chronic illness or disability, the mentally ill and substance dependent, and those with HIV/AIDS, among others. Their solutions focused on large-scale political and economic changes, but they also acknowledged the role of patient-provider communication[21]: "Care must be respectful and culturally competent, including the provision of translation/interpretation services. Patients should be involved personally in the management of their conditions and politically in the governance of their health services."

A 2011 study, however, found that dental students' attitudes toward underserved populations declined across the 4 years of their schooling, suggesting that efforts to enhance attitudes might be warranted.[22] Although many barriers to treatment relate to the inability or unwillingness of stigmatized patients to seek care, other barriers relate to the inability or unwillingness of providers to address and treat stigmatized conditions, even when they are treating stigmatized patients (Box 12-1).

Box 12-1	Barriers to addressing and treating stigmatized conditions

Lack of preparation
- *Barrier:* When the patient discloses or the provider discovers a stigmatized condition, the provider does not know how to respond.
- *Consequence:* The provider ignores the stigmatized condition or responds inappropriately.

Embarrassment
- *Barrier:* The provider is embarrassed or assumes that the patient is embarrassed.
- *Consequence:* The provider ignores the stigmatized condition to avoid (further) embarrassment.

Concern about offending
- *Barrier:* The provider assumes that the patient is unaware of, or is in denial about, the stigmatized condition.
- *Consequence:* The provider assumes that the patient will respond negatively if the stigmatized condition is addressed.

Concern about cultural norms
- *Barrier:* The provider assumes that a stigmatized condition is normative in a patient's cultural background.
- *Consequence:* The provider prioritizes cultural sensitivity over treatment of the stigmatized condition.

First, perhaps the most common provider-related barrier to addressing and treating stigmatized conditions is a lack of preparation on the provider's part. Oral health professionals may not lead sheltered lives, but many of them share similar demographic backgrounds, and their professional status suggests that they share a similar (comfortable) financial status.[23,24] The conditions of some patients may seem unusual, particularly if the patient is new to the practice or different in important respects from other patients treated in the practice. Because such conditions are unexpected, the provider often has no response prepared and therefore simply ignores the situation or responds by saying or doing something inappropriate. Therefore, the provider should prepare for common stigmatized conditions (such as the ones presented in this chapter) and have a ready response for unexpected stigmatized conditions.

Second, disclosure of sensitive conditions can be embarrassing for the patient, the provider, or both. For instance, erectile dysfunction was of little concern to dental providers until the introduction of sildenafil (Viagra, Pfizer) in 1998. Afterward, the condition routinely was implied any time a patient disclosed the medication on the dental health history form. Some patients and providers are embarrassed by the disclosure while others are not, and the sex of the patient and provider may influence any embarrassment felt. A provider who is embarrassed or assumes that a patient is embarrassed by a patient's condition may simply ignore the condition and move on. In some cases, like bulimia, the condition is directly relevant to care. In other cases, such as erectile dysfunction, the condition's relevance to care may seem minimal. Yet if a patient lists Viagra on the health history form and has cardiac health issues or is undergoing oral surgery with sedation, knowledge of whether the erectile dysfunction medication has been taken within the last 36 hours might be important information. The provider should overcome embarrassment about a patient's medical conditions and should never assume that the patient is embarrassed simply because the provider is.

Third, a provider sometimes ignores a patient's conditions because of concerns about offending the patient. This barrier stems from a motive common to several of these barriers: the desire to preserve a good working relationship with the patient. That goal is worthwhile, but the provider must weigh it against a stigmatized condition's relevance to oral health and the potential problems it could cause. Often the provider assumes that the patient will respond negatively if the provider addresses a stigmatized condition revealed or suggested by an examination. This assumption generally presumes that the patient is unaware of the condition, is in denial about it, or wishes to keep it concealed. The provider should never assume that the patient will react negatively if a stigmatized condition is addressed.

Fourth, the provider may avoid addressing a stigmatized condition because he or she assumes that it may be normative and acceptable in the patient's culture. Again, the provider is protecting the patient-provider relationship from possible disruption, but prioritizing relational harmony is acceptable only if the condition is irrelevant to oral health. For instance, khat chewing is associated with compromised periodontal status and increased incidence of oral cancer.[25,26] However, chewing khat is part of the male culture in Yemen and parts of Saudi Arabia. Rather than risk cultural offense, the provider may simply ignore the unhealthy behavior or even the consequences of it. Instead, the provider should discuss unhealthy behaviors in a way that does not disparage the culture of which the behavior is a part.

When to address stigmatized conditions

The previous discussion of provider-related barriers to addressing and treating stigmatized conditions can be summarized in this way: The provider must be prepared for sensitive disclosures and must not assume that a patient is unwilling to discuss a problem. Yet the provider who is prepared and willing to discuss stigmatized conditions should address those conditions at the right time and in the right way.

Although no universal communication rules dictate when and how the provider should address sensitive conditions, we can offer some guidelines. By way of preparation, the provider should have an array of resources and referral options ready for an array of stigmatized conditions. Practically speaking, this means maintaining a supply of brochures explaining specific conditions such as smoking, addiction, eating disorders, and so on. It also means maintaining a file of specialists for consultation and referrals. The dental provider is not expected to treat aspects of a stigmatized condition that are out of his or her area of expertise, but the provider is expected to be part of a health care team that facilitates the patient's return to health. Often the dental provider is in a prime position to facilitate and coordinate care among the various members of the health care team.

When resources and referrals are available, the provider is more prepared to address stigmatized conditions. Deciding when to address them requires some sensitivity and monitoring of the patient's responses. The provider must first know or suspect, based on observation or clinical examination, that a patient has a stigmatized condition or engages in a stigmatized behavior. Such knowledge or suspicion may come about simply by observing the patient. In the close proximity of a dental operatory, a smoker can often be identified by the smell of his or her clothing or the cigarette pack in a shirt pocket. The patient may reveal or imply stigmatized conditions during the health history. Both verbal and nonverbal responses to health history questions can indicate the presence of a condition. Alternatively, clinical evidence may indicate a condition, such as when eroded enamel and swollen parotid salivary glands suggest bulimia.

The provider should usually address stigmatized conditions during the treatment planning phase of the appointment rather than addressing them as soon as they are discovered. Waiting has the advantage of allowing the provider to gather more evidence for the severity of the condition, prioritize treatment relative to other oral health conditions, assess how the patient might respond, and prepare what to say.

In two cases, however, the provider should probably address a stigmatized condition as soon as it becomes apparent. First, if the condition is obvious and cannot be treated casually until the treatment planning phase, the provider should address it immediately. For instance, a patient who is intoxicated or high or a patient who has significant wounds should be asked about the problems.

Second, if the patient seems eager to discuss the stigmatized condition, the provider should not delay. The patient may be more willing to discuss a problem at one time than at another time. Postponing the discussion risks the possibility that the patient may retreat into reticence. Postponement also may lead the patient to believe that the provider is judgmental or uninterested.

The patient may verbalize a readiness to discuss a stigmatized condition, but often the patient does not, challenging the provider to select the time when the patient will be most responsive to a treatment message. In the early 1980s, Prochaska and DiClemente[27,28] began publishing their research into the way smokers successfully quit smoking. Integrating evidence-based concepts from several theoretical models, they proposed the transtheoretical model of behavioral change that proved valid in explaining many types of habitual and compulsive behaviors. The elaborated model involves many more components than can be presented here, but the five stages of change provide a useful framework for determining a patient's readiness to accept treatment (Box 12-2).[29]

Box 12-2	Transtheoretical model's stages of behavioral change*

1. **Precontemplation:** Patient not considering changing within the next 6 months.
2. **Contemplation:** Patient seriously thinking about changing within the next 6 months.
3. **Preparation:** Patient is seriously thinking about changing within the next month.
4. **Action:** Patient has initiated a behavioral change within the past 6 months.
5. **Maintenance:** Patient changed a behavior more than 6 months ago.

*Reprinted from Prochaska et al[29] with permission.

The provider's role is to accurately identify the patient's readiness to change and then facilitate movement toward the next stage. Although conceptually distinct, the transtheoretical model complements the motivational interviewing approach, and motivational interviewing has proven effective in facilitating movement through the stages.[30,31] Both motivational interviewing and the transtheoretical model share the underlying assumption that encouraging behavioral change in a patient who is not ready to change not only is fruitless but also can undermine subsequent attempts to facilitate change. That caveat, however, does not justify ignoring problems. Rather, the patient should be presented with evidentiary findings and a professional prognosis even if he or she is in the earliest precontemplation stage.

If the provider presents information objectively and without judgment, the patient will often respond neutrally or positively, in which case the provider can encourage treatment or at least the contemplation of treatment. The provider should not pressure the patient to change, and even the contemplation of changing should be framed as progress: "I'm going to give you a brochure and ask you to think about it before your next appointment." Refraining from high-pressure tactics can demonstrate to the patient that the provider is trustworthy and increases the possibility that the patient will be receptive to treatment later.

How to address stigmatized conditions

Whether the provider addresses a stigmatized condition when it is first revealed or waits until treatment planning, some general strategies can facilitate the discussion (Box 12-3). First, the provider should react casually to the patient's disclosure of a condition or the discovery of the condition by observation or examination. Because the provider and patient may not share the same sociocultural background, the provider should not assume that a condition that he or she considers stigmatized is perceived that way by the patient. In such cases, a strong reaction (eg, "You did what?!") might make the patient feel self-conscious or guilty and therefore less forthcoming in responding to health history questions. Instead, the provider should acknowledge the response with a nod or other backchannel and then proceed to the next question. Alternatively, the provider might casually ask for more information: "You were drinking before the appointment? How often do you drink alcohol in the morning?"

| Box 12-3 | General strategies for addressing stigma |

React casually to disclosure or discovery
- Say nothing or provide a routine backchannel.
- Ask for more information.

Allow a nondisclosure option
- Lack of response communicates a message.
- Tactfully try to determine if the nondisclosure was intentional.

Offer the opportunity to change a response
- Do not reprimand the patient.
- Casually ask about the change.

List relevant nonverbal responses
- Notice and document nonverbal signs of deception or nervousness when specific questions are asked.

Express concern about symptoms
- Never ignore unhealthy conditions or behavior.
- Frame comments as concern about the patient's health or well-being.

Refer the patient immediately
- State the limits of your training.
- Provide the name of a specialist or facility.
- Offer to coordinate care.

Second, with health history forms and interviews, the provider should allow the patient the option not to respond. The provider should confirm that the omission was not an oversight and then move on: "Did you intend to leave the drug question blank?" A patient may find health history questions intrusive, particularly if he or she does not perceive a question's connection to oral health. Agencies and corporations frequently ask questions seemingly unrelated to their missions, so the patient's small act of rebellion is understandable. The provider should briefly state how the question relates to oral health care but should not force an answer: "We ask about drug use because it can affect blood pressure, which in turn affects your oral health and your response to the treatment you'll receive today. We'll leave the response blank in case you decide you want to answer it later."

Nonresponse communicates a message about the patient's relationship to the question's topic. And a patient may have good reasons for not responding. For instance, the patient may fear criminal prosecution for illegal drug use. By explaining the rationale for the question and by not forcing a response, the provider suggests that he or she can be trusted and does not risk a false response that the patient may never correct.

Third, the provider should allow the patient to change responses. One study found that 32% of patients provide inaccurate or incomplete data on health history forms used in dentistry.[32] If the patient is encouraged to correct inaccuracies, the validity of these forms should be enhanced. A patient may change responses for a variety of reasons:

- Circumstances and conditions may have changed since the previous appointment.
- The patient may have remembered the name of a previously forgotten drug, health condition, or procedure.
- The patient may gain a better understanding of the rationale for a question and therefore decide to answer truthfully.
- The patient who feels ashamed or guilty may decide that a provider can be trusted and therefore decide to change a response.

Whatever the patient's reasons, the provider should never reprimand a patient for changing a response. A reprimand incentivizes a patient to let any other incorrect responses remain incorrect. For the patient who conceals a stigmatized condition because of fear of the responses of others, a negative reaction will only reinforce that fear. At most, the provider should casually ask about the change: "I see that you indicate you have hepatitis C. Can you tell me about that diagnosis?"

 Question of ethics: When patients believe health care providers are acting dishonestly, they have the right to change providers. Yet surveys show that a lot of patients are dishonest when answering health history questions. Should providers have the right to fire patients who are withholding information or providing false responses?

Fourth, the provider should note and document any nonverbal responses that seem unusual. If a given question elicits signs of nervousness or deception cues, the provider may want to flag the question so it can be monitored or explored in future visits. As with a nonresponse, an unusual response may carry information. If the provider does not wish to detail the behavior (eg, "Patient avoids eye contact."), then perhaps some form of shorthand can remind the provider to revisit the question. If the unusual response—such as avoidance of eye contact or nervous laughter—persists, the provider may want to ask the patient about it: "I notice the nervous laughter when I ask about alcohol or drug use. Is there anything I should know?"

Fifth, the provider should express concern about any observations or symptoms. The provider should never simply ignore unhealthy conditions or behaviors, because they can persist for years if the patient either believes they are not harmful or believes nobody notices or cares. This is the case for substance use disorders, compulsive disorders, bulimia, anorexia, intimate partner violence, and other problems. Hearing that something is wrong from a medical professional, who serves as an objective third party, can help the patient move from the precontemplation and contemplation stages of behavioral change toward the preparation and action stages.

The existence of an outside opinion that the patient has a problem reduces the patient's ability to rationalize or deny the problem, and acknowledging the problem is often the first step toward treating it. The provider should avoid dry and clinical verbiage but should present observations and implications with concern: "It is not my job to rat you out to your parents, but I see lots of discoloration on your teeth consistent with cigarette smoking. It concerns me because the next symptoms I often see are plaque and tartar buildup and gum disease, followed by an increased risk for oral cancer. I don't want that to happen to you, so can we discuss smoking-cessation treatment?"

Sixth, when the patient indicates a willingness to discuss a stigmatized condition, the provider should engage the patient in a discussion about referral to the appropriate specialist for needs beyond the scope of the dental provider. The dental provider should discuss aspects of the condition that relate to oral health and propose treatment to address oral health problems, but the provider should also emphasize that the condition requires care coordinated among various trained professionals.

If the provider is prepared, he or she will have the name and contact information of a specialist at hand. If the condition is one the provider has not prepared for, a quick call to a colleague can usually generate a satisfactory referral. The provider should then give the specialist's contact information to the patient, along with any literature on specialized treatment. While the patient is still in the office, the provider should offer to coordinate care by phoning the specialist to make an appointment. Because treatment can seem less urgent after a patient leaves the office, setting up the next step can make the difference between help-seeking and a continuation of the problem: "I'll discuss your treatment options for restoring your teeth and gums, but the methamphetamine addiction requires treatment by substance abuse professionals. I'm going to give you the name of a good treatment professional. If you don't object, I'd like to call her now to set up an appointment."

Patients Who Smoke

Identifying smokers

In developed nations, the changes in social attitudes toward cigarette smoking illustrate perfectly how stigma varies over time. In 1965, 42.4% of US adults smoked.[33] Smoking was very common, even among health care workers, so little stigma was attached to it at the societal level. By 2013, the smoking rate among adults had fallen by more than half, to 17.8%.[34] The reduction corresponds to decades of public health efforts to raise awareness about the health risks of smoking and to legislate cleaner indoor air by banning smoking in most public buildings.[35]

A byproduct of these educational efforts was the psychologic and physical marginalization of smokers from the social mainstream. Today, smokers usually must withdraw from others to satisfy a nicotine craving outdoors, and increasingly they are even pushed away from the doors of buildings. As a result, smoking has acquired a stigma among the mainstream, although it is not as stigmatized among some subpopulations. Dental providers should understand the stigmatized status of smoking and communicate with smoking patients in a way that fosters openness about the habit and encourages help-seeking to stop it.

The variations in smoking rates among groups can be used by dental professionals to identify patients at higher risk for smoking. For instance, 20.1% of adults aged 25 to 44 years smoke, but only 8.8% of adults older than 64 years do.[34] In addition, 26.1% of Native Americans smoke, but only 12.1% of Hispanics and 9.6% of Asians smoke. At 41.4%, adults with a general education development (GED) certificate are seven times more likely to smoke than are those with a graduate degree (5.6%). Poverty is also associated with an increased risk of smoking, and smoking is more prevalent in some regions than in others. Those in the Midwest (20.5%) and South (19.2%) are more likely to smoke than those in the Northeast (16.9%) or West (13.6%).

At the relational level, providers can identify smoking in the three ways mentioned previously: health history responses, observation, and clinical examination. Patients who indicate tobacco use on their health history form are obvious candidates for smoking-cessation treatments. Yet some patients may provide false information or not respond for various reasons. A good patient-provider relationship may increase the likelihood of such false or incomplete responses because the patient may want to avoid disappointing the provider. Alternatively, stigma may lead patients who smoke to not consider themselves smokers. After all, *smoker* has no agreed-on definition, so patients whose cigarette consumption falls under a self-defined threshold may not consider themselves smokers. Therefore, providers might consider asking, "How often do you smoke tobacco?" rather than asking, "Are you a smoker?" or even, "Do you smoke?" Patients also may fear the consequences of self-identifying as a smoker. An adult receiving the nonsmoker's discount on health insurance and the adolescent who smokes illegally have strong incentives not to self-identify as a smoker.[36–38]

Given these reasons for misrepresentation or omission on health history forms and in interview responses, the provider should pay particular attention to nonverbal behaviors when the topic of smoking is mentioned. Laughter, averted gaze, overextended eye contact, vocal uncertainty or overconfidence, and other behaviors that do not conform to a patient's usual communication style may indicate that further exploration of the topic is necessary. Likewise, cigarette packs or lighters in pockets or purses, nicotine stains on hands, and the odor of smoke on clothing can indicate that the patient smokes. Finally, the indicators of smoking that can be identified during clinical examination should be well known to all dental providers.

Addressing smoking

A growing body of evidence shows the efficacy of smoking-cessation programs offered through dental practices.[39] Dental professionals, however, usually do not discuss smoking with their patients who smoke. One reason is that they are not—and do not feel—adequately trained to address tobacco cessation with their patients.[40,41] In fact, dental professionals may be less willing to address smoking than their patients are. A 2004 British study found that 90% of dental team members asked about smoking, but only 30% indicated active involvement in patients' attempts to stop smoking.[42] A 2005 study found that dental hygiene faculty were only moderately confident (3.2 on a 1 to 5 scale) in their ability to discuss tobacco, although 61% of patients who smoke were in the contemplation, preparation, or action stages of change.[43] In other words, providers seem more reluctant than patients are to address this problem that is potentially devastating to oral health. Further, the recent development and usage of the e-cigarette as both a cessation aid and a substitute for actual cigarettes in areas where they are currently banned has been the subject of new and ongoing research regarding safety and legal issues surrounding their use. Providers should not miss an opportunity to provide an informed opinion.

Providers who seek out smoking-cessation training have an advantage over those who lack such skills, but any provider should feel equipped to openly discuss smoking with a patient, because the framework does not vary from the diagnosis-prognosis-treatment discussions that guide any other treatment planning conversation. When the "diagnosis" of smoking is presented by the dentist, the interaction will require extra sensitivity only if the patient is concealing the smoking habit. If the provider strongly suspects smoking in a patient who denies it, the provider should avoid direct confrontation or accusation, which may damage subsequent opportunities to address the issue. Instead, the provider should present the evidence and ask whether the patient would like to review smoking-cessation options: "I see discoloration on your tongue and the enamel of your teeth that suggests tobacco use. May I talk to you about our programs to help patients quit using tobacco?"

This phrasing avoids an accusation of lying and avoids labeling the patient a smoker. The patient in the precontemplation stage can simply decline, whereas the patient in the contemplation stage or a more advanced stage can assent without directly admitting to any deception.

If a patient is uninterested in discussing smoking cessation, the provider has little choice but to drop the subject until the next appointment, when it should be raised again, as the patient may move from one stage to another between appointments. If the patient is willing to discuss tobacco cessation, the provider should first provide a brief overview of the prognosis with and without treatment. The provider should not overwhelm the patient with dramatic stories and visual aids that depict the horror of oral and pharyngeal cancers. Instead, in a few brief phrases, the provider should educate the patient on the oral health risks associated with smoking, presenting statistics for those who can understand them and using simpler terminology for those who cannot. The information should be tailored to the motivating concerns of the given patient—namely, pain, cost, esthetics, and function. The provider should also present the more optimistic prognosis associated with cessation of tobacco use.

The presentation of treatment options depends on the provider's training in addition to the patient's preferences. A number of treatment approaches have proven effective in the dental setting, and we encourage providers to pursue training in one or more of them.[35,44,45] Increasingly, dental providers rely on pharmaceutical treatments in smoking-cessation efforts. Pharmaceutical treatments, however, are most effective when they are combined with behavioral therapy, so providers should at least practice rudimentary motivational interviewing techniques.[46]

Even a provider who has no training in smoking cessation can facilitate treatment by referring the patient to outside programs and following up on the patient's progress. Evidence-based treatment resources are available from the American Dental Association and the National Institutes of Health's National Cancer Institute (for a list of resources, see For More Information at the end of the chapter.) When providers follow up on patients' progress, such referrals constitute a team-based approach that results in a 10% to 15% annual cessation rate.[47,48] A smoking patient will know the challenges, but the provider should inform the patient that many people require multiple attempts before they can stop permanently. Communicating encouragement and support during a patient's attempts to quit smoking may be the most useful treatment the provider can offer.

Activity 12-1

In public health research, smoking is often addressed as a physical dependency—which it is. However, smoking also has social and psychologic components that can tempt people to light a cigarette even if a physical craving is not present. Find a small group of smokers smoking outside a building and conduct an informal focus group, asking them how they started smoking, why they continue to smoke, and what it would take to get them to stop. Do not argue, but instead simply listen to their answers.

Substance-Abusing Patients

Identifying substance abuse and dependence

Alcohol use is popular in the United States, and the use of other drugs is more acceptable than it once was, but addiction remains stigmatized. For many of the same reasons that smokers may not acknowledge their behavior, individuals with a substance use disorder (abuse or dependence) may deny or conceal a problem. For three reasons, dental professionals should be prepared to identify and address substance use disorders. First, substances of abuse can have indirect and direct oral health consequences. Indirectly, the compromised cognitive functioning that results from substance use often entails inattention to self-care behaviors such as tooth brushing and regular dental visits. A 2011 study of substance-dependent individuals found that most had unsatisfactory oral health and most had not visited a dentist within the past year.[49]

Directly, specific drugs may be associated with specific types of oral health problems. The high incidence of missing teeth and oral disease caused by methamphetamine abuse has earned its own name (**meth mouth**) and itself serves as a marker of abuse.[50–52] Excessive and prolonged alcohol consumption is associated with oral cancer and, in combination with tobacco usage (a frequently seen comorbidity), can exponentially raise the risk for oral cancer as well as have an effect on periodontal disease.[53,54] Cannabis use is associated with increased caries risk, and cannabis smoke is associated with lesions of the oral mucosa.[55] In short, the oral health problems associated with addiction make substance abuse a topic meriting exploration by oral health professionals.

Second, on rare occasions, patients may arrive at their appointment drunk or high. Even if they are not a danger to themselves or others, the effects of mood- or mind-altering drugs on their judgment compromise patients' ability to consent to treatment. Intoxication also poses real and significant dangers relating to clinical interactions between common dental anesthetics and substances of abuse such as methamphetamine, cocaine, and ecstasy.[56] Such interactions may induce hypertensive episodes.

Third, it is a near certainty that a portion of the patients dental providers treat will have a substance use disorder. This is a sizable population, with lifetime prevalence of alcohol abuse at 17.8% and of alcohol dependence at 12.5%.[57] The lifetime prevalence of other drug abuse is 7.7% and of other drug dependence is 2.6%.[58] Those with substance use disorders are more likely to be white or Native American, male, younger, and unmarried. Dentists, moreover, may be at risk for substance use disorders, complicating their attempts to identify it in their patients.[59–62] The dental team should therefore work together to share knowledge and observations and to check suspicions of drug or alcohol abuse.

Alcohol and drug abuse can be identified by direct questioning. A provider who has never had a substance use problem may be surprised at the willingness of those who have struggled with addiction—particularly those in addiction recovery—to acknowledge their current or past dependence. If a patient is uncertain and seems willing to discuss his or her substance use, a simple alcoholism screen can help identify a problem to be addressed. The CAGE questionnaire is a four-question screening instrument designed to be administered by health care workers in clinical contexts.[63] **CAGE** is an acronym designed to prompt each of the four questions (Box 12-4). A patient who responds affirmatively to two of the questions likely has a problem with addiction. The dental provider can ask the questions chairside and adapt the instrument to screen for other drugs of abuse.

Box 12-4	CAGE questionnaire*

1. **Cutting down:** Have you ever felt you should cut down on your drinking?
2. **Annoyance:** Have people annoyed you by criticizing your drinking?
3. **Guilty feelings:** Have you ever felt bad or guilty about your drinking?
4. **Eye-openers:** Have you ever had a drink first thing in the morning to steady your nerves or to get rid of a hangover?

Scoring: Two or more "yes" answers suggests a clinically significant substance use problem.

*Reprinted from Ewing[63] with permission.

For a patient who is more reticent to discuss a suspected substance abuse problem, alcohol and drug abuse also can be identified by observation. Clusters of observable symptoms of dependence can be specific to particular drugs. Symptoms of a patient's substance use problem that are more general and observable are listed in Box 12-5.[64]

Box 12-5	Common observable signs of alcohol or drug abuse*

- Tremor, perspiring, tachycardia
- Track marks/injection sites
- Slurred, rapid speech
- Frequent falls, unexplained bruises, or fractures
- Dilated or pinpoint pupils
- Prescription drug–seeking behavior
- Persistent cough
- Frequent hospitalizations
- Skin lesions on face, arms, and legs
- Nonresponsiveness to treatment for diabetes, elevated blood pressure, or ulcers
- Unexplained weight loss
- Marked change in habits or friends
- Inflamed, eroded nasal septum
- Suicide talk/attempt or depression

*Reprinted from Seckman[64] with permission.

Addressing substance abuse and dependence

As with smoking, dental patients often seem more accepting of screening and treatment for addiction than dental professionals do. A 2006 study found that more than 75% of dental patients supported the idea of dental providers screening for alcohol problems and offering advice.[65] Yet providers seem to avoid addressing abuse and dependence even though they are in a position to facilitate treatment for both addiction and the oral health problems associated with it.

We strongly recommend that the provider openly address substance use with any patient suspected of abuse or dependence. A patient with a history of excessive drug or alcohol use has likely been confronted about the issue and may be more forthcoming than the dental professional expects. If the patient is not intoxicated, the discussion can wait until treatment planning, but the issue should be raised. Otherwise, the provider might simply treat the symptoms (oral health damage) without treating the underlying cause (addiction).

To minimize the stigma felt by a patient who may be abusing or dependent on substances, the provider should emphasize his or her role as a medical professional. The patient may be suspicious of questions regarding substance use, particularly if the substances used are illegal. If so, the provider should reassure the patient of confidentiality and clarify the connection between drug use and oral health and treatment: "We need accurate responses to these drug and alcohol questions in order to evaluate your risk for oral health problems and the risk of any negative interactions between our treatment and other substances you may be consuming, whether prescribed, over-the-counter, or recreational. I assure you that anything you disclose is confidential, since I'm legally bound to protect your privacy." The provider should develop the habit of referring to *recreational drugs* rather than *illicit* or *illegal drugs*, terms that only emphasize the stigma and risk of disclosure.

Patients who are dependent on prescription drugs may exhibit drug-seeking behavior.[66,67] Some drug-seeking patients may target dental practices, particularly smaller ones, believing such practices to be less vigilant about monitoring prescriptions. We know an older dentist in solo practice in a resort area who routinely encounters patients claiming to be visiting town, to be in grave pain, to have lost their prescription painkillers, or all of the preceding. Such claims of dire need should alert providers that they may be dealing with an addict. Withholding of opiates that are not medically necessary is in the best interest of addicted patients, but so is addressing the underlying addiction and urging treatment.

The National Institute on Drug Abuse has established the NIDAMED website (http://www.drugabuse.gov/nidamed-medical-health-professionals) to help health care providers screen and refer patients. If a patient acknowledges a problem, the provider should frame it as a health problem rather than a failure of willpower. As a health problem, it can be diagnosed and treated, so the provider should be prepared to provide information and a referral to treatment. The provider should keep addiction and treatment brochures on hand and be prepared to provide contact information for local counselors and treatment facilities. Because alcoholics and addicts seem to waver rapidly among the precontemplation, contemplation, and preparation stages, it is always better to connect the patient to treatment while he or she is in the chair. If possible, the dental provider should telephone a treatment counselor while the patient is in the office and schedule a meeting.

In keeping with the team approach, the provider should address the oral health treatment needs of the patient while other specialists are addressing the addiction treatment needs. Those oral health needs may be significant, but their significance may also serve as motivation for dental and addiction treatment. For instance, a 2010 study of methamphetamine users found that 28.6% were concerned about their dental appearance, suggesting that esthetic restoration could be a motivator for addiction treatment.[51]

The alcoholic or addict—even in early recovery—can be overwhelmed by his or her problems and can be prone to bouts of despair. Therefore, the provider should segment treatment into steps the patient can understand, accomplish, and afford. The provider also should remain upbeat about the patient's prospects for addiction recovery and restoration of oral health. Enthusiasm can be difficult to maintain for the provider, and even more so for the patient when relapse threatens or materializes. At such times, the support of a medical professional can buoy the patient through rough seas.

Activity 12-2

Conduct an Internet search for "addiction recovery podcast" and listen to a couple of addicts or alcoholics discuss their experience with addiction and tell how they got sober. Pay particular attention to two turning points: the moment they realized they had a problem and the moment they sought help. Consider how you, as a health care provider, could help patients realize that they need help and could help patients receive that help.

Patients Suffering Intimate Partner Violence

Identifying intimate partner violence

The US Department of Justice[68] takes a broad view of **domestic violence**, defining it to include violence between family members. By contrast, **intimate partner violence (IPV)** is a subset of domestic violence cases that involves violence between intimates—generally romantic, domestic, or marital partners. Child abuse is a form of domestic violence but not intimate partner violence. Although laws vary, every state has statutes identifying those required to report suspected child abuse.[69] Providers should familiarize themselves with state laws regarding IPV or its consequences, because the intimate partner relationship is not viewed as dependent but instead as consenting. Use of a dangerous weapon, commission of a crime, or suspicion of violence are three common determinants of mandatory reporting of violence in such relationships, and the applicable determinants differ by state. In general, as health care providers, dental professionals are mandatory reporters and legally (and morally) required to report suspected child abuse to the appropriate authorities. Although not irrelevant, communication strategies in such cases are far less important than securing the safety of the child. Identifying and addressing intimate partner violence, on the other hand, requires communication skills because victims may be ambivalent about disclosing the cause of their wounds or unwilling to leave the relationship.

According to the American Dental Association's Code of Professional Conduct, "Dentists shall be obliged to become familiar with the signs of abuse and neglect and to report suspected cases to the proper authorities, consistent with state laws."[9] Research, however, suggests that a substantial number of dental students receive no training in identifying and communicating with patients who are victims of IPV.[70] Yet lack of training is only one barrier to recognizing IPV, a situation that can cause substantial damage to the mouth and teeth. One survey found that 87% of dentists never screened for IPV.[71] Even when they identified patients as victims, dentists responded only minimally to help. In addition to lack of training (68%), they cited the presence of a partner or child (77%), concern about offending the victimized patient (66%), and their own embarrassment (51%) as barriers to intervening. Another study found a general belief among dentists and dental hygienists that they were not responsible for addressing family violence.[72,73]

All of these barriers should be overcome, as the type of physical damage associated with IPV may bring the victim directly to the dental office. Furthermore, IPV can be framed as a dental problem; unless the cause of the oral damage is addressed, the victim's oral health will likely deteriorate.

Dental providers can identify possible IPV through observations, clinical assessment, evaluation of risk factors, and screening. The Massachusetts Dental Society compiled an excellent list of observable signs of IPV (Box 12-6).[74] Several of these are signs of trauma for any patient. Others are signs because they indicate changes in behavioral patterns that are easier to identify if the patient and provider have a common history and a strong relationship.

Box 12-6	Common observable signs of intimate partner violence*

- Does the patient appear to be in pain as he or she walks into the operatory or sits in the dental chair?
- Is the patient's movement restricted? A victim who has fractured bones or ribs may have hindered movement.
- Does the patient seem uncomfortable as he or she sits down? This may indicate sexual abuse.
- Is there swelling or bruising around the face?
- Do hands reveal any type of trauma such as burns from cigarettes, lighters, or "glove-like" burns from scalding water?
- When the patient is in the chair, observe his or her head to detect if there is any swelling of the scalp from trauma or fracture. Are there bald spots where hair was traumatically removed or pulled?
- Are there oval-shaped abrasions or lacerations that indicate bite marks?
- Does the patient appear to be overdressed for the current weather? For example, is he or she wearing long sleeves, long pants, and other heavy clothing during hot summer months? This may be an attempt to cover bruises or injuries to the arms and legs.
- Is the patient dirty or disheveled, or does the patient appear malnourished?
- Was there an obvious delay in seeking dental treatment?
- Have you noticed unexplained bruises, lacerations, burns, fractures, a torn frenum, or several injuries in different stages of healing (for example, bruises that are black and blue or yellow)?
- Does the victim appear embarrassed, vague, anxious, or depressed?
- Is the victim's partner reluctant to leave her or him alone during the interview, domineering, or answering all questions for the patient?
- Have you noticed changes in the patient's routine (for example, a patient who used to come in for regular checkups and who now suddenly stops or who frequently comes late for appointments)?

*Reprinted from the Massachusetts Dental Society Standing Committee to Prevent Abuse and Neglect[74] with permission.

From a clinical standpoint, dental professionals should be adept at identifying facial trauma resulting from violence. In an emergency department setting, research found that 94.4% of domestic violence victims had head, neck, and face injuries.[75] Identifying IPV is facilitated by its prevalence: About 20% of dental students have personal experience with IPV.[70]

The identification of IPV is also facilitated by the risk factors for IPV, which differ from risk factors for other types of injuries. For instance, sports injuries and fistfights between strangers or acquaintances are far more common among young males. Yet for IPV, the stereotype of the adult female victimized by a male partner is grounded in some truth. Females are six times more likely than males to be victims of IPV.[76] Males are also victimized by female partners, however, and those in same-sex relationships may be victimized at a higher rate than those in heterosexual relationships, so dental professionals should, as always, beware of stereotypes.[77]

Although the rate of IPV has been declining, approximately 4.2 of 1,000 women are the victims of nonfatal IPV every year.[76] The rate, however, is much higher for women aged 20 to 24 years (11.3 per 1,000), women aged 25 to 34 years (8.1 per 1,000), and separated women (40.7 per 1,000). IPV also has a negative correlation with household income. Some research has found an association between (nonwhite) ethnicity and

IPV victimization, but a 2003 study found that the association did not remain when data were controlled for income.[78]

Screening instruments for IPV have been developed and validated for use in clinical settings, including the Woman Abuse Screening Tool, the Abuse Risk Inventory, and the Composite Abuse Scale.[79–81] In 2006, Halpern and Dodson[82] validated a three-item predictive model for identifying IPV victims in a dental setting. Their model consisted of younger, nonwhite ethnicity, and one or more "yes" answers to the three-question Partner Violence Screen[83]:

1. Have you ever been hit, kicked, or punched in a relationship?
2. Have you ever felt unsafe in a relationship?
3. Do you feel safe now?

Perhaps because they anticipate defensiveness, because they feel embarrassed, or because a partner or child is present, nearly half of dentists who suspect abuse never express any concern.[71] Patients, however, express a strong preference for screening for physical abuse in medical settings.[84] A dental professional who suspects abuse should screen for IPV. When signs of abuse are acknowledged, the patient feels validated.[85] However, the patient may be reluctant to disclose abuse in the presence of the abuser or other family members, so the provider should ask family members to leave the operatory: "We need the presence of just the staff and the patient, so I'm going to ask you to wait in the reception area. I'll let you know when we are through." If the provider senses reluctance on the part of the family members or volatility on the part of the suspected abuser, it may be safer to say, "I need to take some x-rays now, and we will return momentarily." This is a time when everyone should know that only the patient and the provider are allowed in the area of treatment.

An abuse victim may also disclose more when fewer staff are present, so staff should be restricted to one or two during the IPV screen. If possible, the person screening should be the same sex as the patient. The provider can also enhance the perception that the office is a safe place to disclose abuse by hanging posters in the operatory or in the bathrooms that ask patients to telephone an abuse resource line or notify the hygienist or dentist if they have been bullied or abused.[86]

Activity 12-3

To those who have never been in a relationship characterized by violence, IPV can be very difficult to understand. To enhance your understanding of why people remain in relationships that are physically or emotionally unhealthy, conduct an online search for "domestic violence stories" and read several of the linked narratives. Afterward, summarize similarities in the stories. Were the victims similar in (prerelationship) background? How did the violence begin and escalate? What reasons were given for remaining in the relationship? How did they finally end the relationship, if they did end it?

Addressing intimate partner violence

Unless he or she has specialized training, a dental provider has neither the appropriate background to treat an IPV victim's psychologic needs nor the resources to secure a victim's safety. Attempting to do so could even be dangerous to the staff or make the victim's situation worse. Instead, the provider's role should be limited to identifying the victim, proposing and providing dental treatment, and referring the patient to specialists who can help. The identification and referral process can be carried out in four steps proposed by Gerbert et al[87]: (1) ask, (2) validate, (3) document, and (4) refer.

First, the provider should ask the patient about the suspected abuse. Observation, clinical examination, risk factors, and screening can indicate that a patient is likely the victim of abuse, but the presence of abuse must be made explicit through verbal communication. Asking the patient about suspected abuse may reveal that the provider's suspicions of abuse are mistaken. In some cases, the provider will be correct, but the patient will be unwilling to disclose abuse. In either case, the patient will not be a candidate for immediate referral to an IPV specialist or shelter.

The questions should always be asked in private, with nonjudgmental language and tone. Questions may start out more generally: "How are things at home?" or "Do you feel safe in your home?" Eventually, questions should become specific, while remaining empathetic: "People who have been physically abused often end up in the dental office, and we can help. I'm seeing symptoms of physical abuse (in your behavior, in your mouth, etc), so please tell me, is someone hurting you?" If a language barrier is present, the provider should not ask about IPV through a family member acting as an interpreter.

Second, the provider should validate the experience of abuse. Doing so does not depend on direct disclosure of IPV by the patient. Instead, it is a two-part acknowledgement by the provider that (1) abuse is wrong and (2) the patient has worth. Thus, the provider can say: "Physical violence has no place in a relationship, and no one deserves to be hit." If the patient does not confirm that abuse has taken place, the validating messages nevertheless reinforce the idea that the dental office is a safe place to go for help. Patients who have been victims of IPV report that hearing validation repeated over time finally motivated them to seek help.[88]

Third, the provider should document his or her observations.[89] Only 36% of dentists who suspect abuse ever document it.[71] Yet documentation can be of tremendous legal help when a victim is seeking to end an abusive relationship. Isaac and Enos[90] offer several recommendations for health care workers who are documenting suspected abuse in a patient's chart:

- The provider should take photographs of injuries.
- The provider should indicate the patient's own words, particularly when identifying the perpetrator, through quotation marks or verbal markers such as, "Patient says...."
- The provider should use medical terminology, avoiding legal terms (eg, *alleged* and *perpetrator*), ambiguous words, and abbreviations (eg, *domestic violence* and *IPV*).
- The provider should document details of the patient's demeanor and time since the abuse occurred.

Finally, the provider should refer the patient to a specialist in domestic violence. Laws and resources vary, so the provider should be aware of the availability of assistance in his or her locality. In many ways, this referral is similar to referral for other problems such as smoking or addiction, except that it is perhaps more urgent, given that abuse can escalate if the patient does not immediately seek help. Therefore, the provider should have brochures and contact information on hand for IPV specialists. Perhaps more important, the provider should contact a specialist while the patient is in the office and attempt to schedule a meeting as soon as the patient leaves the office. The provider may have to arrange transportation. Fortunately, most shelters are equipped to handle referrals 24 hours a day. The provider must remember, however, that change must occur on the patient's timetable.

Question of ethics: With the other stigmatized conditions mentioned in this manual (eg, smoking, substance abuse, and eating disorders), the person engaging in the unhealthy behavior is primarily the one who suffers. With IPV, however, children may also be involved, either as witnesses or as fellow victims. If you were treating a patient you strongly suspected was a victim of IPV, would the presence of children in the household influence the likelihood you would address the suspected IPV? If the patient were unwilling to acknowledge the IPV and seek help, would the presence of children influence your response to the patient's refusal to seek help?

Chapter Checklist ☑

Overcoming barriers
❑ Prepare for common stigmatized conditions and have a ready response for unexpected stigmatized conditions.
❑ Overcome embarrassment about a patient's medical conditions.
❑ Never assume that the patient is embarrassed simply because you are embarrassed.
❑ Never assume that the patient will react negatively if you address a stigmatized condition.
❑ Discuss unhealthy behaviors in a way that does not disparage the culture of the patient.

When to address stigmatized conditions
❑ Address conditions at the right time and in the right way.
❑ Keep an array of resources and referral options ready for a wide range of stigmatized conditions.
❑ Maintain a supply of brochures for common conditions and a list of specialists for consultation and referral.
❑ Remain part of the health care team that facilitates a patient's recovery by addressing oral health needs and coordinating care.
❑ In most cases, address stigmatized conditions during the treatment planning phase.
❑ Address stigmatized conditions immediately if the condition is obvious or interferes with scheduled treatment or if the patient is eager to discuss it.
❑ Understand the transtheoretical model's five stages of change: precontemplation, contemplation, preparation, action, and maintenance.
❑ Accurately identify the patient's readiness to change and facilitate movement toward the next stage.
❑ Present evidentiary findings and a professional prognosis, even if the patient is in the precontemplation stage.
❑ Do not pressure the patient to change.
❑ Frame even the contemplation of changing as progress toward improved oral health.

How to address stigmatized conditions
❑ React casually to a patient's disclosures or discovery of stigmatized conditions by observation or examination.
❑ Do not assume that the patient perceives the stigmatized condition the same way you do.
❑ React casually: When a patient discloses a stigmatized condition, respond with a backchannel response and proceed with the next question or respond with a casual request for more information.
❑ Allow nondisclosure: Confirm that the nonresponse was not an oversight.
❑ Allow nondisclosure: State how the question relates to oral health.
❑ Allow nondisclosure: Never force an answer the patient is reluctant to provide.
❑ Allow the patient to change answers: Never reprimand a patient for changing a response.
❑ Allow the patient to change answers: Casually ask about the change.
❑ Record nonverbal responses: Document the nonverbal response and ask the patient about it.

❑ Express concern: Note observations and symptoms with concern.
❑ Express concern: Never ignore unhealthy conditions or behaviors.
❑ Refer: Refer the patient immediately to a specialist.
❑ Refer: Discuss aspects of the condition that relate to oral health.
❑ Refer: Emphasize that the condition requires care coordinated among professionals.
❑ Refer: Keep contact information on hand and give the specialist's contact information to the patient along with information on treatment.
❑ Refer: Offer to telephone the specialist, coordinate care, and make the first appointment.

Smoking patients
❑ Understand that smoking is now stigmatized in the broader culture.
❑ Foster openness about tobacco use and encourage help-seeking behavior.
❑ Identify smoking via health history, observation, or clinical examination.
❑ Realize that a patient may provide false information or nonresponses to questions on tobacco use.
❑ Ask about the frequency of smoking instead of asking whether the patient "is a smoker."
❑ Attend to nonverbal behaviors when the topic of tobacco use is mentioned.
❑ Follow the diagnosis-prognosis-treatment discussion framework when addressing smoking.
❑ Diagnosis: Avoid direct confrontation or accusation when addressing smoking with a patient who denies tobacco use.
❑ Diagnosis: Avoid accusations and labeling by presenting the evidence and asking whether the patient would like to discuss cessation options.
❑ Prognosis: Provide a brief overview of the prognosis with and without smoking-cessation treatment.
❑ Prognosis: Do not overwhelm the patient with dramatic stories or visual aids.
❑ Treatment: Present treatment options tailored to the concerns of the patient (ie, pain, cost, esthetics, and/or function).
❑ Treatment: Emphasize the optimistic outcomes associated with successful treatment.
❑ Treatment: Practice motivational interviewing techniques.
❑ Treatment: Refer the patient to outside programs and follow up on the patient's progress.
❑ Treatment: Inform the patient that multiple attempts may be required before he or she can quit successfully.
❑ Treatment: Communicate encouragement and support during the patient's attempts to quit smoking.

Substance-abusing patients
❑ Work with other members of the dental team to identify or confirm the patient's potential drug or alcohol abuse.
❑ Identify alcohol and drug abuse through the health history, an addiction screening instrument such as the CAGE questionnaire, or observation.
❑ Openly address substance use in the treatment planning discussion, unless the patient is under the influence, in which case it should be addressed immediately.
❑ Emphasize the provider's role as a medical professional.

❑ Reassure the patient of confidentiality.
❑ Clarify the relationship between drug use and oral health.
❑ Refer to *recreational drugs* instead of *illicit* or *illegal drugs*.
❑ Consider a patient's urgent claims of needing painkillers as potential drug-seeking behavior by an addict.
❑ Frame alcohol or drug abuse as a health problem requiring medical treatment.
❑ Provide information and referral by keeping on hand addiction and treatment brochures and contact information for local counselors and treatment facilities.
❑ Address the patient's oral health treatment needs while coordinating care for addiction treatment needs.
❑ Segment oral health treatment into steps the patient can understand, accomplish, and afford while in early recovery.
❑ Remain optimistic about the patient's prospects for addiction recovery and restoration of oral health.

Identifying intimate partner violence

❑ Identify possible IPV through observations, clinical assessment, evaluation of risk factors, and screening.
❑ Be familiar with common observable signs of IPV: pain, discomfort, restricted movement, bruises, etc.
❑ Be able to identify facial trauma resulting from violence.
❑ Avoid stereotyping IPV victims by gender or sexual orientation.
❑ Use IPV screening instruments: the Woman Abuse Screening Tool, the Abuse Risk Inventory, the Composite Abuse Scale, or the Partner Violence Screen.
❑ When interviewing a patient suspected to be a victim of IPV, ask family members to leave the operatory and minimize the number of staff members present.
❑ Have a provider who is the same sex as the patient administer any screening questions.
❑ Place posters or fliers in the operatory or bathrooms informing patients of IPV resources and encouraging patients to notify a dentist or hygienist if they need help.

Addressing intimate partner violence

❑ Limit your role to identifying the victim, proposing and providing dental treatment, and referring the patient to IPV specialists.
❑ Use the four-step ask-validate-document-refer process.
❑ Ask: Confirm suspected abuse through explicit verbal communication.
❑ Ask: Never ask about IPV through a family member acting as interpreter.
❑ Ask: Ask about IPV in private, using nonjudgmental language and tone.
❑ Ask: Ask specific questions, but remain empathetic.
❑ Validate: Confirm that abuse is wrong and that the patient has worth.
❑ Validate: Repeat validations over time, even if the patient does not seek help.
❑ Document: Note objective observations in the patient's file.
❑ Document: Photograph injuries.
❑ Document: Record the patient's own words, particularly when the patient identifies the perpetrator.
❑ Document: Use medical terminology and avoid legal terms, ambiguous words, and abbreviations.

❑ Document: Note details of the patient's demeanor and the elapsed time since the abuse.
❑ Refer: Keep on hand IPV brochures and the contact information for specialists in IPV and refer the patient immediately.
❑ Refer: Contact an IPV specialist while the patient is in the operatory or office.
❑ Refer: Attempt to schedule a meeting between specialist and patient as soon as the patient leaves the office.
❑ Refer: Remember that an adult patient determines his or her readiness to leave a relationship affected by IPV.

For More Information

Stigma
- http://www.reseaufranco.com/en/research/best_of_crosscurrents/page51891.html
- http://www.icrw.org/files/publications/suspending-judgment-a-report-from-stigma-reduction-for-health-care-workers-workshop.pdf
- http://www.rcpsych.ac.uk/about/campaigns/changingmindscampaign1997-.aspx
- http://www.heart-intl.net/HEART/Stigma/Comp/OnStigma&itspublichealthimplicions.htm

Transtheoretical model
- http://dhonline.chattanoogastate.edu/modules/prevention/Health%20Behavior%20Models%20%20Review%20JDH%202004.pdf
- http://fataids.org/assets/pdf/00002703-200707000-00012.pdf
- http://www.dentalcare.com/media/en-US/education/ce74/ce74.pdf
- http://www.nature.com/bdj/journal/v187/n6/full/4800266a.html
- http://www.dimensionsofdentalhygiene.com/ddhright.aspx?id=9280

Smoking
- http://www.ab.lung.ca/sitewyze/files/Discussing_oral_health_Barbara_Gitzel.pdf
- http://rochester.edu/uhs/healthtopics/Tobacco/AssessmentFiles/rediness.html
- http://www1.umn.edu/perio/tobacco/Intervening_with_Tobacco_Patients.pdf
- http://www.smokefree.gov
- http://www.cancer.gov/cancertopics/tobacco/smoking
- http://www.ada.org/2615.aspx

Substance abuse
- http://www.drugabuse.gov/nidamed
- http://www.ada.org/en/member-center/oral-health-topics/meth-mouth
- http://www.ada.org/en/member-center/oral-health-topics/drug-use
- http://www.ada.org/en/member-center/member-benefits/health-and-wellness-information/substance-abuse-disorder

- http://www.dentalgentlecare.com/drug_use_&_oral_clues.htm
- http://www.rdhmag.com/index/display/article-display/161716/articles/rdh/volume-22/issue-11/feature/the-oral-clues.html
- www.deltadentalmn.org/content/files/Oral_Health_Education/082108_ddmn_meth_booklet_.pdf

Intimate partner violence
- http://www.msnbc.msn.com/id/44678589/ns/health-oral_health/t/after-abuse-shattered-smiles-bring-shame-stigma
- http://media.dentalcare.com/media/en-US/education/ce338/ce338.pdf
- http://media.dentalcare.com/media/en-US/education/ce49/ce49.pdf
- http://www.ihs.gov/doh/portal/feature/DomesticViolenceFeature_files/CoverStory_June08.pdf
- http://www.massdental.org/stop-violence.aspx
- https://www.ncjrs.gov/pdffiles1/nij/188564.pdf
- http://www.childwelfare.gov/systemwide/laws_policies/state

References

1. Givens JL, Tjia J. Depressed medical students' use of mental health services and barriers to use. Acad Med 2002;77:918–921.
2. Beach MC, Sugarman J, Johnson RL, Arbelaez JJ, Duggan PS, Cooper LA. Do patients treated with dignity report higher satisfaction, adherence, and receipt of preventive care? Ann Fam Med 2005;3:331–338.
3. Laine C, Davidoff F. Patient-centered medicine. JAMA 1996;275:152–156.
4. Robinson JH, Callister LC, Berry JA, Dearing KA. Patient-centered care and adherence: Definitions and applications to improve outcomes. J Am Acad Nurse Pract 2008;20:600–607.
5. Agne RR, Thompson TL, Cusella LP. Stigma in the line of face: Self-disclosure of patients' HIV status to health care providers. J Appl Commun Res 2000;28:235–261.
6. Norton C. Nurses, bowel continence, stigma, and taboos. J Wound Ostomy Continence Nurs 2004;31:85–94.
7. Corrigan P. How stigma interferes with mental health care. Am Psychol 2004;59:614–625.
8. Magliocca KR, Jabero MF, Alto DL, Magliocca JF. Knowledge, beliefs, and attitudes of dental and dental hygiene students toward obesity. J Dent Educ 2005;69:1332–1339.
9. American Dental Association. American Dental Association Principles of Ethics and Code of Professional Conduct. Chicago: American Dental Association, 2012. http://www.ada.org/~/media/ADA/About%20the%20ADA/Files/code_of_ethics_2012.ashx. Accessed 26 February 2015.
10. American Dental Hygienists' Association. Bylaws: Code of Ethics. Chicago: American Dental Hygienists' Association, 2014. http://www.adha.org/resources-docs/7611_Bylaws_and_Code_of_Ethics.pdf. Accessed 26 February 2015.
11. ABIM Foundation, ACP–ASIM Foundation, European Federation of Internal Medicine. Medical professionalism in the new millennium: A physician charter. Ann Intern Med 2002;136:243–246.
12. Friedlander AH, Mahler ME. Major depressive disorder: Psychopathology, medical management and dental implications. J Am Dent Assoc 2001;132:629–638.
13. Fiscella K, Meldrum S, Franks P, et al. Patient trust: Is it related to patient-centered behavior of primary care physicians? Med Care 2004;42:1049–1055.
14. Earnshaw VA, Quinn DM. The impact of stigma in healthcare on people living with chronic illnesses. J Health Psychol 2012;17:157–168.
15. Livingston JD, Boyd JE. Correlates and consequences of internalized stigma for people living with mental illness: A systematic review and meta-analysis. Soc Sci Med 2010;71:2150–2161.

16. Kopera M, Suszek H, Bonar E, et al. Evaluating explicit and implicit stigma of mental illness in mental health professionals and medical students [epub ahead of print 23 December 2014]. Community Ment Health J.

17. Richmond JA, Dunning TL, Desmond PV. Health professionals' attitudes toward caring for people with hepatitis C. J Viral Hepatitis 2007;14:624–632.

18. van Boekel LC, Brouwers EPM, van Weeghel J, Garretsen HFL. Stigma among health professionals towards patients with substance use disorders and its consequences for healthcare delivery: Systematic review. Drug Alcohol Depen 2013;131:23–35.

19. Hart JT. The inverse care law. Lancet 1971;1(7696):405–412.

20. Watt G. The inverse care law today. Lancet 2002;360(9328):252–254.

21. Fiscella K, Shin P. The inverse care law: Implications for healthcare of vulnerable populations. J Ambul Care Manage 2005;28:304–312.

22. Habibian M, Seirawan H, Mulligan R. Dental students' attitudes toward underserved populations across four years of dental school. J Dent Educ 2011;75:1020–1029.

23. Solomon ES. Dental workforce. Dent Clin North Am 2009;53:435–49.

24. American Dental Education Association. Students. Washington, DC: American Dental Education Association, 2012. http://www.adea.org/publications/tde/Pages/Students.aspx. Accessed 18 May 2015.

25. Mengel R, Eigenbrodt M, Schünemann T, Florès-de-Jacoby L. Periodontal status of a subject sample of Yemen. J Clin Periodontol 1996;23:437–443.

26. Soufi HE, Kameswaran M, Malatani T. Khat and oral cancer. J Laryngol Otol 1991;105:643–645.

27. DiClemente CC, Prochaska JO. Self-change and therapy change of smoking behavior: A comparison of processes of change in cessation and maintenance. Addict Behav 1982;7:133–142.

28. Prochaska JO, DiClemente CC. Stages and processes of self-change of smoking: Toward an integrative model of change. J Consult Clin Psychol 1983;51:390–395.

29. Prochaska JO, Velicer WF, Rossi JS, et al. Stages of change and decisional balance for 12 problem behaviors. Health Psychol 1994;13:39–46.

30. DiClemente CC, Velasquez MM. Motivational interviewing and the stages of change. In: Miller WR, Rollnick S (eds). Motivational Interviewing: Preparing People for Change, ed 2. New York: Guilford Press:201–216.

31. Miller WR, Rollnick S. Ten things that motivational interviewing is not. Behav Cogn Psychother 2009;37:129–140.

32. Brady W, Martinoff J. Validity of health history data collected from dental patients and patient perception of health status. J Am Dent Assoc 1980;101:642–645.

33. Centers for Disease Control and Prevention. Trends in current cigarette smoking among high school students and adults, United States, 1965–2010. Atlanta: Office on Smoking and Health, National Center for Chronic Disease Prevention and Health Promotion, 2011.

34. Centers for Disease Control and Prevention. Current cigarette smoking among adults—United States, 2005–2013. MMWR Morb Mortal Wkly Rep 2014;63:1108–1112.

35. Burns DM. Reducing tobacco use: What works in the population? J Dent Educ 2002;66:1051–1060.

36. Hennrikus D, Rindal DB, Boyle RG, Stafne E, Lazovich D, Lando H. How well does the health history form identify adolescent smokers? J Am Dent Assoc 2005;136:1113–1120.

37. Ingram JD. Misrepresentations in applications for insurance. U Miami Bus Law Rev 2005;14:103–118.

38. Tarr JAR. Disclosure in insurance law: Contemporary and historical economic considerations. In: Kinsler J, Jones R, Moens G (eds). International Trade and Business Law Annual. Sydney: Routledge-Cavendish, 2001:209–225.

39. Carr AB, Ebbert JO. Interventions for tobacco cessation in the dental setting. A systematic review. Community Dent Health 2007;24:70–74.

40. Gordon JS, Albert DA, Crews KM, Fried J. Tobacco education in dentistry and dental hygiene. Drug Alcohol Rev 2009;28:517–532.

41. Monson AL. Barriers to tobacco cessation counseling and effectiveness of training. J Dent Hyg 2004;78(3):5.

42. Watt RG, McGlone P, Dykes J, Smith M. Barriers limiting dentists' active involvement in smoking cessation. Oral Health Prev Dent 2004;2:95–102.

43. Davis JM, Stockdale MS, Cropper M. The need for tobacco education: Studies of collegiate dental hygiene patients and faculty. J Dent Educ 2005;69:1340–1352.

44. Gordon J, Severson H. Tobacco cessation through dental office settings. J Dent Educ 2001;65:354–363.

45. Ramseier CA, Fundak A. Tobacco use cessation provided by dental hygienists. Int J Dent Hyg 2009;7:39–48.

46. Kotlyar M, Hatsukami DK. Managing nicotine addiction. J Dent Educ 2002;66:1061–1073.

47. Warnakulasuriya S. Effectiveness of tobacco counseling in the dental office. J Dent Educ 2002;66:1079–1087.

48. Johnson NW. The role of the dental team in tobacco cessation. Eur J Dent Educ 2004;8:18–24.

49. D'Amore MM, Cheng DM, Kressin NR, et al. Oral health of substance-dependent individuals: Impact of specific substances. J Subst Abuse Treat 2011;41:179–185.

50. Shaner JW, Kimmes N, Saini T, Edwards P. "Meth mouth": Rampant caries in methamphetamine abusers. AIDS Patient Care STDs 2006;20:146–150.

51. Shetty V, Mooney LJ, Zigler CM, Belin TR, Murphy D, Rawson R. The relationship between meth-amphetamine use and increased dental disease. J Am Dent Assoc 2010;141:307–318.

52. Venker D. Crystal methamphetamine and the dental patient. Iowa Dent J 1999;85(4):34.

53. Ogden GR. Alcohol and oral cancer. Alcohol 2005;35:169–173.

54. Tezal M, Grossi SG, Ho AW, Genco RJ. Alcohol consumption and periodontal disease. J Clin Periodontol 2004;31:484–488.

55. Cho CM, Hirsch R, Johnstone S. General and oral health implications of cannabis use. Aust Dent J 2005;50:70–74.

56. Diago S. When your patient is an addict. AGD Impact 2003;33(9).

57. Hasin DS, Stinson FS, Ogburn E, Grant BF. Prevalence, correlates, disability, and comorbidity of DSM-IV alcohol abuse and dependence in the United States: Results from the National Epidemiologic Survey on Alcohol and Related Conditions. Arch Gen Psychiatry 2007;64:830–842.

58. Compton WM, Thomas YF, Stinson FS, Grant BF. Prevalence, correlates, disability, and comorbidity of DSM-IV drug abuse and dependence in the United States: Results from the National Epidemiologic Survey on Alcohol and Related Conditions. Arch Gen Psychiatry 2007;64:566–576.

59. Coombs RH. Addicted health professionals. J Subst Use 1996;1:187–194.

60. Fung EY, Lange BM. Impact of drug abuse/dependence on dentists. Gen Dent 2011;59:356–359.

61. Kenna GA, Wood MD. The prevalence of alcohol, cigarette and illicit drug use and problems among dentists. J Am Dent Assoc 2005;136:1023–1032.

62. Underwood B, Fox K, Nixon PJ. Alcohol and drug use among vocational dental practitioners. Br Dent J 2003;195:265–268.

63. Ewing JA. Detecting alcoholism. The CAGE questionnaire. JAMA 1984;252:1905–1907.

64. Seckman CH. The oral clues. RDH 2002;22(11):66–68, 99.

65. Miller PM, Ravenel MC, Shealy AE, Thomas S. Alcohol screening in dental patients: The prevalence of hazardous drinking and patients' attitudes about screening and advice. J Am Dent Assoc 2006;137:1692–1698.

66. Balevi B, Breen L, Krasnowski J. The dentist and prescription drug abuse. J Can Dent Assoc 1996;62:56–60.

67. Denisco RC, Kenna GA, O'Neil MG, et al. Prevention of prescription opioid abuse: The role of the dentist. J Am Dent Assoc 2011;142:800–810.

68. US Department of Justice. Domestic Violence, 2014. http://www.justice.gov/ovw/domestic-violence. Accessed 18 May 2015.

69. Child Welfare Information Gateway. Mandatory reporters of child abuse and neglect. Washington, DC: US Department of Health and Human Services, Children's Bureau, 2014. https://www.childwelfare.gov/pubPDFs/manda.pdf. Accessed 15 February 2015.

70. Connor PD, Nouer SS, Mackey SN, Banet MS, Tipton NG. Dental students and intimate partner violence: Measuring knowledge and experience to institute curricular change. J Dent Educ 2011;75:1010–1019.

71. Love C, Gerbert B, Caspers N, Bronstone A, Perry D, Bird W. Dentists' attitudes and behaviors regarding domestic violence: The need for an effective response. J Am Dent Assoc 2001;132: 85–93.

72. Tilden VP, Schmidt TA, Limandri BJ, Chiodo GT, Garland MJ, Loveless PA. Factors that influence clinicians' assessment and management of family violence. Am J Public Health 1994;84:628–633.

73. Chiodo GT, Tilden VP, Limandri BJ, Schmidt TA. Addressing family violence among dental patients: Assessment and intervention. J Am Dent Assoc 1994;125:69–75.

74. Massachusetts Dental Society Standing Committee to Prevent Abuse and Neglect. A guide to family violence for the dental team [brochure]. Southborough, MA: Massachusetts Dental Society. https://www.massdental.org/uploadedfiles/guide%20to%20family%20violence.pdf. Accessed 16 February 2015.

75. Ochs HA, Neuenschwander MC, Dodson TB. Are head, neck and facial injuries markers of domestic violence? J Am Dent Assoc 1996;127:757–761.

76. Catalano S. Intimate partner violence in the U.S. Washington, DC: United States Bureau of Justice Statistics, 2007.

77. Messinger AM. Invisible victims: Same-sex IPV in the National Violence Against Women Survey. J Interpers Violence 2011;26:2228–2243.

78. Rennison C, Planty M. Nonlethal intimate partner violence: Examining race, gender, and income patterns. Violence Vict 2003;18:433–443.

79. Brown JB, Lent B, Brett PJ, Sas G, Pederson LL. Development of the Woman Abuse Screening Tool for use in family practice. Fam Med 1996;28:422–428.

80. Yegidis BL. Abuse Risk Inventory Manual. Palo Alto, CA: Consulting Psychologist Press, 1989.

81. Hegarty K, Sheehan M, Schonfeld C. A multidimensional definition of partner abuse: Development and preliminary validation of the Composite Abuse Scale. J Fam Violence 1999;14: 399–415.

82. Halpern LR, Dodson TB. A predictive model to identify women with injuries related to intimate partner violence. J Am Dent Assoc 2006;137:604–609.

83. Feldhaus KM, Koziol-McLain J, Amsbury HL, Norton IM, Lowenstein SR, Abbott JT. Accuracy of 3 brief screening questions for detecting partner violence in the emergency department. JAMA 1997;277:1357–1361.

84. Friedman LS, Samet JH, Roberts MS, Hudlin M, Hans P. Inquiry about victimization experiences. a survey of patient preferences and physician practices. Arch Intern Med 1992;152:1186–1190.

85. Gerbert B, Abercrombie P, Caspers N, Love C, Bronstone A. How health care providers help battered women: The survivor's perspective. Women Health 1999;29:115–135.

86. Bair-Merritt MH, Mollen CJ, Yau PL, Fein JA. Health care providers' opinions on intimate partner violence resources and screening in a pediatric emergency department. Pediatr Emerg Care 2006;22:150–153.

87. Gerbert B, Moe J, Caspers N, et al. Simplifying physicians' response to domestic violence. West J Med 2000;172:329–331.

88. Zink T, Elder N, Jacobson J, Klostermann B. Medical management of intimate partner violence considering the stages of change: Precontemplation and contemplation. Ann Fam Med 2004;2:231–239.

89. Taliaferro E. Domestic violence: The need for good documentation. Action Notes (Physicians for a Violence-Free Society newsletter) 1997;23(1).

90. Isaac NE, Enos VP. Documenting Domestic Violence: How Health Care Providers can Help Victims. Washington, DC: US Department of Justice, Office of Justice Programs, National Institute of Justice, 2001.

Index

Page numbers followed by "t" indicate tables; those followed by "b" indicate boxes.